# SURF
# SURVIVAL

## SECOND EDITION

T0111986

# Praise for *Surf Survival*

"Nobody has thought more, studied more, or cared more about the lifelong health and survival of surfers than Mark Renneker. *Surf Survival* brings together all that priceless knowledge, along with invaluable contributions from Nathanson and Everline, to make a must-have volume for every surfer everywhere. From surf-specific wilderness first aid—critical on any serious surf trip, anywhere on earth—to big-wave safety and even the very real scourge of surfer's ear, it's all here. Don't even think about it: if surfing plays any role in your life, you need this book."

—Daniel Duane, author of *Caught Inside,*
*A Surfer's Year on the California Coast*

"Good medicine, and a fun read in the bargain. Read this book and surf until you're 100."

—Matt Warshaw, author of *The History of Surfing*

"These days, 'playing hurt' among professional athletes is usually only after being worked over by a fleet of trainers, PT's, and docs. The most unbowed of bloodied athletes has to be surfers—ever self-sufficient, all about self-care. This book will help surfers do an even better job of taking care of themselves."

—Bruce Jenkins, sports writer with the *San Francisco Chronicle,*
and author of *North Shore Chronicles*

"This thorough, authoritative, and oddly enjoyable book tells you not only how to treat surfing's myriad ailments, but also how to prevent them. For that reason alone, it might be the most important piece of surf literature you ever buy. All that, plus lots of photos of gnarly injuries."

—Steve Hawk, former editor of *Surfer* magazine

"I've read over 100 surfing-related books, but *Surf Survival* is the first one that I'll carry with me on every surf trip."

—Drew Sievers, *The Waterman's Library*

"Great book by great doctors. What a great combo: smart and hard-core surfers who care deeply about people and their health!"

—Greg Noll, legendary big wave surfer,
author of *Da Bull, Life Over the Edge*

# SURF
## SURVIVAL

### THE SURFER'S HEALTH HANDBOOK

#### SECOND EDITION

**Andrew Nathanson, MD**
**Clayton Everline, MD**
**Mark Renneker, MD**

Foreword by Gerry Lopez

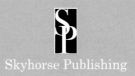

Skyhorse Publishing

Skyhorse Publishing books may be purchased in bulk at special discounts for sales promotion, corporate gifts, fund-raising, or educational purposes. Special editions can also be created to specifications. For details, contact the Special Sales Department, Skyhorse Publishing, 307 West 36th Street, 11th Floor, New York, NY 10018 or info@skyhorsepublishing.com.

Skyhorse® and Skyhorse Publishing® are registered trademarks of Skyhorse Publishing, Inc.®

www.skyhorsepublishing.com

10 9 8 7 6 5 4 3 2

Library of Congress Cataloging-in-Publication Data available on file.

Cover design by Daniel Brount
Cover photograph by iStockphoto

ISBN: 978-1-5107-4090-7
Ebook ISBN: 978-1-5107-4904-7

Printed in China

To my father, who took me to the sea
To my mother, who encouraged my spirit of creativity
And to Cheryl and Nainoa, my two favorite surf
buddies. —Andrew

I would like to dedicate this book to my wife, Kristina,
for her support. —Clayton

To Jessica, and the legions of the jazzed.
—Mark

# CONTENTS

ACKNOWLEDGMENTS IX

FOREWORD BY GERRY LOPEZ X

INTRODUCTION XII

1 BASIC LESSONS OF THE SEA 1

2 FITNESS FOR SURFERS 24

3 NUTRITION AND HYDRATION 64

4 SURFING INJURIES AND INJURY PREVENTION 71

5 CHRONIC SURFING INJURIES: AVOIDANCE AND REHABILITATION 95

6 SURVIVING THE SUN 116

7 SKIN PROBLEMS OF SURFERS 130

8 SURFER'S EAR, NASAL, AND SINUS PROBLEMS 142

**9** EYE AND VISION PROBLEMS      156

**10** WILDERNESS FIRST AID FOR SURFERS      162

**11** DANGEROUS MARINE ANIMALS      207

**12** SURVIVING BIG SURF      232

**13** STAND-UP PADDLE SURFING      248

**14** SURF TRAVEL MEDICINE: THE SURFARI      262

**15** SURF TRAVEL-RELATED INFECTIONS:
PREVENTION, DIAGNOSIS, AND TREATMENT      271

**16** THE SURFER'S MEDICAL KIT      288

**17** SEAFOOD POISONING      296

**18** SURFIATRICS      309

ADDITIONAL READING AND ONLINE RESOURCES      324
INDEX      326
ABOUT THE AUTHORS      332

# Acknowledgments

## Andrew Nathanson

I would like to thank Chris Vantilburg and Michael Jacobs from the Wilderness Medical Society for their encouragement and support for this book. Many thanks to illustrator Aria Marcos and to map designer and icon guy Carter Skemp for his great design concepts. Much gratitude to my little brother Nicholas at Quiksilver, who gave me the thumbs-up on every request, and to Jason Murray at Quik who provided some super-high-quality photos. Special thanks to Norm, Vinn, DO, longtime SMA member for stepping up to the plate to write the lion's share of the Surfiatrics chapter. To Mike Mello, Janette Baird, and the rest of the crew at the Injury Prevention Center at Rhode Island Hospital. A big aloha to Dave Skedeleski, owner and mastermind of SurfCo Hawaii who is one of the few manufacturers out there trying to make surfing a safer sport. Another big aloha to Jan and Donna Asuncion who always set us up with wave-riding vehicles on Oahu. To my surf gurus Kurt and Diane Vogelman and, of course, their surf gurus Gene and Susan Bagley. And lastly a big thank-you to my co-authors. Clay, for getting the ball rolling, and Mark, for his wise counsel and superb editorial skills.

## Clayton Everline

Acknowledgments go to my family and ardent supporters: Chris Boni, DO; David Ross, MD: David Kruse, MD; Bill Rosenblatt, EdD; Warren Kramer, MD; Tim Brown, DC; Scott Adams, CSCS; Blake Wylie, DO; Chip Martoccia and Hunter Joslin; Paul Frediani, Suzie Cooney, and Simone for the fitness photos; Leland Dao, DO; the crew at Waves of Health providing medical care in Dajabon and Haiti; Mark and the Surfer's Medical Association for the inspiration, and Andrew for his dedication to detail and execution. Thank you to the Wilderness Medical Society for your support of Surfing Medicine and the network of individuals who share our common interests.

## Mark Renneker

To Jessica: sorry you had to be in New York City that week, but by going along with you, I got to meet Andrew Nathanson, and then Jennifer McCartney and the Skyhorse folks (who mightily impressed me by having already published six different zombie books, some of which I didn't yet own, and then gave us less than six months to write this book).

For helping pave the way for this book: Geoff Booth and Kevin Starr, ever stalwart surf docs.

For their careful review of select chapters: Dave Parmenter, Dick Underwood, Douglas Hetzler, and Mark Bracker.

For his offer to translate this book into Portuguese: Joel Steinman.

For his pioneering work on surfer's physiology: Brian J. Lowdon; he would be so proud to see how his field has grown!

# Foreword

## Surf to Surf Tomorrow

Some might think "Surf to Surf Tomorrow" is a cryptic coded message, like a secret handshake. Actually, it is nothing more than a simple way to deal with surfing in today's world.

The Sport of Kings began centuries ago in Old Hawaii, and while it did favor the ali'i or royalty, it also was enjoyed immensely by the common folk. The modern age of surfing from the time of Duke Kahanamoku in the 1930s to the present day has seen an unprecedented growth in popularity. This has had the effect of increasing the number of surfers in the water to a point where tensions get hot and the thrill of surfing can get lost in the shuffle. For surfers who have been at it for a long time and remember better days, sometimes it just seems easier to give up and find another pastime.

To me, one of the biggest mistakes a surfer can make is to quit surfing. One of my main ground rules is to always surf to surf again tomorrow, no matter what that takes. As bad as today might seem, the sun will come up again tomorrow, we get to paddle back out once more, and we can start fresh all over.

Surf to Surf Tomorrow came from our early days at the surf camp in G-Land. Located on the southeastern tip of Java in the Blambangan Jungle Preserve, it was the most remote surf location anywhere. We boated in from the fishing village of Gradjagan, twelve miles across the bay to our makeshift camp that was built to last only that surf season. The monsoons and rainy season would begin late October or early November and that would be the end of our bamboo huts. The next April, we would rebuild everything. The fishing boat would drop us off on the beach with our supplies, turn around and leave us. There were no cell phones or any way to contact anyone. It was a camping trip; anything we needed, we had to bring with us, including our drinking and wash water. The surf was some of the most challenging I have ever found anywhere in Indonesia and, when the waves were big, it was hairy. None of us could afford to get hurt; we weren't equipped to deal with injuries. Eventually we brought out suturing gear and I stitched up plenty of lacerations. Nowadays, there are staple guns, surgical super glue, and other alternatives that *Surf Survival* will elaborate on in some detail. But back then, the thought that a major injury could occur was really quite frightening.

That was where I would have a serious talk with anybody new we brought into the camp with us. The waves were great and inspired high performance, edge of the envelope surfing, but I would warn everyone to never surf here like there was no tomorrow. I would try to instill in everyone the lesson to always surf to surf again tomorrow.

In 1981, during a wipeout at the Pipeline, my single fin pierced my colon, causing a lot of internal bleeding. While recovering, I realized that had this injury occurred at the G-Land camp, chances are I wouldn't have made it.

Surf to surf tomorrow has become my mantra for more than just surfing. Metaphorically, it is about balance and pacing myself in all things. Some people like to go through life, splashing and making a lot of noise. For me, I like leaving as small a wake as possible.

—Gerry Lopez,
Bend, Oregon
February 28, 2011

*Gerry Lopez is a legendary surfer and shaper, snowboard enthusiast, actor (co-starred in* Conan, the Barbarian*), and author (*Surf Is Where You Find It*, Patagonia Books, 2008).*

# Introduction

For those who may think that a book on the health problems of surf-ers couldn't possibly be needed in this digital age, go ahead and "surf" the Internet for even the most basic surfer's medical problems: Surfer's Ear, Surfer's Eye and Skin problems, Surf Travel Medicine. Wikipedia has zip, except a short blurb on Surfer's Ear. Surfing web-sites have a smattering of gobbledygook. Conventional medical sites? Hopeless. But worry not (Dick Dale guitar blast here!): Surf Docs TO THE RESCUE!

We three surfers who put this book together come from diverse surfing subcultures and medical backgrounds but share in common a longtime fascination with surf medicine. Mark, who hails from San Francisco, was the first of us surf docs to make the drop and contin-ues to lead the charge as both a world-traveling big-wave kahuna and founder of the Surfer's Medical Association. Andrew is an ER doc at Brown with an academic interest in marine medicine who spends summer and winter plying the nooks and crannies of Rhode Island's fickle coastline in search of quality surf. And Clay, the young gun based in Hawaii, is a sports-medicine doc and fitness guru who trains some of the top names in the sport. As we've been out there for years getting battered ourselves by the surf, giving beachside consul-tations, and providing care to legions of injured and ailing surfers, we've learned a thing or two along the way. This book is our tell-all on the subject.

The surfer's life is not without risks. Indeed, some would argue that the risks involved are part of the sport's allure. The rush we get from taking a late drop or pulling under a heavy lip is fueled in part by fear, fear that any misstep could lead to a serious thrash-ing (or worse). The vast majority of the time, we manage to emerge unscathed from even the ugliest wipeouts, but occasionally things don't turn out so well. *Surf Survival* was written to help you patch yourself back up when you get dinged, particularly when surfing in remote areas where medical care is nonexistent, and help may be hours or even days away.

However, the health issues faced by surfers aren't just limited to getting dragged over a coral reef or sliced open by a surfboard's fin. A lifetime of exposure to heat, cold, seawater, and sun can take its toll on a surfer's skin, eyes, and ears. Surf travel to the tropics opens up yet another medical can of worms, with the very real possibility of contracting life-threatening diseases such as malaria, dengue, and yellow fever, never mind a gut-busting case of Montezuma's revenge, which may not kill you, but will definitely put a serious downer on your trip.

As surfers, we know that self-care is the goal. When far off the beaten path, self-care is often your only option. Say you're out in the middle of nowhere and you or one of your surf mates dislocates a shoulder, gets bitten by a sea snake, suffers a major wound, or spikes a high fever. Would you know what to do? This book offers practical advice on how to deal with the medical emergencies you are most likely to encounter as a surfer and shows you how to improvise medical care in wilderness settings by using everyday items you are likely to have with you when medical supplies are not available. We also lay down some guidelines to help you decide if the problem can be safely handled on scene or whether you should bail on the trip and seek help.

Even when modern medical care is available, most surfers discover early on that having to buckle down and go in to a doctor can be particularly discouraging, particularly if that doctor knows nothing about surfing. Regardless of whether they figure out what is wrong with you, the usual advice comes down to: "Stop surfing!" To cut down on these frustrations, we include in-depth discussions that cover a vast array of ailments that afflict surfers and tell you how you can treat the majority of these at home; for those issues that will require a doctor's care, you'll have the advantage of being well versed in the treatment options available.

Ultimately, this book was written by surfers for surfers to help encourage the long-standing surfing traditions of independence and self-sufficiency. We hope you keep it conveniently close to you in your wave pursuits, whether that be in the glove compartment of your car or deep in the innards of your dry bag when you travel.

Cowabunga,

Andrew, Clay, and Mark

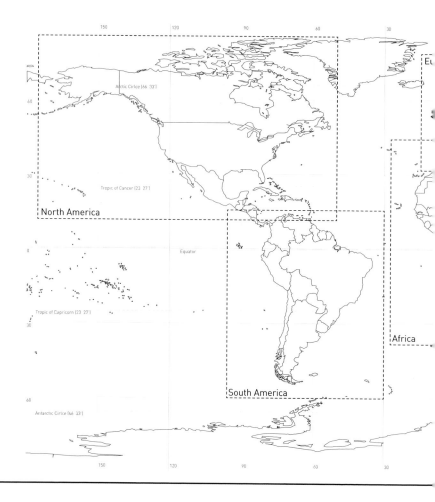

I.   North America
II.  South America
III. Europe

IV.  Africa
V.   Asia
VI.  Australia/Oceania

# INDEX TO SURFING
# RISKS WORLDWIDE

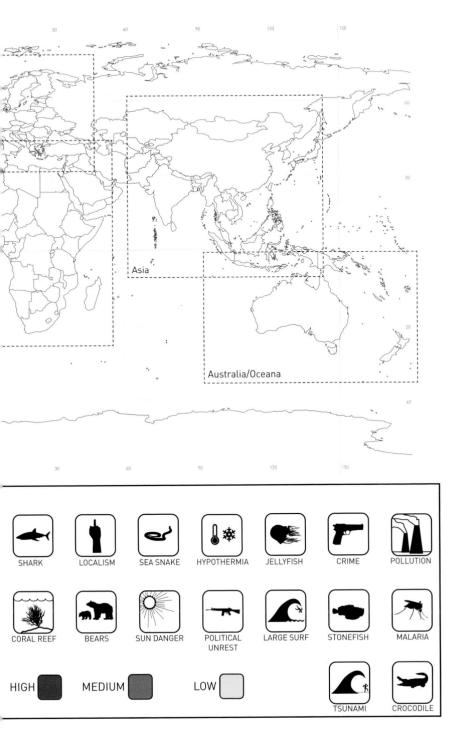

Asia

Australia/Oceana

| | | | | | | |
|---|---|---|---|---|---|---|
| SHARK | LOCALISM | SEA SNAKE | HYPOTHERMIA | JELLYFISH | CRIME | POLLUTION |
| CORAL REEF | BEARS | SUN DANGER | POLITICAL UNREST | LARGE SURF | STONEFISH | MALARIA |

HIGH ☐    MEDIUM ☐    LOW ☐

TSUNAMI    CROCODILE

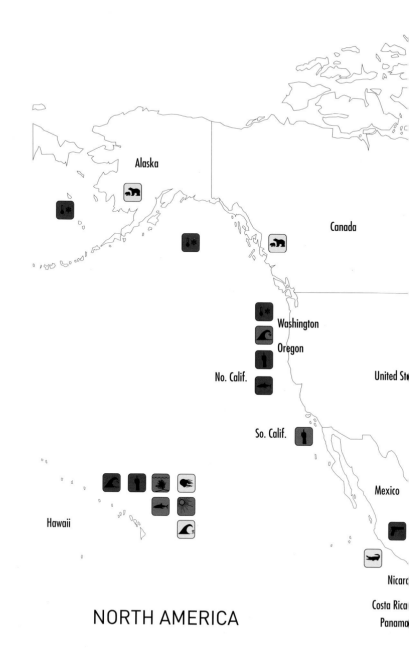

Alaska

Canada

Washington

Oregon

No. Calif.

So. Calif.

United St

Mexico

Hawaii

Nicara

Costa Rica

Panama

NORTH AMERICA

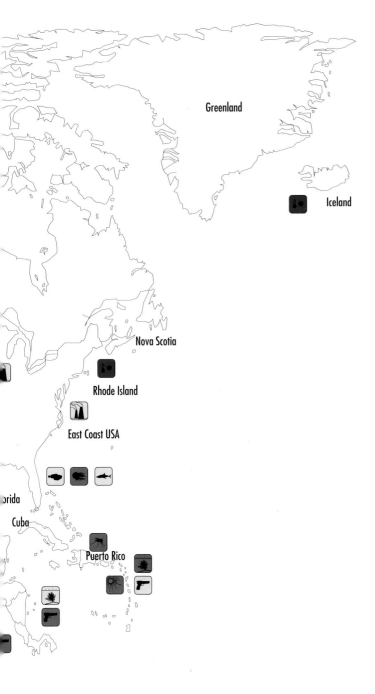

Greenland

Iceland

Nova Scotia

Rhode Island

East Coast USA

orida

Cuba

Puerto Rico

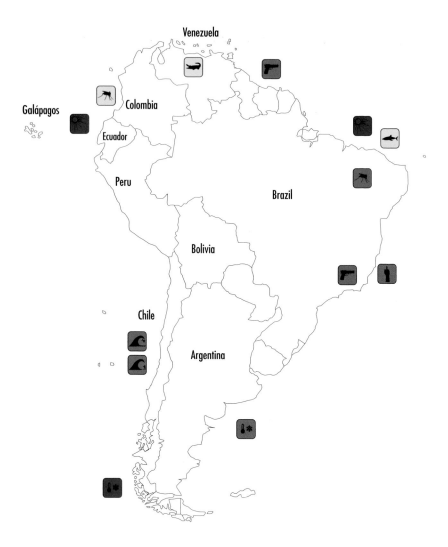

SOUTH AMERICA

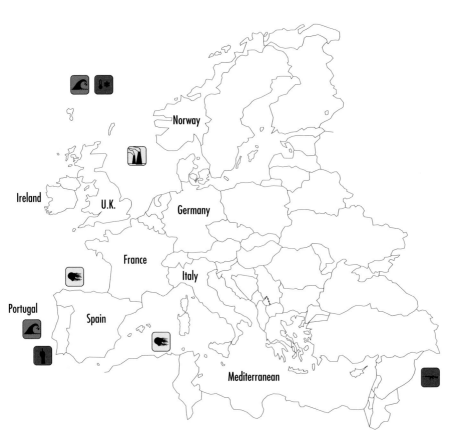

Ireland

Norway

U.K.

Germany

France

Italy

Portugal

Spain

Mediterranean

EUROPE

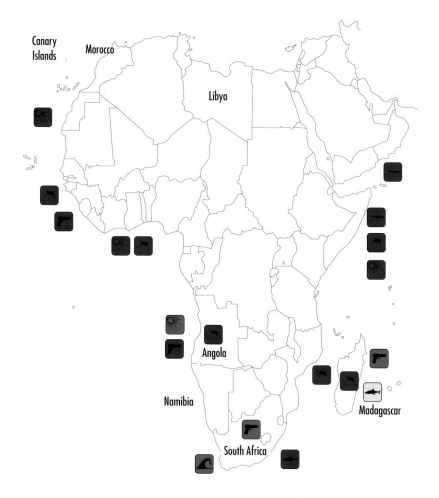

Canary
Islands

Morocco

Libya

Angola

Namibia

Madagascar

South Africa

AFRICA

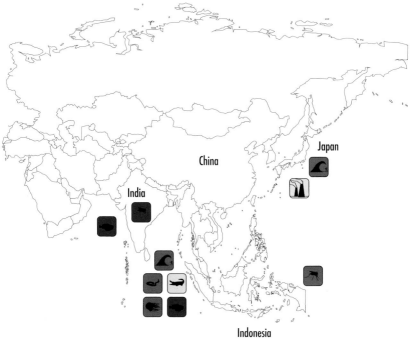

China

Japan

India

Indonesia

ASIA

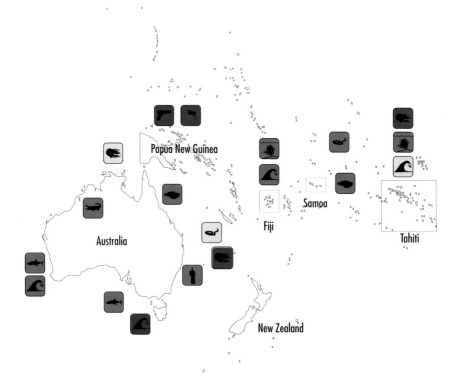

Papua New Guinea

Australia

Fiji

Samoa

Tahiti

New Zealand

AUSTRALIA
AND
THE SOUTH PACIFIC

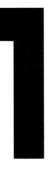

*Roll on, thou deep and dark blue Ocean—roll!*
*Ten thousand fleets sweep over thee in vain;*
*Man marks the earth with ruin—his control*
*stops with the shore.*

—**Byron**

# Basic Lessons of the Sea

The ocean is vast and powerful, in a constant state of flux, and its moods are unpredictable. As surfers, we have the opportunity to harness some of its awesome power and witness its beauty from a unique perspective that few others will ever get to see. However, we must also be respectful of the ocean's power—aware that it can be an unforgiving environment for those who are ill prepared.

Humans have little natural buoyancy, are poorly insulated from the cold, and can survive but a few minutes underwater. As such, any activity that takes place in the surf zone carries inherent risks and leaves little margin for error. Understanding and respecting the power of the ocean and learning one's limits are the most basic and important tenets of surfing safety.

## RESPECT THE OCEAN

 This chapter discusses some of the fundamental principles of ocean safety, including the science of waves and currents, surfing etiquette, and ocean swimming skills. The basic information presented here should be studied closely by beginners and will serve as review for more experienced watermen.

### Swim like Your Life Depends on It

It's easy to be lulled into a false sense of security in the water by becoming overly reliant on your board as a flotation device. In the preleash era, surfers were strong swimmers by virtue of the fact that swimming after one's board was a routine occurrence, but there is little doubt that most of today's surfers lack the swimming prowess of their predecessors. However, strong swimming skills should be an absolute requirement for

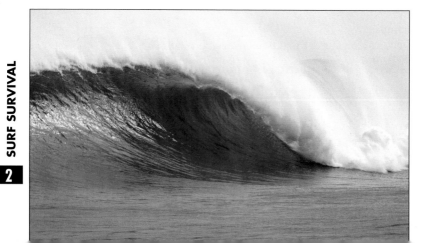

participation in the sport because inevitably your leash will break, you'll lose your board, and you'll need to rely solely on your swimming abilities to make it back to shore. Odds are pretty good that this will happen at a most inopportune time, in powerful surf when the stress on your leash is greatest, and the swim to shore most challenging, so the importance of confident ocean swimming skills and overall physical fitness cannot be overstated. Simply put, swimming is your best defense against drowning.

## SURF-SURVIVAL TIP

**Don't paddle out if you don't think you could swim in.**

Being a strong swimmer not only helps inspire confidence in all ocean conditions, but also helps develop the upper body strength needed to be a good surfer. If you have access to a swimming pool or, better yet, the ocean, make swimming a priority in your fitness routine. Incorporate short underwater swims, sprints, and long-distance endurance swims so you'll be adequately prepared for a worst-case scenario.

Open-ocean swimming is intimidating to some people and requires a slightly different technique than lap-pool swimming. Lack of underwater visual cues as well as currents and waves make swimming in a straight line a challenge. To maintain a steady course and avoid zigzagging, line up two points of reference on land (flagpole and house) in the direction you want to go and look up at them every four strokes or so. Another useful skill that requires some practice is to alternate your breaths between your left and right sides when swimming freestyle, giving more symmetry to your stroke, which will help you swim a more direct course.

The uneven surface of the ocean also requires some modification of the traditional freestyle stroke. Most open-water swim experts recommend reaching higher out of the water with each stroke because when using the traditional (bent-arm recovery) stroke, your arm tends to slap the water's surface before it is fully extended, slowing you down and hampering your rhythm. A more pronounced body roll in rough conditions can help avoid an inadvertent gulp of water that can trigger a choking reflex and needs to be avoided at all costs.

Next time you drive to the beach and the surf is flat, make the best of it and go for a long swim parallel to the shoreline to work on your technique and gain experience. Or if you are out in lackluster surf, roll off your board and head off for a swim, trailing your board on its leash. Consider this truth: if swimming in the ocean spooks you, you shouldn't be out there surfing. If need be, practice with a partner and go for incrementally longer swims until you are completely comfortable being out there alone.

## Never Let Your Tank Run Low

Managing your energy reserves out on the water can be challenging and is important for ensuring your safety. Surfing safely and effectively requires the ability to generate short bursts of paddling power at all times, not only to catch waves but also to get out of harm's way. It is critically important that you always keep some juice in reserve should you need to paddle hard to deal with a big set, survive an unexpected holddown, or sprint-paddle to avoid an oncoming surfer. Surfing to exhaustion is foolhardy and a sign of inexperience—not only won't you catch any waves, but you'll leave yourself exposed, like a piece of driftwood, at the mercy of the elements.

A good rule of thumb is that at any given moment you should be able to hold your breath for at least thirty seconds, which is about the maximum amount of time you can expect to get held under in all but the biggest surf. Heavy arms and labored breathing are certain signs that it's time to take a break. Heed your body's warnings by heading back in to the beach or paddling to a safe zone outside the lineup where you can rest and allow your heart rate and breathing recover before getting back into the mix.

## Understand the Motion of the Ocean

Good conditioning and swimming skills alone are not enough to keep you out of trouble; physical fitness needs to be coupled with a complete

SURF SURVIVAL

4

understanding of waves and currents, because even the fittest swimmers and surfers will struggle when trying to confront the power of the ocean head-on. Many a swimmer has panicked and drowned because they tried to swim back to shore against a rip, rather than swimming (or even drifting) back to shore in an area where the flow of water is shoreward.

The experienced surfer understands the complex interactions between swell, wind, tide, and bathymetry (underwater contour), and conserves energy by traveling with the flow of water, whenever possible, rather than against it. Understanding how water flows through a surf break is hugely important in terms of efficiently getting from point A to point B because the fastest and safest route is rarely the most direct and often depends on using rips and other near-shore currents to maximum advantage. Each surf break is unique, and surface currents at a given break can change, sometimes dramatically, depending on the tide, wave size, swell direction, wind speed, wind direction, and other factors. An intimate local knowledge of water flow becomes particularly critical if you find yourself in the predicament of having lost your board and need to swim in or are getting pinned against a dangerous shoreline and need to escape.

Though the seasoned waterman almost intuitively recognizes the dynamics of a new spot after just a cursory surf check, the subtle visual cues indicating rip currents, side-shore drift, tide, wind direction, and other important features of a break are likely to be lost on the novice. While a full discourse on wave science and currents is beyond the scope of this book, the following is a brief primer.

## Wave Formation

The ocean's waves are formed by the friction of wind over the water's surface, and the size of those waves is determined by three factors—namely, the wind strength (wind speed), the length of time that the wind blows (wind duration), and the span of open water over which the wind is blowing (fetch). Quality waves are usually generated by distant offshore storms (sometimes several thousand miles away), blowing over a large fetch, for a prolonged period of time and aimed in a favorable direction (toward your home break!). Near the center of such a storm, the seas are large, steep, closely spaced, and chaotic (which is why surfing in close proximity to a storm is so unrewarding and potentially hazardous). However, as waves propagate away from the storm center, they gradually "clean up" and organize into a smooth, widely spaced pattern of waves called a "swell." The largest of these waves are also the fastest and tend to travel together in "sets" away from the slower waves, like groups of elite runners in a marathon. These swells move across the ocean in a predictable fashion at between fifteen and thirty plus miles per hour, and though they gradually fade, given enough initial energy, they can travel thousands of miles before finally breaking—and dissipating their energy on a distant shoreline.

The *time interval* between two successive wave crests (the time it takes two successive crests to pass a fixed object in the water such as a buoy) is termed the "wave period," and the *distance* between successive peaks is termed "wavelength." Because automated offshore buoys measure wave period rather than wave length, surfers generally refer to the period of a swell as opposed to its related wavelength. A long period swell (greater than thirteen seconds) contains more energy, can travel farther, and will create bigger surf than shorter-period swell of equal height.

Contrary to appearance, waves in deep water do not actually "carry" water with them; rather, they transmit energy along and beneath the ocean's surface. A surfer floating in the deep water outside of a break will simply bob up and down (following a circular motion) with the passing of each wave, no matter what its size. As swells approach the shallower water of a shoreline, they drag along the bottom, slow down, and the distance between waves decreases (but the period remains the same). Waves begin to "feel" the bottom at a depth equal to half their *wavelength*, at which point the bottom of a wave will slow down while the top of the wave continues to move forward, which increases a wave's height and steepness. Once a wave reaches water of a depth that is equal to 1.3 times its *height*, the top of the wave will in effect trip over the bottom of the wave and break, spilling over as a rush of moving white water. At this point, there *is* a net movement of water toward the shoreline, and a surfer in this area will get forcefully pushed shoreward by the white water.

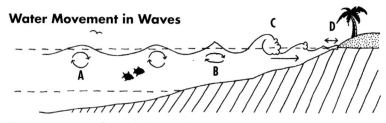

**Water Movement in Waves**

Water at points A and B moves in a circular motion.
Water in the surf break C flows shoreward, and in the wash zone D, it flows shoreward and seaward.

## A Swell Approaching Shallow Water

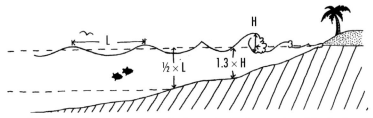

Waves begin to "feel" the bottom at a depth equal to ½ the wavelength L. As they are slowed by the bottom, the wavelength L decreases, but the wave height H, increases. At a depth of approximately 1.3 × H a wave will begin to break.

# The Importance of Wave Period and Refraction

Wave period has a big effect on how waves travel across the ocean and how those waves behave when they approach shallow water and break. Long-period swells carry a large proportion of their energy underwater and have gentle (as opposed to steep) wave faces, so they are less susceptible to wind resistance and can travel greater distances than short-period swells, which are quickly knocked down by opposing winds. Because they carry their energy deep underwater, long-period swells begin to feel the bottom at great depths. For example, a "ground swell" (so called because it feels the ground beneath it) with a period of eighteen seconds will begin to drag on the bottom in 830 feet of water, whereas a similarly sized "wind swell" (caused by local winds) with a period of eight seconds will only feel the effect of the bottom at a depth of 164 feet. As a result, long-period ground swells respond to changes in underwater contour (bathymetry) at a greater distance from shore than short-period wind swell and will "wrap" around curved coastlines, whereas shorter-period swells will be very near shore and almost ready to break before they feel the bottom.

Just like light waves and sound waves, ocean waves refract (bend) when they encounter resistance (in this case the seafloor). Reefs and underwater canyons can bend waves in such a way that their energy becomes focused and their size magnified in much the same way that a magnifying glass can focus beams of sunlight on a leaf and set it aflame. The unique bathymetry at spots like Mavericks and Jaws act as very efficient wave magnifiers and explain why, given the right swell, the waves at those breaks might have sixty-foot faces, while just a few miles up the coast, the surf will be less than a third of that height.

## Wave Shape

Waves breaking in an area where the seafloor has a gradual slope will be gentle, crumbling waves ideal for beginners (e.g., Waikiki, San Onofre), whereas waves breaking over a steeply sloping seafloor will have hollow, plunging, more powerful waves better suited to experts (e.g., Pipeline, Puerto Escondido). Wind direction also has a significant effect on wave shape; onshore winds cause wave crests to topple early, creating unfavorable conditions with mushy waves and a bumpy surface, while offshore winds prop up the face of a wave, producing steeper waves with smooth surfaces. Note that a steeply sloping seafloor and offshore winds cause waves to break in water that is slightly less than 1.3 times their height, whereas the opposite is true for onshore winds, and gently sloping bottoms.

### SURF-SURVIVAL TIP

Though often mistakenly called *undertows*, rip currents will not pull you under, just out. If you find yourself caught in a rip and are trying to head in to shore, *do not* panic and *do not* try to fight the rip. Simply paddle (or swim) parallel to the shore, even if in doing so you are being pushed away from shore, until you get to an area of breaking waves where the flow of water will carry you shoreward.

## Rip Currents and Side-Shore Drift

Rip currents are infamous for drowning swimmers, but can be a surfer's best friend if properly understood. The dynamics are simple. Waves breaking over a reef or sandbar push white water shoreward where it accumulates, slightly above sea. The water that has piled up toward shore is then forced by gravity to drain back out to sea. The course of this outflowing water follows the path of least resistance and often will run in "gutters" inside the break and parallel to the shoreline until it reaches a deeper channel where it can drain back out to sea through a gap in the reef or sandbar. In sand-bottom breaks, the outflow or rip current scours the seafloor, further deepening the channel and creating an even better conduit for outflow of water. A surfer floating above such a channel or "rip" will be carried out to sea as if on a conveyor belt, making the channel an ideal place to paddle out, but a very difficult place to paddle or swim in. Note in the figure (rip current) that at the offshore end of a rip, there is often a plume of turbulent water where the rip dissipates and that the direction of the current there may curl back around toward the shore.

## Rip Current

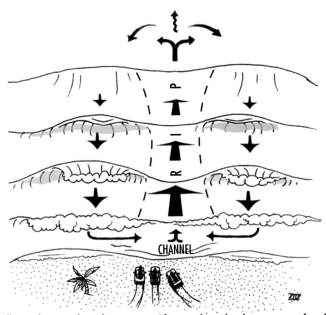

Water flows shoreward in white water. After reaching the shore, water often flows parallel to the shoreline in a gutter between the surf break and the shore. Finally, water is funelled seaward in a deeper channel to form a rip current.

In breaks with hard bottoms, notably point breaks and reef breaks, these channels (and their corresponding rips) are distinct, stationary, and well defined. However, at sand-bottom beach breaks, where sandbars are constantly being reshaped by the action of storms and currents, the channels are shifty and ill defined, making the identification of rips and the paddle out from a beach break substantially more challenging. Rips at beach breaks can be pretty subtle and are generally no more than twenty to forty feet wide, so it is not uncommon to see a surfer just a few feet away (but in a rip) scooting past with little effort as you struggle to make headway. The ideal situation is to be in a rip when paddling out and to take advantage of the onshore flow of breaking waves in the middle of the surf break when heading in.

It is important to note that rip currents get stronger and wider in bigger surf. As more water pours over a surf break in a big swell, there is an increased volume of water needing to squeeze out through the channel to make its way seaward. The current in a rip will even fluctuate with sets, temporarily strengthening just after a big set and then settling down between sets.

Rip currents can often be recognized by looking for areas of slightly discolored, foamy, or choppy water where suspended particles of sand or seaweed are being carried out to sea. The surface texture of a rip is usually subtly different than that of surrounding waters. Because rips usually form in areas of deeper water, you will often see a break in the normal wave pattern. Fixed obstructions such as piers, jetties, and headlands are often associated with fixed outflowing currents, and surfers with local knowledge use these rips to advantage when paddling out.

Whereas rip currents tend to pull a surfer out to sea, side-shore currents, as the name implies, tend to drag a surfer down a coastline, parallel to shore. These currents are primarily caused by swells sweeping into the shoreline at an angle and pushing water down the length of the beach in the direction they are breaking. The more prominent the swell size, the more angled the swell direction; and the longer and straighter the beach is, the more powerful the side-shore current tends to be. Side-shore currents can also be influenced or even caused by tides and side-shore winds.

## Side-Shore Current

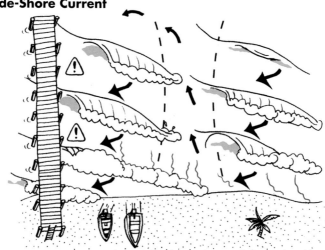

When waves are approaching a shoreline at an angle, a side-shore current will form. In this illustration, a surfer will drift to the left. Winds and tides can also cause side-shore currents.

Side-shore currents usually extend from the beach to just outside the surf zone and can be dangerous because they make returning to one's original launching spot difficult and may sweep surfers down the beach into piers, jetties, or other hazards. Some breaks have a persistent side-shore drift that always flows in the same direction, while others have a drift that may fluctuate from one direction to the other depending on the direction of the swell, tide, or wind. Maintaining your position in the takeoff zone in these conditions requires constant paddling (which can be tiring) and often requires triangulating your position by using fixed objects on land. (For more on triangulation see chapter 12.)

## Know before You Go

Prior to the advent of weather satellites, weather radar, and automated offshore buoys, finding good surf was based on local knowledge, intuition, and karma—in other words, it was largely a crapshoot, and unless you lived right at the beach, getting skunked was commonplace. Though some of the mystery (and excitement) of the hunt is gone, buoy reports, surf forecasts, and webcams are considered invaluable tools by today's surfers and certainly save a lot of time and energy in the quest for favorable conditions.

The science of surf forecasting has progressed enormously in the last two decades, primarily due to the improvement of remote monitoring instruments and computer-modeling tools. Near-term (one to four days) surf forecasts are remarkably accurate, particularly when it comes to the prediction of long-period swells, which march across the ocean at predictable speed and direction with little decay. If the surf forecasts are favorable, the buoys show swell, and the wave cams look good—it should be a rare thing indeed to get to the beach and find it completely flat. The experienced surfer checks out the wave and weather forecasts and takes a quick look at real-time wind, buoy data, and wave conditions (if available) before committing to a session. Keeping a tide table in the car as a reference is also a good idea, as tides can be predicted with 100 percent accuracy and may dictate the safety of a given spot. In areas with significant tidal ranges, a given break, which may be fun at high tide, may have exposed rocks or reef and be super sketchy or even unrideable at low tide. Knowing when a given swell is supposed to peak and its height, period, and direction is also important information from a safety perspective. If you arrive at the beach and the conditions are at the upper limit of your comfort zone, you may not want to paddle out knowing the swell hasn't peaked yet, whereas you may choose to go out if you know that the swell is fading.

There is a vast array of data on the Internet that pertains to surf and weather forecasting, much of it compiled by the US government and available for free. Some sites are better for real-time and predicted wind conditions, while others may be better for surf, tides, water temperature, etc. A savvy surfer develops a list of go-to sites for the best available information for his or her local waters and consults them before heading out the door.

## Surf-Check 101: Look before You Leap

The wise surfer takes a few minutes to assess conditions before paddling out, waiting for a couple of sets to roll through before reaching any conclusions about wave size. Many a surfer has made the mistake of rushing out prematurely only to find that the waves are significantly larger than what they bargained for, and that they are undergunned, or in over their heads. Know, too, that waves viewed from above and at a distance—for instance, when looking down from a cliff—can appear to be deceptively small but are always much bigger when seen up close and personal from the deck of your board. Also, keep in mind that set waves are often more than twice the size of the average waves on a given day, particularly at the beginning of a long-period swell when it can be nearly flat between sets. As you wax your board and warm up, pay particular attention to the timing between sets and the wave count in each set so you can paddle out during a lull. Keep in mind that the number of waves in each set is relatively constant at any given time, so if there are seven waves to a set, you may not want to paddle for the first one because a botched takeoff will mean taking the next six waves on the head. Experienced surfers often stash a set of binoculars in the car, which they can use to get a better sense of wave size and offshore conditions.

If you forgot to check the tide tables, check the shoreline to see if the tide is high or low, flooding (coming in), or ebbing (going out). Exposed barnacles and seaweed indicate that the tide is low, and if the beach above the surge line is dry, the tide may be rising (because the beach has had time to dry out); but if the upper beach is wet, it is more likely that the tide is ebbing. Get a sense of the strength and direction of any rips or side-shore currents, of wind speed, wind direction, and swell direction. Look to see where the ideal takeoff spots are, how the waves are lining up, and how crowded it is. Surfers often have a herd mentality, and the most crowded spot is not necessarily the best.

When surfing an unfamiliar break for the first time, get as much local knowledge about the place as you can before venturing out—preferably from an experienced local surfer. It takes a lifetime to acquire local knowledge, and local surfers are by far the best sources of information regarding where to go in a given wind-swell combo and, just as importantly, where not to go. Recognizing that the locals wouldn't want to give you the real keys to their kingdom, you have to earn that kind of knowledge, but they will generally give you the basics if you ask them respectfully. Ask about where the safe entry and exit points are—and what they'll look like at high and low tides. Is there a rip? Where is the best place to paddle out? Are there any hidden underwater hazards you should know about? (You don't want to discover the submerged remnants of a long-forgotten pier the hard way.) How about the local crowd—is the vibe friendly or aggro? And how about the local marine critters? Are *they* friendly or aggro?

Be aware that nonsurfers are notoriously poor sources of information when it comes to surfing conditions. Remember that even fishermen and others who spend a lot of time on or around the ocean are generally fearful of breaking waves and take great pains to avoid them. Nonsurfers have little understanding of what makes a good surfing wave, where there may be good channels in a reef, etc., and their judgment regarding surf conditions and rideability is hardly worth soliciting.

## Entering and Exiting the Water

Oftentimes the most perilous moments of a surfing session occur not out in the break, but rather when getting in and out of the water. From thumping shore pound, to precarious balancing acts over seaweed-slick rocks, to jumps off wave-slammed ledges, to razor-sharp coral reefs, the hazards vary according to the locale. Entering or exiting the water safely is often trickier than it looks, particularly at an unfamiliar break, so we've included a few tips to help you avert disaster.

### Beach Breaks

The main risk here is getting pounded into the sand by a large shore break on the way in or on the way out. If you get knocked off your feet or trip on your leash in the shore break, the situation can turn ugly very quickly, as the backwash will invariably drag you back into the

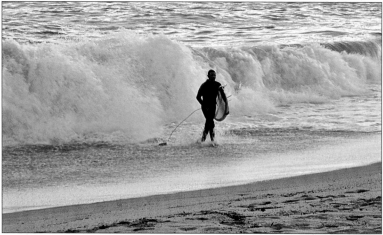

**A meaty shore break requires a good exit strategy. Note: leash has been removed before exiting the water.**

impact zone where the next wave will have its way with you. Before jumping in, closely study the wave pattern along the beach and look to see where others are coming in and out of the water. Steeply sloped beaches create conditions for a heavy shore break and should be avoided if possible. Often the best place to enter will be in a channel where the shore break may be less powerful, and the rip current will carry you out. Stand at the water's edge, waiting for a lull and then sprint into the water, jump over the top of the first small breaking wave landing prone on your board, and sprint-paddle until you are well past the shore break and away from immediate danger. Timing is everything here; it pays to be patient so as to avoid a dangerous situation where you get tossed into the shore pound and lose your board.

To exit the water, find a place where most of the wave energy has been dissipated offshore and the shore break is less violent. This may be directly in front of the surf break and not in front of the channel where you paddled out. Again, timing here is everything. Wait offshore, just outside of the shore break. When there is a lull, paddle quickly toward the beach *following* a wave in to shore. You want to be *behind* the wave, not in front of it. As the wave you follow in breaks, get carried by the surge up the beach until you are in water that is less than thigh deep. Roll off your board just before the backwash starts sucking out, stand up quickly, grab your board, and raise it up high, then scamper up the beach like a sandpiper. The backwash will be pulling hard against you as you attempt to run up to dry sand, so a little bit of high-stepping may be needed for optimal forward progress. Don't dawdle around and always keep a wary eye behind you for incoming waves.

## Rocky Shorelines

In order to avoid a long paddle out, advanced surfers will often jump in off a rocky ledge, but this may not be the best option for you if you don't have your duck-dives nailed or have the wrong equipment. Beware that cliff-strewn shorelines are dangerous because waves often haven't yet dissipated any energy in the deeper water offshore, so the rocks take the full brunt of impact. When you are at the base of a cliff, "sneaker" waves may reach higher than the others, and rocks or difficult terrain may make a speedy retreat impossible. In Hawaii, more people die from being swept off cliffs by unexpectedly large waves than are killed in shark attacks. If you are unfamiliar with a particular break, particularly if the surf is big, a longer paddle out from a protected cove is always smarter than taking a more perilous shortcut.

If you do decide to launch off rocks or a low cliff, spend a good five minutes carefully observing the situation from the safety of high ground. Watch how and where other surfers are getting in and out and note which areas are submerged by the largest waves. Look at the launch zone to see where your path of retreat would be and to assess other hazards such as offshore rocks. Note that launch zones that work well at high tide may not work well at low tide and vice versa and that places that are easy to jump into may be very difficult to get out of. Make sure to coil your leash in preparation so it won't get snagged. When a lull arrives, walk briskly down to the water's edge (being careful not to slip) and jump in horizontally, landing prone on your board, and paddle out quickly beyond the point of any breaking waves.

If you find yourself stranded on rocks at the base of a cliff and it looks like a breaking wave might be threatening your safety, you have a couple of options. Retreating to higher ground is the safest bet if you are sure you can outrun the wave. If retreating is not a viable alternative, you can crouch behind a large boulder and hold on like a limpet, hoping to be shielded from any direct impact. Lastly, depending on size of the wave and your exact predicament, you can face the music directly by jumping over the approaching wall of white water and landing prone on your board or diving through the oncoming wave and trailing your board behind.

## Lightning

Every year approximately one hundred people in the United States are killed by lightning strikes, and more than half of them are engaged in outdoor recreational activities. As with shark attacks, Florida (the Sunshine State) leads the way, with over ten lightning-related deaths annually. Other surfable coasts notable for their thunderstorm activity are the Gulf of Mexico, the northern Caribbean, the Pacific Coast from Mainland Mexico through Central America, as well as much of Indonesia. Because lightning bolts tend to strike the highest object in the vicinity and are attracted to objects that conduct electricity (like salty, wet surfers), surfers both in the water and on the beach are at risk. A single lightning strike at Shonan Beach near Tokyo hit a surfer wearing a gold chain, killing him and four others in the lineup. If you are out on the water when a thunderstorm hits, paddle in and seek shelter in a low-lying area on land. If stranded on the beach, stay low and sit on your board to minimize direct contact with the ground. Avoid standing under tall trees (which are likely to get struck) and near metal objects such as fences or flagpoles. Getting in a car or building provides a safe shelter. If on a boat, avoid proximity to the mast and any metal objects (e.g., wheel, rigging, electronics). Go below decks if possible and stay low when on deck.

To calculate your approximate distance from a thunderstorm, count the seconds between the flash and the crash. For every five-second interval between when you see lightning and when you hear thunder, the storm is one mile away. The coast is generally clear for return to outdoor activities thirty minutes after the flash-to-crash interval has increased to thirty seconds (i.e., the storm is six miles away).

Lightning kills in two ways. Sometimes the victim suffers from severe internal burns, which may not be survivable. Others die because their diaphragms (breathing muscle) and hearts are temporarily stunned, rendering them pulseless and unable to breathe. For these people, a minute or two of CPR is sometimes all that is needed before the spontaneous return of respirations. If you approach a scene where a number of people have been struck by lightning, attend to those that are apparently dead first, as resuscitation is often successful (see CPR).

## Beginners Only

Okay, admit it, you're a kook, a barney, a hodad even. You are such a rookie that you thought that surf wax went on the bottom of the board, like skis, not on the top. Good, then read on (so long as no one is looking over your shoulder), 'cause this little section has a few pointers just for you. You reeeeeally want to get a shiny new surfboard, something that will fit smartly under your arm and you can put on the roof of your car. You think that just buying a board is going to improve your chi (energy flow). If you've already bought a board, you know this to be true. But before you paddle out into the great blue yonder, there are a few important things you need to know so you don't kill yourself or anyone else on your first outing. First of all, don't even *think* about learning to surf before you are a confident swimmer (see minimum swimming requirements above). You also need to be in reasonable physical shape, and if you are over fifty years old or have any serious medical conditions, you should consult a doctor to clear you for splashdown.

Okay, so you can swim, and your body is in passable condition. If you did not grow up playing in waves, you should start in the ocean without a surfboard. Wade out at a sandy lifeguarded beach with gentle crumbling surf that is waist high or smaller, avoiding areas where the waves are hollow or plunging. *Feel* the waves. Get a sense of how they push you around after they have broken and how they move you in a circular fashion outside (seaward) of the breakers. Practice diving through waves, just under the surface and parallel to the bottom, being extremely careful not to hit bottom. Get a sense of how much easier it is to duck under breaking waves as opposed to crashing through them.

In order to get a basic sense of how waves break and how to catch them, spend some time bodysurfing or bodyboarding. The more time spent doing these complementary wave sports, the faster you will progress as a surfer. When taking off on a wave, make sure to always keep one or both arms extended in front of you so you can fend off the bottom, and learn how to angle off along the wave face so you don't get your head pile-driven into the sand (which can result in a broken neck). You will initially catch more waves than on a stand-up surfboard because you have the added propulsion of swim fins and don't need to pop up to a standing position. Furthermore, bodyboards are soft and have no sharp pointy edges, so it is difficult to get injured by your board. In fact, both bodysurfing and bodyboarding are excellent sports in their own rights, and both sports run competitions at the famed Banzai Pipeline in Oahu, the contest wave by which all others are judged. Advanced bodysurfing is a full-contact mano-a-mano sport and is an integral component of the basic skill set possessed by all true watermen. Skilled surfers will bodysurf in toward shore if they lose their boards in the surf. Bodyboarders can excel at tube riding. They can take off steeper and deeper than stand-up surfers, and they tackle shore break and other heavy waves that most surfers shy away from.

If you are surfing for the first time, it is probably best to rent a big, stable, foam long board nine plus feet long with rubber fins whose impact-absorbing properties will be much appreciated during the innumerable collisions between you and your board, which are an inevitable part of the learning process. Most beginners will quickly outgrow the sluggish performance characteristics of such a board and within five to ten sessions will want to progress to a "real" (fiberglass or epoxy) surfboard, which is why we recommend you rent or buy a cheap used foam board for your first few sessions. Most will graduate to a hard fiberglass board, and a nine-foot long-board shape is a safe bet for learning. Invest in a quality leash. If you have a young child, go out and buy them a foamie, as it will provide years of fun and can be used by less experienced friends when your child progresses to a real board.

Another essential piece of gear is a wet suit for cool or cold water, or a rash guard if the water is very warm. A wet suit not only keeps you warm but also protects you from chafing against the deck of your board, protects you from the sun, and provides a bit of flotation. If you opt for a rash guard, we recommend you buy one made of sun-blocking fabric.

Now that you've got the gear, you need to find a suitable place to learn. The ideal beginner spot is an uncrowded sandy beach break with gentle, crumbly small waves, preferably near a lifeguard tower. Either take a couple of lessons or find a mentor willing to teach you the basic techniques of paddling, wave selection, popping up, and riding.

After a while you will have noticed that all of the "real" surfers are packed in a few relatively small areas and are getting some nice long rides, while you get only a few short dumpy rides in your uncrowded spot. The surfers in the good spots are not all congregated together because they are good buddies, but rather they are clustered in good takeoff spots where the waves peak and then peel in a continuous fashion, allowing for longer rides. You have taken your licks on the dumpy waves inside, you've bought yourself a board, and naturally figure it is time to go and join them—whoa! Before you even *think* about getting out in the actual lineup, you need to (1) make sure you have the skills to maintain control of your board (so it doesn't hit someone) and (2) you are familiar with the rules of surfing etiquette. If you don't follow steps 1 or 2, you will be immediately banished from the lineup by a local heavy and sent doggy-paddling with your leash between your legs back to your uncrowded spot.

As a beginner, avoid the common mistake of succumbing to peer pressure from your more experienced friends and venturing out in spots that are clearly beyond your abilities. Surf breaks that may be veritable surfing playgrounds for the experienced surfer can prove extremely hazardous for the novice who doesn't have the skill set to "read" a break, duck-dive large waves, or paddle with power and efficiency. Surfing in such conditions not only jeopardizes your safety, but also poses a risk to those around you.

## "My Wave!"—the Rules of Surfing Etiquette

Before we get too far with this, a few observations are in order. Surfing is all about freedom. There are no surf police, and no property lines or road signs out on the water. The rules of surfing etiquette have evolved over time to minimize the risk of collisions between surfers and to ensure that a surfer who is up and riding on a favorable section of a wave is free to surf the entire length of the wave without interference from other surfers. To some extent, these rules also allow the most skillful surfers (those who can take off steep and deep) to catch the best waves.

Remember, these are *unwritten rules* and they may vary from place to place according to the traditions of the local surfing subculture; they may even vary depending on where you are in the pecking order of the lineup. Localism has always been somewhat of an issue, particularly at crowded quality surf breaks, and just as with the pigs in George Orwell's *Animal Farm*, at some heavily localized spots, some piggish surfers feel like they are *more* equal than others. Local surfers (that is, anyone who has been in town a few months longer than you) may use subtle or not-so-subtle forms of intimidation to discourage others from surfing "their" break. However, with rare exception, a combination of good surfing and good manners (like waiting your turn in the lineup) will earn you respect in such places. Beginners will do better by avoiding these highly competitive localized breaks and should sacrifice wave quality in favor of smaller crowds, a mellower vibe, and most importantly, the opportunity to catch more waves.

## Never Drop In

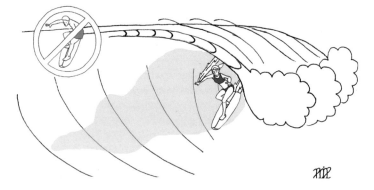

The surfer up and riding, closest to the curl, has right of way, and all others must stay clear. The male surfer must exit the wave and should not "drop in."

## Avoid Interfering with Those Riding a Wave

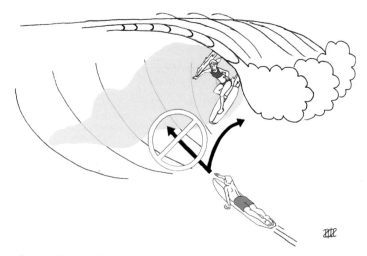

Surfers paddling out should paddle clear of those riding a wave, even if it means getting "stuffed" by the white water. Those paddling out should stay well clear of the break.

# Rule 1

The first surfer up and riding closest to the peak of the wave has right of way, and all others must stay clear. It follows then that if two surfers are paddling side by side for the same wave, the surfer closest to the peak has priority.

There is some ambiguity (and we're just on rule 1!) as to whether it is the first surfer standing or rather the surfer closest to the peak who has priority. Usually the first one up *is* closest to the peak, but occasionally a long-boarder may be the first one up because of their board's greater planning capability, but then a short-boarder will catch the wave deeper, closer to the curl. Local customs vary on the interpretation of this scenario, and you'll just have to get a feel for it in your own locale.

Occasionally you will be riding a wave, and someone who does not see you will attempt to "drop in" in front of you. If someone is attempting to drop in on you, hoot or whistle to make your presence known so they can kick out of the wave.

Surfers who are caught inside and making their way out to the lineup should make every effort to avoid a rider, even if it means they have to paddle into white water and get stuffed by the wave. In order to avoid paddling across the path of oncoming surfers, always try to paddle well around the surf break and through a channel (if one exists). There are occasions when, despite everyone's best intentions, the rider's preferred line will place him or her on a collision course with a paddling or swimming surfer. Because of the rider's superior speed and maneuverability, it is ultimately his or her responsibility to avoid such collisions (in fact, despite the rules of surfing etiquette, in most courts of law it is the *rider*, not the paddler, who has been held liable for damages resulting from collisions).

The paddling surfer who has interfered should immediately offer an apology to the rider, which is generally sufficient to maintain a positive vibe in the lineup. If there is even a small chance that you *may* have interfered with someone's ride, apologize anyway—it's just good karma.

When paddling for a wave at an A-frame peak, which can be ridden both left and right, it is courteous to make your intentions clear to those around you by stating something like, "I'm going right," so that another surfer can ride the wave in the opposite direction.

# Rule 2

Always control your board. Control it when paddling out, sitting in the lineup, catching waves, and when you finish a ride. When you end a ride, don't just let your board shoot away where it may. Never throw your board by abandoning it so you can swim under a large wave. Remember, even on its leash, your loose board poses a serious hazard to anyone within about a twenty-foot radius.

If you find yourself consistently unable to hang on to your own board, then the conditions are probably too big for you to handle safely. That being said, even the most accomplished surfers will sometimes resort to letting the board go and diving under a wave in *really* big surf. This should only be done as a last resort and only after making absolutely sure that no one is behind you.

## Rule 3

No snaking. If a surfer is perfectly positioned and paddling to catch a wave, do not paddle around and "inside" of them at the last second to claim priority. This is termed "snaking." Ideally there is a general understanding that if you wait your turn, you will gradually make your way through the rotation, progress to the ideal takeoff spot, and when the next wave comes, it is yours for the taking. In reality, this idealized system only occurs when there is a small group of surfers who know one another. In most cases, the best surfers snag the most waves. In some places, if a surfer is up and riding and you take off inside of him or her, this, too, is considered a form of snaking. This latter version of snaking can be bent a bit. For example, in a lineup consisting of long-boarders, SUP'ers, and short-boarders, those on bigger boards have a distinct paddling advantage and can catch waves much earlier than a short-boarder who requires a steeper section for taking off. If the long-board riders are hogging all the waves, it may be okay for a short-boarder to occasionally catch a wave inside of the already-up-and-riding long-boarder and claim priority. Ideally everyone plays well in the sandbox; the short-boarders are allowed their fair share of waves and no snaking occurs.

## The Buddy System

A buddy system is a standard procedure for many water sports like scuba diving and has been advocated for surfing as well. Should you become injured, exhausted, or lose your board, a buddy can let you rest on their board and escort you back to terra firma. However, do not go surfing with the *expectation* that others will quickly come to your aid should you get into trouble. Surfing is a solo sport, and once you commit to paddling out, you are pretty much on your own. To begin with, it may be a couple of minutes before anyone even realizes that you are in trouble; it will then take a while for them to reach you, and depending on the circumstances, they may have limited options once they get there.

Though many find surfing alone to be a peaceful, almost-mystical experience, like other guilty pleasures, it carries with it some measure of risk, and surfing alone should be discouraged from a pure-safety perspective. That being said, if you happen upon clean, empty waves and are unable to resist the temptation of a solo session, be wary that without the potential help of others, you have less margin for error, so it behooves you to take a few extra precautions: if you have a helmet, use it; use your heavy-duty leash; and only go out if the conditions are well within your comfort zone. It is also always a good idea to make sure someone on land knows where you are and when you expect to return (so at least they can find your body).

Children under the age of fourteen, however, should *never* surf alone and *must* be supervised by a responsible, undistracted adult at all times. It often works best to have one adult watching the *keikis* on land, while another keeps an eye on things from the water. One scary moment in the water may be all it takes to dissuade a young child from surfing for many years to come.

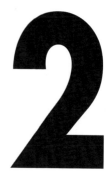

# Fitness
# for Surfers

Success in some sports like long-distance running and bike racing requires significant amounts of stamina. Other sports like sprinting and weight lifting favor those with the ability to generate short bursts of strength. Surfing, however, demands elements of both. Considerable stamina is needed simply to make it out to the lineup through a heavy beach break or when caught inside during a particularly long set, and quick bursts of paddling power are necessary to generate the speed required to catch waves or to avoid oncoming surfers. Quality wave riding, particularly at the elite levels of the sport, also calls for a combination of flexibility, core strength, balance, and reaction time. These traits are not only essential ingredients for good surfing, but are also necessary to meet the demands of an unpredictable and potentially dangerous ocean environment, where there is a real risk of drowning from heavy wave action and strong currents, and risk of injury from collisions with surfboards, other surfers, and the seafloor.

While surfing is an excellent workout in its own right and is the best and most specific way to stay in shape for paddling, lack of swell or lack of free time prevent many of us from depending on surfing as our only workout. Furthermore, time-motion studies have demonstrated that while 50 percent of one's time spent surfing is devoted to paddling, less than 5 percent is actually spent riding waves—so unless you are lucky enough to be riding the mile-long point break in Chicama (Peru) every day, it is hard to effectively build strength in the muscles that you actually use to ride waves solely by surfing. Relying exclusively on surfing as a means of physical fitness can also lead to muscle and postural imbalance by over-developing the paddling muscles in the chest and shoulders and neglecting the legs and core. Moreover, a well-rounded waterman or woman should develop a balanced physique that works not only for surfing but also for swimming, SUP (stand-up paddling), running, and free diving. Professional surfers, who generally have access to good surf year-round, almost universally supplement their time in the water with some form of dynamic warm-up, post-surf stretching, and land-based strength training for peak performance.

Effective surf-specific training regimens focus not only on improving aerobic capacity and upper body strength, but also include an emphasis improving posture, stability, flexibility, and balance. We describe how to achieve these fitness objectives by dividing your workouts into five major components: pre-surf dynamic warm-ups, post-surf stretching and massage, aerobic exercise, strength training, and balance training. We've included surfing-specific workouts and stretching routines from a number of the sport's leading fitness and training authorities that incorporate the principles of modern sport medicine in combination with a variety of Eastern practices. Unlike many traditional weight training routines, which work muscles in isolation (and can ultimately compromise flexibility), these exercises allow you to move your body naturally using your muscles in many of the same functional groups that are used when you surf. Most rely simply on your own body weight and do not require specialized equipment, so they can be performed anywhere and have the added advantages of helping to improve your balance as well as your proprioception (sense of body position).

Your own fitness program should be tailored to your unique surfing goals and aspirations. If you are a weekend warrior with limited free time who at most surfs once or twice a week and during the off-season may go for a few months without riding any waves at all, your top priority should be to maintain aerobic paddling capacity. When you take your yearly surf trek, you want to be able to pick up where you left off at the end of your last trip, not waste the first few precious days sucking wind. For the competitive surfer who consistently surfs a few times a week and wants to bump it up to the next level, the emphasis will be on core strength, harnessing explosive power from balanced positions, and incorporating leg strength into rail-to-rail turns.

An exercise program is no good if you don't stick with it, so make sure to set realistic goals that are achievable and compatible with your schedule. Keep things fresh by mixing up your activities, training with a partner, and surfing whenever possible. Also, remember to keep the fundamentals of surfing in mind when you are training. Visualize duck-diving and pop-ups when doing push-up–type exercises and imagine bottom turns, snaps, airs, and cutbacks when performing squatting and trunk-twisting maneuvers. It is ultimately up to you to generate surf specificity into your training.

## Dynamic Warm-ups

"You pull up to your local break and it is firing. Winds are light, and the crowds aren't on it. So you add a little wax to your board, race across the beach, and drop your board on the sand. You reach to touch your toes (man, those hamstrings are tight), do a few arm circles, and hit the water. Sound familiar?" —Scott Adams, CSCS (founder of Surf Stronger)

Most surfers are so eager to make the most of their limited free time that they often skip a pre-surf warm-up altogether. However, if muscles are not properly warmed up, then power cannot be successfully harnessed, sprains and strains become more common, and your peak potential in surfing will never be achieved.

So what constitutes a good pre-surf warm up? It all depends on the kind of surfing you'll be doing. A competitive surfer with good wave-selection skills will be paddling less and attempting aerial maneuvers that stress the ankles, knees, and hips more than the shoulders. So if you're a young gun, you'll want to concentrate on loosening up your lower body with hip knee and ankle circles, shakeouts, and hip bridges. Conversely, a more novice surfer will be paddling more and stressing the shoulders more than the lower body, and should concentrate on warming up the upper body. Regardless of what kind of a surfer you are, a good warm-up gradually increases your heart rate, lets you break a light sweat, and moves in a manner that looks like surfing. When stretching, bear in mind that your body has plastic qualities. Stretch it slowly, and it will adapt; but force it quickly (particularly when cold), and it might break. Try visualizing your body as a kinetic chain of synchronously moving bones, tendons, and muscles from the soles of the feet to the top of the head. Most routines should take about five minutes and should be performed while facing the beach, allowing you to assess conditions while you warm up.

Contest surfers often seek myofascial release via massage, acupuncture, osteopathic, or chiropractic manipulation before and after their heats as a means of improving elasticity and preventing painful muscle spasms. For those of us without a personal manual therapist, a proper dynamic warm-up before surfing and a good post-surf stretch with some self-massage can go a long way toward preventing the chronic neck, back, and shoulder overuse injuries that are so common among surfers.

# Here Are Some Dynamic Warm-up and Breathing Exercises to Choose From

Remember to warm up to the point of breaking a light sweat. The goal with these warm-ups is to use momentum to propel each body part fluidly through a full range of motion.

## Shoulder to Arm to Trunk, Hip, Knee, and Ankle Circles

Stand upright, slowly rotate your shoulders in a forward circular motion five times, then reverse the movement, and rotate your shoulders in a backward circular motion five times.

## ARM CIRCLES

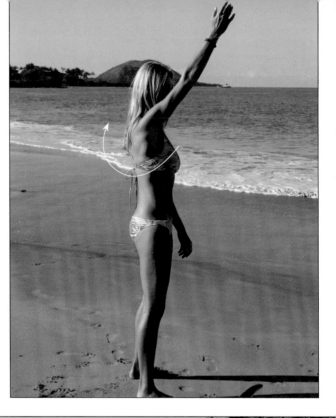

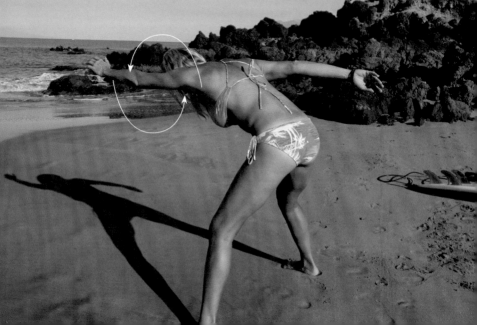

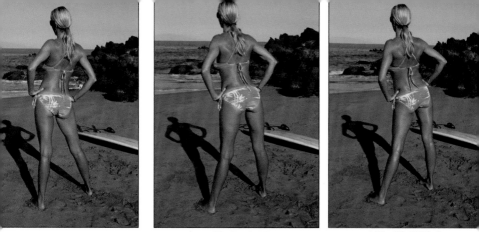

HIP CIRCLES 1      HIP CIRCLES 2      HIP CIRCLES 3

    Do the same with some big, wide arm circles twenty to thirty times in both directions. Avoid violent or jerky movements. Try to mimic the paddling motion as best as possible with full extension of the arms to adequately warm up the appropriate muscles. You can also incorporate the core and hamstrings by bending at the hips and relaxing your knees with feet double-shoulder width apart while performing these arm circles.

    Progress to trunk twists with the arms fully relaxed. Actively twist your trunk from side to side and let your arms flail passively. This technique is used extensively in Eastern therapies such as Tibetan rite 1 and Chinese Qigong as well as modern sports medicine and is quite popular with professional surfers before their heats to warm up the muscles and increase the flexibility of the joints. Passive circular movements of the knees, hips, and shoulders help preserve joint range of motion by maintaining elasticity. Once the series is complete, go back up the kinetic chain, from ankle to knee, hip, trunk, and shoulders and back down one more time.

    Breathe normally.

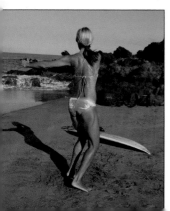

TRUNK TWISTS

## Neck Stretches and Circles

Stand upright, tilt your head sideways toward your left shoulder, and hold it for five seconds, then tilt your head toward your chest, and hold it for five seconds. Then tilt your head toward your left shoulder and hold it for five seconds, and lastly, tilt your head backward and hold it for five seconds. Return your head to a normal position.

For breathing, exhale as you move your head around, and inhale as you return to the upright position.

Incorporate a smooth rolling neck warm-up by performing gentle circles twenty to thirty times in each direction. Also, perform chin tucks by retracting head back like a cobra twenty to thirty times. Chin tucks during paddle outs can also prevent hyperextension neck strain.

## Shake Outs

Shake outs just involve loosening up the limbs by shaking them gently with the muscles completely relaxed. This is another warm-up technique common to both Qigong and sports medicine. Start at the bottom of the kinetic chain by shaking out the ankles and then knees, hips, shoulders, elbows, and wrists.

### Shoulder Protraction and Rotational Mobility

For the shoulders, stand upright with your arms just below shoulder level, your elbows bent, and your hands together in front of your chest, with your fingertips touching and palms apart. Press inward on your fingers until their inside surfaces are almost touching. Your palms should not be touching. Release and press your fingers again. Repeat twenty times.

For breathing, breathe normally.

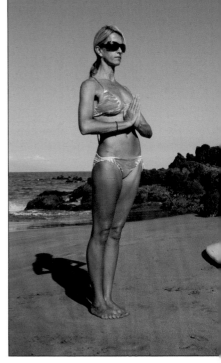

ISOMETRIC SHOULDER
PROTRACTION

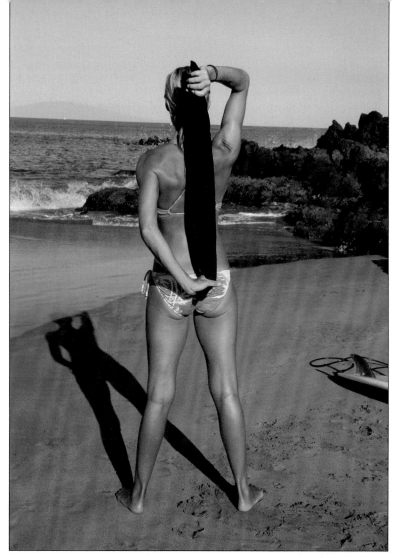

Take a rash guard, T-shirt, surf leash, or towel and, holding it in your left hand, flip it over your left shoulder. Catch the loose end of the towel behind your back with your right hand by smoothly reaching up as far as possible. Repeat with the towel in your right hand catching the loose end with your left hand. This exercise is important for internal and external rotational mobility of the shoulders.

For breathing, breathe normally.

## Scapular Retraction Squeezes

Practice the important shoulder-preserving technique of scapular stability by squeezing the shoulder blades together. Scapular movement asynchrony has been implicated in the sports medicine literature as the most common cause of shoulder pain and overuse injury. You may perform these scapular retraction exercises with or without holding a towel, leash, or rash guard in your hands, or you may incorporate them into an active chest stretch with lunges. The variations are endless, pick what you like best, but always maintain proper form. Do these squeezes about twenty times. You can also do these while waiting for waves in the lineup.

Breathe normally.

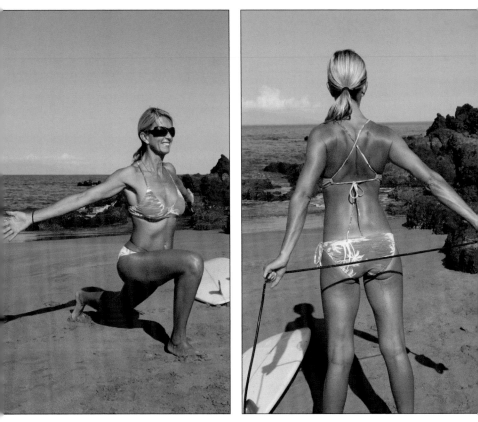

SCAPULAR RETRACTION SQUEEZE WITH
LUNGE

SCAPULAR RETRACTION SQUEEZE

Note scapular asynchrony, and scapular winging. This is due to weak scapular stabilizing muscles, and can result in chronic shoulder pain.

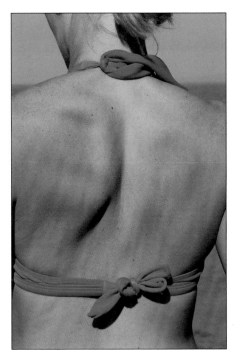

## Hip Bridges, Spinal Mobilization, and Warming Up the Core

**Tibetan Rite 2**

Lie flat on the ground face up. Fully extend your arms along your sides and place the palms of your hands against the ground, keeping fingers close together. Lift your legs, knees straight, into a vertical position. If possible, extend the legs over the body toward your head. Do not let the knees bend. Then slowly lower the legs to the ground, always keeping the knees straight. Allow the muscles to relax and repeat. This movement pattern, activating the core muscles, is also known as Tibetan rite 2.

This maneuver should be approached cautiously by those with chronic lower back or neck problems, trying to avoid strain and over-arching of the the lumbar spine, always making sure the lower back stays flat on the ground; it may be more easily done by raising one leg at a time.

Breathe normally.

FITNESS FOR SURFERS

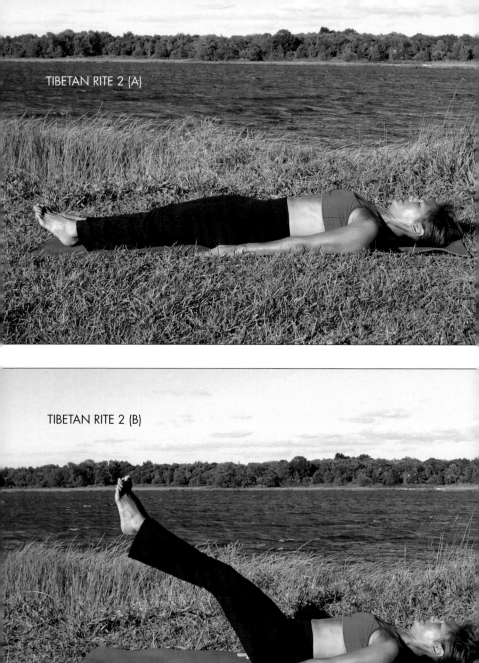

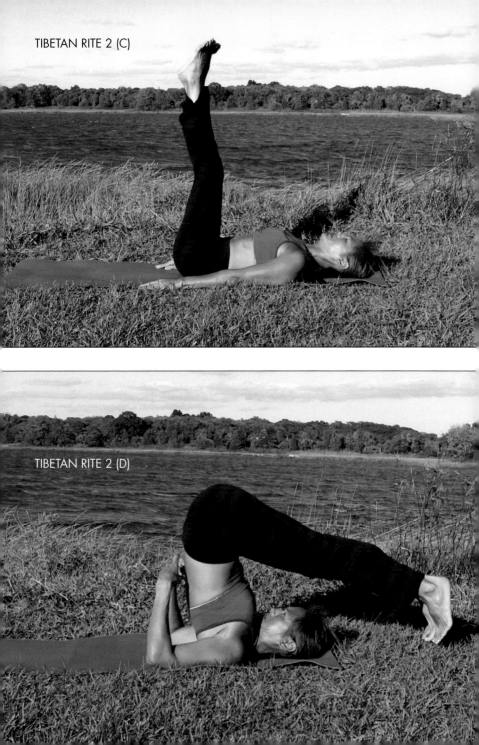

TIBETAN RITE 2 (C)

TIBETAN RITE 2 (D)

## Tibetan Rite 3

Progress to a similar movement lying on the ground with just the upper back and shoulders touching, feet flat on the ground, and butt lifted up in the air. Lift your left foot off the ground for one set and then your right. Finish by relaxing the back and allowing the knees to fall to the left while turning your head to the right. Repeat this motion in the opposite direction. Repeat this set five times. This will open up often-tight muscles of the hips and lower back. It is a modified combination of Tibetan rite 3 and Qigong for warming up the core muscles essential for surfing.

For breathing, breathe in deeply as you lift your legs and exhale as you lower your legs.

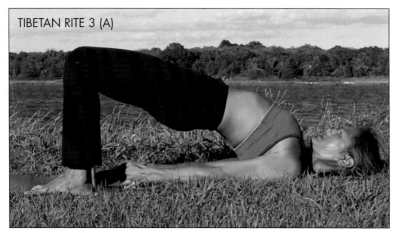

TIBETAN RITE 3 (A)

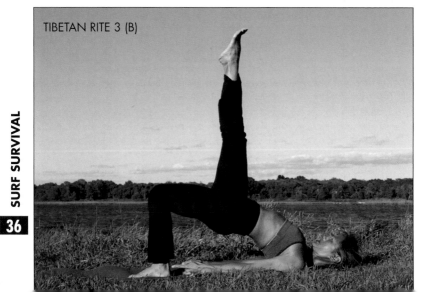

TIBETAN RITE 3 (B)

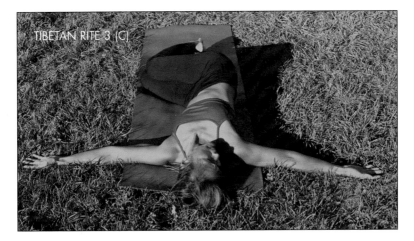

TIBETAN RITE 3 (C)

## Tibetan Rite 4

Sit down on the ground with your legs straight out in front of you and your feet about twelve inches apart. With the trunk of the body erect, place the palms of your hands on the floor alongside your buttocks. Then tuck the chin forward against the chest. Now drop the head backward as far as it will go. At the same time, raise your hips so that the knees bend while the arms remain straight. Let the muscles relax as you return to your original sitting position. Rest before repeating this exercise adapted from Tibetan rite 4.

For breathing, breathe in as you raise the hips up and breathe out fully as you come down.

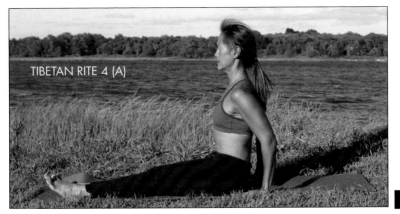

TIBETAN RITE 4 (A)

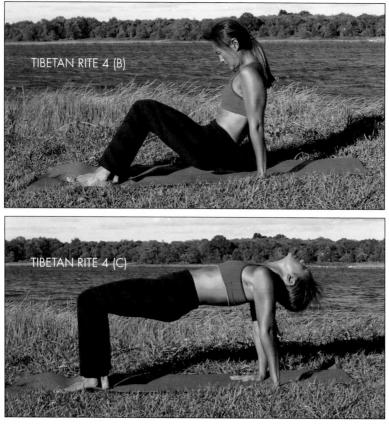

TIBETAN RITE 4 (B)

TIBETAN RITE 4 (C)

**Tibetan Rite 5**

Assume the plank (push-up) position with elbows extended but not locked, facing the sand. The hands and feet should be kept straight. Next, arch your spine into an upward-dog position, like you are craning over your surfboard looking for those outside set waves. Bending at the hips, bring the body up into an inverted V or downward-dog position like duck-diving a large wave with both feet at the tail of the board (no duck-diving on your knees!).

For breathing, breathe in deeply as you raise the body and exhale fully as you lower the body.

This movement is adapted from Hindu push-ups, Qigong, and Tibetan rite 5. It also reflects the body motion of a successful duck-dive: feet at tail of board, breathing in as you push the board under the water, exhaling as you push the board forward underwater, following its buoyancy up and out the back of the wave.

Note that the dynamic warm-up does not involve static stretching (the kind of stretch where you lengthen the muscle and hold the position). Save this type of stretching for after surfing.

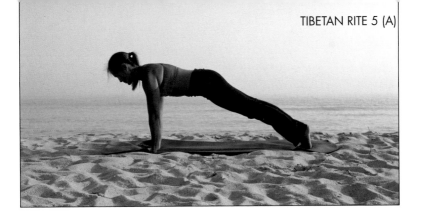

TIBETAN RITE 5 (A)

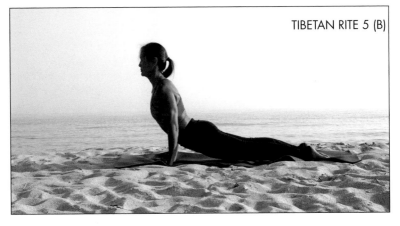

TIBETAN RITE 5 (B)

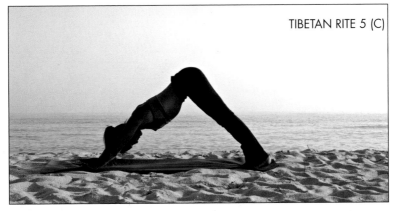

TIBETAN RITE 5 (C)

"Keep the pre-surf stretching active. The slower-paced and longer-held stretches hinder your reaction time by reducing the elasticity of your muscles. A slower reaction is the last thing you want as you drop in under a pitching lip!" —Scott Adams, CSCS

# Apres Surf: Stretching and Flexibility

> "Stretching trains the muscles to perform at their normal full-length and allows your joints to move at full range of motion. When joints move freely, you actually use less energy to surf because you move with efficiency and fluidity—which translates directly to less stress on the joints most commonly injured in surfing."
> —Tim Brown, DC (Surfline.com Health and Fitness Column)

With apres-surf stretching, the idea is to increase the length of the muscles that have been contracting during the surf session. A good way to do this is to perform slower-paced, static stretches and use myofascial-release and self-massage techniques such as foam rollers and assisted stretching with a partner, therapy bands, or using a heat source like a hot tub, steam room, or sauna. The best time to stretch like this is after surfing, because that is when you want your muscles to relax and lengthen. Before you start stretching, make sure your body is warm; then, follow these guidelines to get the most out of your practice. Ultimately, those of us who neglected flexibility in our youth will be behind the curve and have to work much harder to achieve satisfactory flexibility in middle age and beyond.

Move into each stretch slowly. Hold your stretch for twenty to thirty seconds. Breathe evenly and don't strain. The idea is to be relaxed. Come out of the stretch slowly and repeat if necessary. Note: do not attempt headstand poses on soft sand.

## Iron Cross and 90-90 Stretches

Iron Cross and 90-90 stretches are compound stretches that stretch multiple muscles and help greatly with the hip mobility crucial for progressive surfing.

The Iron Cross stretches the gluteals and piriformis of the butt, vastus lateralis and iliotibial band of the thigh, scalenes of the neck, biceps of both hamstrings and arms as well as the peroneals of the calves.

The 90-90 stretch involves flexing both hips and knees ninety degrees (hence the term "90-90"). Alternate leaning forward on each flexed hip. This alternately stretches both the internal hip rotators, such as the obturator muscle, and external hip rotators, such as the piriformis muscle, that are stressed from surfing.

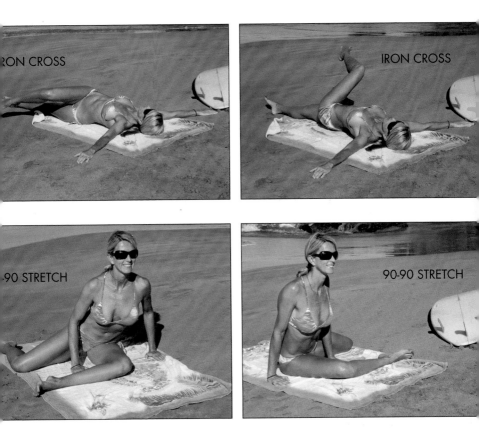

IRON CROSS

IRON CROSS

90-90 STRETCH

90-90 STRETCH

## Chest Stretch

Open your arms facing a wall or your car and lean in so your cheek almost touches the surface. Lunge slightly with one leg until you feel a stretch in the opposite chest muscle, hold for thirty seconds, and repeat on the other side. These stretches are beneficial immediately and within hours after a surf session and only take a minute and can be done in a hot shower, which is a plus in colder climates.

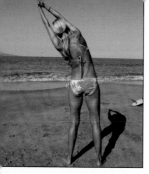

At home, you may continue to perform the following static stretches for the often-tight surfing muscles. Such stretches include the following:

## Latissimus Stretch

Pull upward while leaning straight over toward your left side. Keep your lower body straight. You should feel the stretch along your right side. Hold fifteen to thirty seconds and then switch sides. Repeat two to four times for each side.

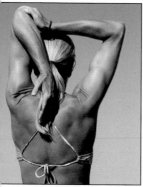

## Triceps Stretch

Bring your left elbow straight up while bending your arm. Grab your left elbow with your right hand and pull your left elbow toward your head with light pressure. If you are more flexible, you may pull your arm slightly behind your head. You will feel the stretch along the back of your arm. Hold fifteen to thirty seconds and then switch elbows. Repeat two to four times for each arm.

## Calf Stretch

Place your hands on a wall, car, tree, or lifeguard tower for balance. Keep your right leg straight and press your right heel into the floor. Press your hips forward, bending your left knee. Feel the stretch in your left calf. Hold for fifteen to thirty seconds. Repeat two to four times for each leg.

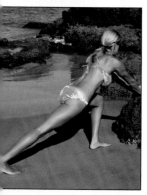

## Groin Stretch

Grab your ankles while sitting butterfly style and gently pull your legs toward you. Use your elbows to press your knees toward the floor. Feel the stretch in your inner thighs. Hold fifteen to thirty seconds and repeat two to four times.

## Hamstring Stretch (not pictured)

Lie on the ground. Extend your left leg out straight with your toes pointing up. If your back is uncomfortable, use a rolled towel for support. Gently pull your left leg toward you as you straighten that knee. You should feel a gentle stretch down the back of your right leg. Hold the stretch fifteen to thirty seconds and repeat two to four times for each leg.

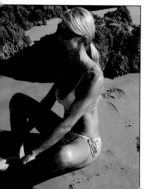

# Yoga and the Sun Salutation

Surfing and yoga have been tied together in many books on surf training because yoga is a great way to increase strength, balance, and flexibility. The core sequence to take away from this literature is Surya Namaskar, the sun salutation, a series of twelve postures that are performed in a graceful single flow.

Each movement is coordinated with the breath. Inhale through your nose as you extend or stretch and exhale through your nose as you fold or contract. This type of breathing is known as oceanic breathing (and no, we didn't just make that up for the book). Different styles of yoga perform the sun salutation with their own variations, however, the flow presented below covers core steps used in most styles.

For the series below, a single round consists of two complete sequences: one for the right side of the body and the other for the left. Try to perform the sun salutation as part of your daily stretching routine.

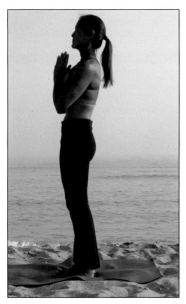

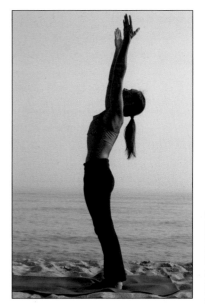

1. Mountain
Begin by standing in mountain pose, feet about hip-width apart, hands in prayer position. Take several deep breaths.

2. Hands Up
Inhale slowly while extending arms. Do not overarch the back but rather try to lengthen the spine by reaching up.

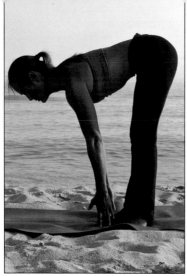

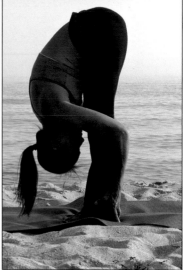

3. Flat Back
Exhale, hinge at the hips, and touch your toes. Keep your back flat; do not overbend at the spine. Hold the position and inhale.

4. Head to Knees
Exhale. Bending at the hips, bring your head toward your knees. Place your hands on the backs of your heels to gently pull inward.

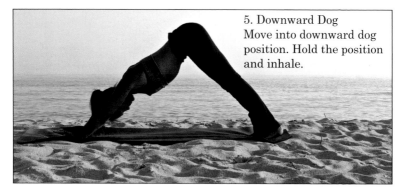

5. Downward Dog
Move into downward dog position. Hold the position and inhale.

6. Low Plank
Exhale and lower yourself as if coming down from a push-up. Only your hands and feet should touch the ground.

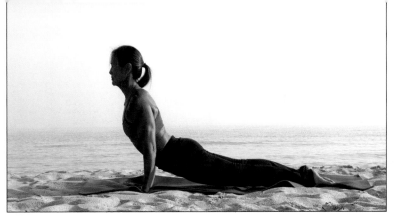

7. Upward Dog
Inhale and stretch forward and up, bending at the waist. Use your arms to lift your torso, but only bend back as far as it feels comfortable and safe. Lift your legs up so that only the tops of your feet and your hands touch the ground.

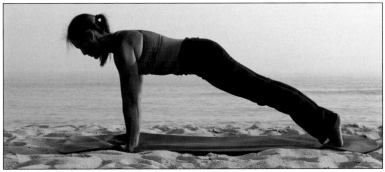

8. Plank
Exhale, lift from the hips, and push back and up as if coming through a wave during a duck-dive.

9. Warrior
Inhale and lunge the right foot forward as your arms reach up toward the sky; keep your back straight.

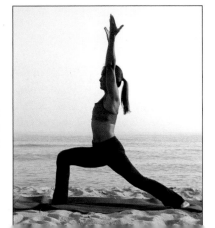

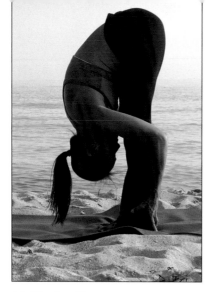

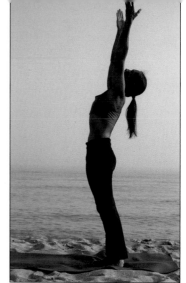

10. Head to Knees
Exhale as you bring the left foot forward and step into head-to-knee position. Hinge at the hips and do not overbend at the spine.

11. Hands Up
Inhale and rise slowly while keeping arms extended. Do not overarch the back.

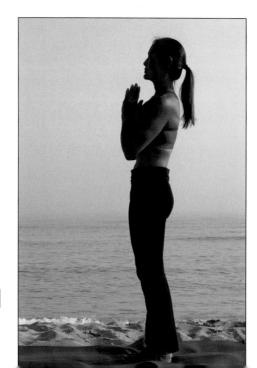

12. Mountain
Exhale, and in a slow sweeping motion, lower your arms into a prayer position. Repeat the sequence.

# Strength Training: Building Up from the Basics

Strength training increases fitness by increasing muscle strength and endurance and maintaining the body's fat within acceptable limits. It should be an important component of your fitness and surf-training program, regardless of your age or gender, and will improve your surfing, as well as your overall sense of well-being.

A common mistake, particularly among younger male athletes, is to concentrate predominantly on limb strength (look at my pipes!) while neglecting core strength, which often leads to injuries stemming from a weak core. To avoid being sidelined by injury, begin by building a solid core as your foundation, then work on training your balance, and finally progress to building limb strength.

## Core Region Circuit Training Exercises

The core is comprised of the hip, pelvic, and spinal muscles up to the base of the skull. It is essential to have good core strength before moving on to any other type of strength training or even progressing toward more aggressive surfing. The core muscles are the balance muscles. Balance is a trained skill! The more you train your balance and posture, the better your balance, posture, and, ultimately, your surfing will become. Once you have achieved a solid core, then you can begin stability training by performing rotational maneuvers. Try the following exercises when the waves are flat to develop the core muscles, and you will see similarities to the dynamic warm-ups:

### Spine Flutter

Lie on your back with knees bent comfortably and feet flat on the ground. Extend the arms straight back with the biceps next to the ears and hands about an inch off the ground. Keep a slight bend in the elbows and the back of the head on the ground. Press the ribs downward using the abdominal muscles and keep the low back in contact with the ground. Raise and lower the hands a few inches from the ground for ten to twenty repetitions. When it feels like the ribs are lifting from the ground, use the abdominal muscles to counteract this. To increase resistance, straighten the knees in increments as tolerated.

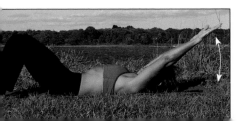

## Supermans

Lie facedown on ground or with chest on foam roller with hands in front of you like Superman. You may place a rolled towel under the forehead to clear the face from the ground. Raise the chest and head off the floor keeping feet in contact with the floor. Do not raise head past eight to twelve inches off the ground, as excessive hyperextension may cause injury.

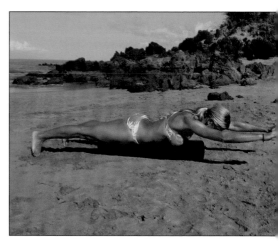

## Push-up Superman Alternating Arms

Start the movement in a plank (push-up) position. Holding that position, raise your right arm and left leg off of the ground. Return to the starting position and repeat with the other arm and leg. Hold each lift for one to two seconds. Use a foam roller or Indo board for more of a challenge.

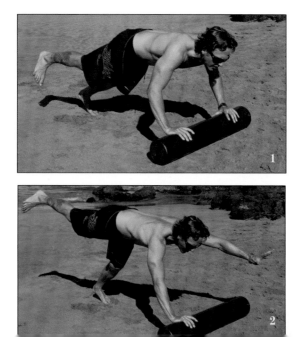

## Hip Bridge

Lie on your back with your legs bent ninety degrees at the knees. Make sure that the low back is not arched. Slowly lift your hips off the floor and toward the sky. Lower your hips to the floor and repeat for the prescribed number of repetitions.

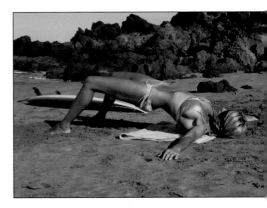

## Single-Leg Split Squat

This is one of the more difficult core body exercises—even with just your own bodyweight; however, it is essential to training for surfing and stability. Make sure you build gradually up to this one and be sure to sit back so that knees stay over the feet. Knees that are an inch or more beyond the toes during a squat are more prone to injury. For balance you can hold on to your surfboard.

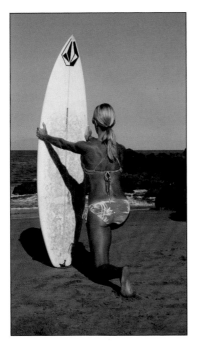

To recruit the core muscles during this exercise, exert diagonal downward pressure on the surfboard in a direction opposite the dropping knee (left knee drops, hands grip the board, and drive the tail into the sand in front of right foot; the board does not move at all but the core muscles contract isometrically). Once your thigh is slightly above parallel, return to start position. Keep most of the movement through the hips. Remember to keep head and back straight in a neutral position—hyperextension or flexion may cause injury. Keep weight over the middle of foot and heel, not the toes. Keep abdominals tight throughout exercise by drawing stomach in toward spine. This exercise can cause knee pain if the knee is flexed greater than ninety degrees.

## Prone Plank to Duck-Dive

Hold a plank position. Lift one leg up as if duck-diving on a surfboard while performing a push-up. Repeat with alternate leg ten times. Perform on sand or, for more of a challenge, on an unstable surface such as the Indo board. Use your surfboard with the Indo Giganté cushion for a more surfing-specific excercise. Don't cheat on the exercise by resting a knee down when you perform the duck-dive push-up. Unless you keep the back foot planted on the tail of the board with your body driving the nose of the board forcefully underwater, your duck-dive will be weak.

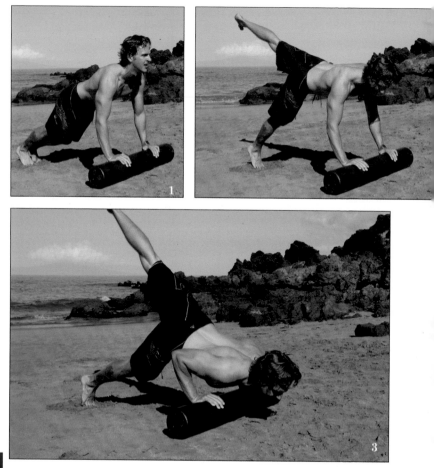

# Balance, Stability, Agility, and Regenerative Training

Balance must be trained consistently, or it will be lost. The same applies for stability. While many believe that balance and stability are the same, for purposes of sports medicine, balance is the ability to keep an unstable position, while stability is the ability to perform dynamic and explosive maneuvers from an unstable position. Therefore, balance must be mastered before stability.

Training on an unstable surface such as the Indo board (balance board on a roller), foam roller, or exercise ball is an excellent method of improving the body's balance and stability systems. Incorporating these accessories with body-weight training described above will guarantee a progression in core strength and stability. Cross-training with other board sports such as stand-up paddling, windsurfing, and kiteboarding is also a great way of improving one's balance and agility. On land, skateboarding and snowboarding are probably the best ways to simulate the dynamics and flow of surfing and are excellent ways to keep yourself in shape during the off-season. Don't forget to practice proper postural exercises as a lifestyle. Keep the shoulders back and pelvis tilted forward during daily activity.

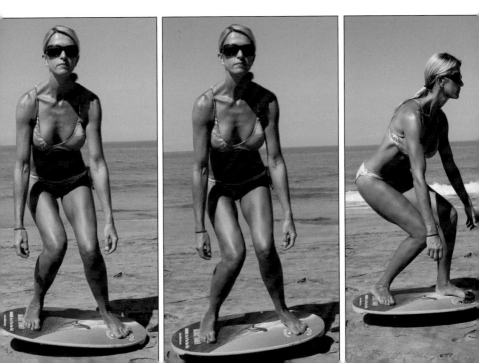

Practice balancing on a foam roller or Indo board by lying on it like a surfboard to find your body's center of gravity. Practice maintaining proper pitch (front to back), roll (side to side), and yaw (twist about a vertical axis) by adjusting the position of the roller. Once balanced in this method, work on stability. Try some paddling motions. Then try a pop-up. Progress slowly and at your own risk; the landings will be a lot harder than in the ocean!

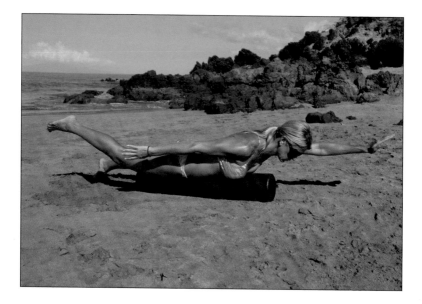

Massage of muscle knots and tight myotendonous complexes (where muscles merge into tendons) after workouts is considered regenerative training because it helps tendons and muscles repair themselves. Recent studies have shown that acute muscle inflammation also decreases with prompt massage. Whether you can afford a personal masseuse after each workout or give yourself a self-massage with a foam roller, it does a body good to engage in post-workout regenerative training. The variations are endless. Just remember the fundamentals of proper form and attention to all muscle groups.

# CORE STABILITY EXERCISES USING A FOAM ROLLER

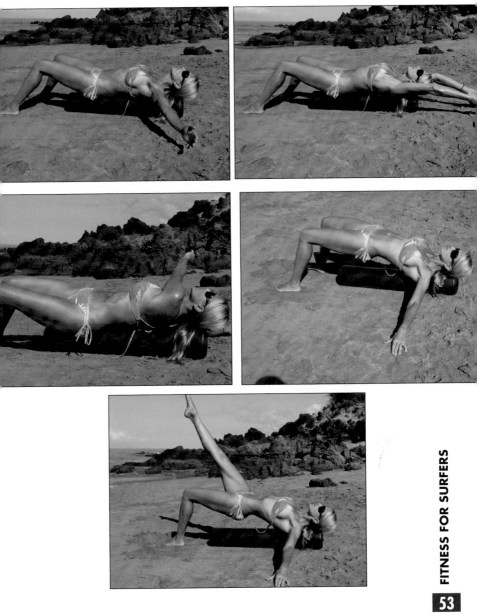

# High-Impact Explosive Body-Weight Training

High-impact exercise, while shown to increase the explosive strength beneficial for surfing, can accelerate or worsen arthritis, the bane of aging athletes. This technique has been highly touted as a means of training for the aerial maneuvers, which are pushing the boundaries of high-performance surfing above and beyond the wave face. Be aware that some of these ballistic-type exercises carry risks of severe muscle strain, arthritis, and tendon injury if done improperly. Only athletes who have already achieved high levels of strength through traditional training should consider this type of "plyometric" training and these drills should not be performed when surfer is fatigued or on consecutive days. Many of these exercises are done in high-intensity intervals, progressing in circuit fashion from speed and agility drills to jumps, push-ups, and medicine ball training.

## Squat Jumps

Stand with feet shoulder-width apart and trunk flexed forward slightly with back straight in a neutral position. Arms should be in the ready position with elbows flexed at approximately ninety degrees. Lower body where thighs are parallel to ground. Explode vertically and drive arms up. Land on both feet and repeat. Prior to takeoff, extend the ankles to their maximum range (toes pointing down) to ensure proper mechanics.

This exercise can cause patellar femoral syndrome (front-of-knee) pain if the knee is flexed greater than ninety degrees. Improper landings also stress the patellar tendon, just below the kneecap, causing jumper's knee. This is why perfect form is necessary. Once squat jumps lose their challenge, you may perform variations using trunk-twisting and single-leg maneuvers to attain surf specificity.

## Burpees

Start in a standing position, then bend your knees, and place your hands on the ground. Quickly hop back by extending your legs back into a push-up position. Hop back into a squat so your knees come into your chest and jump back up. This should be one continuous fluid motion.

This exercise can also cause knee pain if the knee is flexed greater than ninety degrees. Once standard posture is perfected, one may perform variations using medicine balls, Indo boards, exercise balls, foam rollers, and foam pads in a gym or at home.

BURPEE 1

BURPEE 2

BURPEE 3

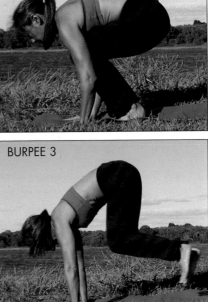

BURPEE 4

BURPEE 6

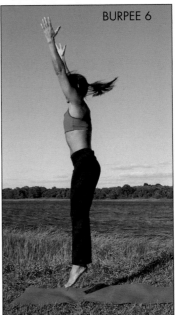

BURPEE 5

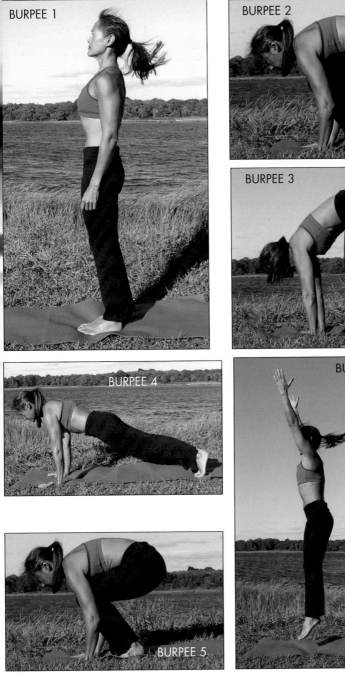

## Squat Thrusts

In a push-up position, bring both knees in toward your chest and then explode out again so they are fully extended. Repeat in a smooth, rhythmical fashion. These exercises are great especially if you keep banging your rear-foot big toe on the board, which indicates that during pop-ups you are not completely getting your feet on the board and under your body. Once standard posture is perfected, one may perform variations on an unstable surface as previously mentioned.

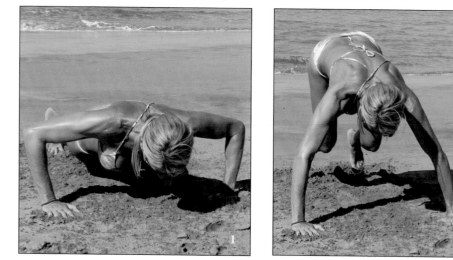

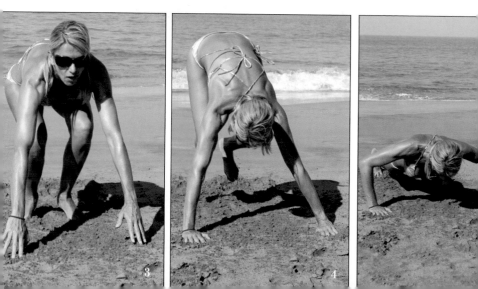

## Mountain Climbers

Mountain climber is similar to squat thrusts, only alternate your feet. In the push-up position with legs extended, bring one knee into your chest and then quickly switch to bring the other knee into your chest. The action should be a smooth running motion as your arms stay fixed. To increase the challenge, place your arms on an unstable surface (Indo board, etc.).

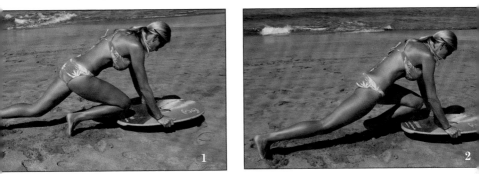

## Push-ups

To make regular push-ups functional, keep your core muscles engaged by tightening the abs and prevent the low back from arching or swaying. Tilt the pelvis up with those tightened abs to engage the core muscles. Hold the head straight in line with the back and do not let the upper back round out. Do not lock out any motions, meaning shoulders and elbows should have a slight bend at the end range of motion. Increase difficulty and functionality by walking hands forward on the ground past your shoulders to eye level. Again, you can increase the challenge and improve your proprioception by placing your arms on a wobbly surface such as an Indo board, which mimics the instability of a surfboard when popping up or duck-diving.

## Aerobic and Anaerobic Conditioning In and Out of the Water

Prolonged strenuous activities such as surfing are dependent on aerobic metabolism to power muscular contraction. This form of metabolism derives its energy from burning the sugar-fuel glycogen by combining it with oxygen in the miniature power plants found in muscle known as mitochondria. During periods of high workload—like when you are paddling out through a long set—the rate-limiting step in this energy-producing process is not glycogen, but oxygen. It follows then that the more oxygen-rich blood that your heart can pump through your lungs and into your muscles, the longer and faster you should be able to paddle without becoming fatigued.

The purpose of so-called aerobic exercise is to hone your heart and lungs to maximum capacity so as to increase the efficiency of this energy-generating system. The heart is a muscle, and just like other muscles, the harder you work it, the bigger and stronger it gets. A stronger heart can pump more blood to your muscles, which in turn translates into better endurance. Regularly engaging in just about any continuous form of activity which consistently raises your heart rate for twenty minutes or more, will do the job. From chopping wood to running, swimming, or biking, the exercise you choose really does not matter, so long as heart and lungs are working hard. Not only will regular aerobic training serve to increase your wave count, but it also comes with the added bonus of lowering your blood pressure and cholesterol and decreasing your risk of heart attack, stroke, and diabetes.

## Getting in the Zone

Exercise physiologists have created three so-called "zones" of exercise, which are based on achieving a percentage of one's maximum heart rate during physical activity. Traditionally, maximum heart rate was calculated by subtracting one's age in years from the number 220, but this formula has been challenged. Recent sports medicine studies have found that the maximum heart rate for male athletes can be more closely calculated using the formula $202–(0.55 \times age)$, and for female athletes, using $216–(1.09 \times age)$.

Poorly conditioned individuals, those that are winded paddling out at a two-foot beach break, should start their aerobic training programs at 50–60 percent of their maximum heart rate or zone 1. With improved conditioning, target heart rates of 70–80 percent of maximum or zone 2 should be able to be tolerated for twenty minutes or more with only minimal discomfort. It is in this aerobic training zone where the greatest improvements in endurance are achieved. After just four to six weeks of regular zone 2 exercise, beneficial adaptations to the cardiovascular system occur; your heart transforms itself into a more effective pump, your lungs deliver more oxygen to your bloodstream, and new blood vessels form in your muscles. At the cellular level, the density and efficiency of mitochondria in your muscles increases, and more glycogen is stored away. Though the maximum amount of oxygen that your body can burn per minute—your so-called VO$_2$ max—is to some extent genetically pre-determined (go ahead, blame your parents), the good news is with as little as twenty minutes of aerobic exercise three days a week, you can boost the performance of your body's engines and increase your current VO$_2$ max by as much as 20 percent from pre-exercise levels. As well as improving aerobic capacity, this type of exercise also shortens the time it takes your heart rate recover (to resting rates) after a bout of exertion. Shorter recovery times translate into more waves ridden. Instead of huffing and puffing as before while you watch that first set roll by after a long paddle out to the lineup, in short order you'll be fully recharged and ready to paddle for a set wave.

When exercising in zone 3 or 81–90 percent of your maximum heart rate, you are really red lining it. These all-out efforts can only be tolerated for a few minutes because at this point you overwhelm your body's ability to burn oxygen and are relying on anaerobic metabolism to make energy. With these intense bursts of maximal exertion, lactate, a by-product of anaerobic metabolism, builds up in your muscles and you start to "feel the burn." Interspersing brief intervals of maximal-effort sprints with lower-intensity zone 1 or zone 2 exercise (known as high-intensity interval training) is a technique used by many elite athletes to build strength. For example, occasionally pretending that a cleanup set just appeared on the horizon when swimming laps or even working out on a rowing machine will go a long way to improving anaerobic capacity. Though zone 3 exercise does little to build endurance, it is essential for building the muscle mass and strength necessary to generate the intense bursts of paddling power required to catch waves.

## Forms of Aerobic Exercise: Different Strokes for Different Folks

Aerobic exercise can be achieved through a wide variety of activities. In cold climates you may find it convenient to go to the gym and use a standard stationary bicycle or elliptical trainer with a built-in heart rate monitor. Conversely you may prefer to be outdoors and go cross-country skiing, running, or hiking with a portable heart rate monitor. If the weather is warmer, you can bike, run, or skateboard outdoors. These forms of exercise are recommended because they work the quadriceps and gluteus muscles (thighs and butt), which are some of the largest muscle groups in the body for effecting successful aerobic training. Remember, you are conditioning your heart and lungs, so this training need not be surfing specific. A rowing machine is also excellent for cardio respiratory training and helps balance out the paddling muscles by strengthening the back and legs. Running outdoors or on a treadmill is perhaps the most effective way to burn calories but over the long haul carries a higher risk of knee pain and arthritis.

Swimming is yet another great form of aerobic exercise, particularly if you go for a couple of weeks or more between surfs. Being a strong swimmer is part and parcel of being a skilled surfer, and many of the muscles used while swimming the crawl are also used for paddling a surfboard. That being said, if you suffer from shoulder tendinitis or rotator cuff problems, you may want to limit the frequency and intensity of your swim workouts so as to preserve your shoulders for surfing.

## Customizing Your Own Program

In this chapter we have included what is essentially a broad menu of exercises that can be used to build your own fitness program. Try to include an element of aerobic training, stretching, strength training, and balance training into your fitness routine at least once a week. The natural tendency for most athletes is to gravitate toward their strengths and avoid their weaknesses. Those with good aerobic capacity will go for long bike rides or swims but may avoid flexibility training because they find it difficult or uncomfortable. Athletes who are very strong but get winded after an hour of surfing will favor push-ups and squats over aerobic activities. Try to avoid this natural inclination and devote some of your time to upgrading those aspects of your fitness that are most in need of improvement.

If you are just starting a fitness program, seek to improve endurance at about 10 percent per month. This can be accomplished by increasing the intensity of your workout, for example, incrementally increasing the pace at which you ride your bike over a set distance, or by increasing the volume of your workouts by biking at the same pace, but for a longer distance. Work out for at least half an hour three to five days a week for best results, but don't overdo it. Our bodies need time to rest and recuperate. The improvements that occur as a result of regular exercise occur not during exercise, but after your workout, as you are recovering. It is during this period that damaged muscle fibers are repaired, new muscle is built, and glycogen stores are replenished.

Most fitness experts recommend mixing up your routine by cross-training in a variety of different activities to keep from getting bored and to avoid overuse injuries. Whichever forms of exercise you choose, be it going to the gym, yoga, swimming, biking, or rowing, you are most likely to stick with your fitness program if you set realistic goals, incorporate exercise into your weekly schedule, and do activities that you find enjoyable. Included below are some sample workouts, but you'll need to customize a program that fits your schedule and addresses your unique needs and aspirations. Good luck!

A sample workout by Dr. Tim Brown, the North America Division of the Association of Surfing Professionals' Sports Medicine director, incorporating interval, balance, and stability training, looks like this:

- Three sets of thirty-second, twenty-second, ten-second pull-ups, as many as can be done without sacrificing form.
- Three sets of thirty-second, twenty-second, ten-second push-ups on balance board or ball.
- Three sets of balance board squats. (Or begin without balance board, doing squats with back flat and sliding against the wall for support.) First set is full up and then down movement; second set is holding still in balance for thirty seconds and then back up and down for thirty seconds.

## Hawaiian Lifeguard Standards

More than just surfing, you are training to be a waterman or one that can handle just about any ocean conditions. Physical fitness standards for the surfing world's best watermen, the Hawaiian Lifeguard, are illustrated here:

- *Cardiovascular fitness.* Run one thousand yards on the beach and swim one thousand yards in calm ocean water in less than twenty minutes.
- *Burst speed and agility.* Run one hundred yards on the beach, swim one hundred yards in the ocean, and then run back one hundred yards on the beach in under three minutes.
- *Upper body strength, balance in the ocean, and familiarity with surfboards.* Paddle one hundred yards in calm ocean waters, make a 180-degree turn, and then repeat three times under four minutes.

A training schedule for Hawaiian Lifeguards looks something like this:

- *Day 1.* Half-mile run, twenty-five-foot hill run × five, one hundred yards of lunges on beach, ten push-ups, and ten pull-ups, fifteen-minute cooldown. Increase the distances of runs, hill runs, and swims incrementally. Also, aim for ten sets of ten push-ups and five sets of ten pull-ups by the third week.

- *Day 2.* Half-mile swim, twenty-five-foot hill run × five, one hundred yards of lunges on beach, twenty push-ups, and twenty sit-ups, fifteen -minute cooldown.

- *Day 3.* Yoga class.

- *Day 4.* Half-mile run, twenty-five-foot hill run × five, fifty yards of breath-hold lunges on beach, ten push-ups, and ten sit-ups, fifteen-minute cooldown.

- *Day 5.* Three-mile bike ride and surf.

- *Day 6.* Yoga class.

- *Day 7.* Rest.

# Special Considerations: Overtraining

Training for competitions, as well as for improved free-surfing sessions, is important for growth in the initiative and confidence necessary to progress a novice surfer toward the elite level. Confidence must stem from superior physical condition, technical prowess, and adequate rest. A tapering period is essential after periods of heavy training and before contests. Many archetypal methods of training for surfing have been glorified in surf magazines and movies but have little scientific basis.

For example, in a recent advertisement, a pro surfer is quoted as saying, "You don't just wake up one morning and decide to qualify for the World Surf League (WSL). You wake up every morning for a year before dawn and drag yourself out of bed and into a life of discipline and physical and mental anguish. What doesn't kill you only makes you stronger." The advertisement illustrates several points, psychologically and physically.

It illustrates the perils of overreaching and overtraining when goaded on by the competitive mentality. Recognition and avoidance of overreaching and overtraining is important. Overreaching is physiologic fatigue, with increased resting heart rate and unsatisfying workouts, but it resolves with two weeks of rest. Overtraining is pathologic and, without quick resolution, could lead to daily fatigue, depression, and increased frequency of illness as well as muscle and ligament injury and breakdown.

With a contest mentality, surfer athletes may push themselves beyond their body's limits. Overreaching is the first step in the continuum but may progress to overtraining if ignored. There are several blood markers of the overtraining cascade that physicians can test such as testosterone levels. Other causes of pathologic fatigue include thyroid disorders, substance abuse, and mood disorders such as depression. Focus on hydration, nutrition, sleep, rest, relaxation, emotional support, and stretching for a two-week period. If no better, see your doctor.

Professional surfers at the highest levels may have full-time personal and athletic trainers, therapists, and psychologists to guarantee peak performance. Some swear that they do nothing but surf. Surfers, ultimately, are athletes whether or not they want to be considered such and deserve, in kind, the best form of sports medicine care and supervision. A multidisciplinary approach to training and prevention of injuries is important for peak performance.

# Conclusions

While no perfect regimen exists for optimal surf training, this chapter is an effort to cull effective and well-studied methods of improving physical conditioning from a wide range of available techniques with relative specificity to surfing. Consistency and diligence are required in training as in surfing itself. Training has a focus of improving muscle strength and endurance to tolerate longer and more rewarding surfing sessions. Confidence in one's own physical condition remains an important element of successful surfing.

Know your personal limits of ability and physical fitness and adapt them to your workouts and surf sessions. Learn how long you can hold your breath in a struggle, safely (on land). Learn how fast you can sprint-paddle. Allow your body to rest adequately, from twenty-four to forty-eight hours between workouts of similar muscle groups; eat a balanced diet with fruits, vegetables, and protein (especially after a surf session); and avoid fad diets, processed foods, drugs, alcohol, and tobacco. Warm up prior to surfing. Stretch after surfing. Respect your body. Have fun surfing and training and maintain a positive attitude. If this is impossible, take a break from training, nourish the body, and rest until it is possible. Remember that the best surfer out there is the one having the most fun!

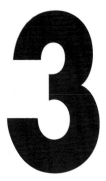

# 3

## Nutrition and Hydration

Low carb, carbo loading, high protein, low fat, Atkins diet, South Beach diet, vitamin E, vitamin D, blah, blah, blah. With this ever-rising mountain of information about diets, much of it conflicting, how is a surfer supposed to know what to eat these days? Despite a large body of research regarding nutrition, there is surprisingly little concrete evidence as to which types of diets are good for you and which types are bad. One thing we know for certain is that for most athletes, a well-balanced diet containing a broad variety of fruits and vegetables should be sufficient to meet all their nutritional needs. Contrary to the claims touted by the manufacturers of many health supplements, unless you suffer from a medical condition such as anemia or are unable to absorb certain nutrients, you probably don't need to take supplemental vitamins or minerals to stay strong and healthy. In fact, the excessive consumption of some dietary products such as protein powders, vitamin A, and vitamin E carry a potential health risk.

 But what constitutes a well-balanced diet? Although the variety of healthy foods is nearly endless, the Mediterranean diet has often been touted as typifying a well-balanced, wholesome diet. Such a diet consists of pasta, cheese, olive oil, fresh fruits and vegetables, nuts and grains, fish, and modest amounts of lean meats. This Mediterranean cuisine is close to the land, meaning that locally grown fruits and vegetables are eaten in season and the meals are freshly prepared and contain few processed ingredients. Over the long term, eating in this way is associated with a longer life expectancy and a lower risk of cardiovascular disease, diabetes, and cancer than is a modern Western diet, which is substantially lower in fiber and higher in processed foods, saturated fats, and calories.

## Major Nutrients

Most aerobic exercise is fueled by carbohydrates and fat. High-intensity aerobic exercise predominantly relies on carbohydrates whereas low-intensity aerobic exercise mostly burns fat. Surfing is a form of high-intensity interval exercise, so surfers depend on a mix of carbohydrates and fats to meet their energy needs. While protein can be converted to sugars during periods of starvation, its primary nutritional role is to build and maintain muscle and to synthesize enzymes (used in chemical reactions), antibodies (used to fight infection), and hormones (think sex!). But what is the proper mix of these three major food groups?

While nutrient profiles are constantly being researched by dieticians and exercise physiologists, a general rule is that carbohydrates should constitute roughly 65 percent of one's caloric intake; fats, 20 percent; and proteins, 15 percent. In theory, glycemic indices further complicate the consumption of carbohydrates. For optimal carbohydrate fueling, high-glycemic carbohydrates such as table sugar, white bread, and cereals, which cause a quick spike in glucose levels, should be balanced with low-glycemic fruits, vegetables, and whole grains, which release sugars into the bloodstream more slowly. To avoid headaches with this, focus on eating a rainbow of colors in fruits, vegetables, and grains.

Raw fruits, vegetables, and grains are also beneficial because they are important sources of dietary fiber, which is sorely lacking in the typical Western diet. While the US Department of Agriculture (USDA) recommends that we should eat 25–35 grams of fiber a day, the average fast-food junkie in American consumes only 12 grams of this important foodstuff. Though relatively indigestible, plant fiber is extremely important because it has been shown to help absorption of nutrients, naturally lower cholesterol levels, and reduce the incidence of colon cancer. Fiber also creates a feeling of satiety while adding nearly zero calories and, therefore, helps minimize unwanted weight gain. White rice, bread, and flour tend to be less rich in nutrients and fiber than their whole-grain counterparts and fall into a category of processed foods that should be avoided when possible. Also, try to avoid an excess consumption of simple sugars with high-glycemic indices that are so ubiquitous in the Western diet, including corn syrups and fructose, often used as sweeteners in sodas and sports drinks.

Proteins are made from twenty-two amino acid building blocks, eight of which are considered essential because they cannot be synthesized by the human body. Fortunately, natural food sources containing all these essential amino acids are abundant, and despite muscle-building advertisements to the contrary, protein need not be supplemented by specially formulated shakes, powders, or bars. Lean meats, fish, milk products, nuts, and egg white are all excellent sources of protein and provide the full complement of amino acids. Even strict vegetarians can easily get enough protein by eating a wide variety of foods such as bean curd (tofu), buckwheat, or the combination of rice and beans or hummus and pita bread. While dietary protein is generally not an issue for vegetarians, they should occasionally take a vitamin $B_{12}$ supplement, as this important nutrient is lacking in most vegetable sources. For those who have little time for food preparation or prefer to take their protein in a drink, a scoop or two of whey powder in a fruit smoothie makes an excellent choice for a quick protein-rich meal.

Though fats always seem to get a bad name in the press, they too are an important food group as they aid in the absorption of fat-soluble vitamins (A, D, E, and K), and provide fuel for endurance activities. In terms of fat consumption, the healthiest sources are unsaturated fats such as olive oil, canola oil, and avocados, as well as polyunsaturated fats, such as nuts, cheese, and seeds. Limit the consumption of saturated fats found in fatty beef, pork, egg yolks, coconut oil, palm oil, and many dairy products. These foods are high in triglycerides and LDL cholesterol (bad cholesterol) and are thought to lead to clogging of the arteries and heart disease. Trans fats, found in processed foods (and now banned in the US and other developed countries), are also to be avoided, as they, too, raise levels of LDL cholesterol, lower levels of HDL cholesterol (good cholesterol), and have been strongly associated with premature death from coronary artery disease. Fish oils, on the other hand, are quite important to the nutrient profile as they contain omega-3 fatty acids and are high in HDL cholesterol. These omega-3 fatty acids are found in cell membranes and are utilized by all of the body's systems, including cardiovascular, immune, and nervous systems. Unless you are currently eating fish rich in fatty acids (e.g., salmon, striped bass, sardines) at least twice a week, you are probably not getting enough omega-3s in your diet.

# Refueling the Engines

Surfing burns approximately five hundred calories an hour, and an active athlete may need to consume up to ten grams per kilogram of body weight of quality carbohydrates daily to support their caloric needs. As opposed to eating three large daily meals as most of us are accustomed to, the majority of sports nutritionists recommend dividing one's caloric intake into five or six small meals, which is thought to minimize excessive weight gain and more closely approximate the way our hunter-gatherer ancestors ate. The key to doing this successfully without overeating is to eat small portions of nutritious, low-fat foods every three or four hours.

Fueling up properly before a long surf is important as you'll need energy to power you through the session, and once you're out there on the water, snacks are hard to come by. This meal should be eaten at least two hours before you paddle out, so it has time to get adequately digested and doesn't come back up to haunt you. Your pre-surf meal can consist of something like a turkey and avocado sandwich on whole wheat bread with an apple and a piece of cheese. Meals such as this contain fat and protein, which slow digestion, and slow absorption of carbohydrates, so as to maintain a steady level of blood sugar over time. The complex carbohydrates found in whole wheat and fruit have low glycemic indices and, thus, will release sugar into the bloodstream slowly and help endurance. If eating hours before a session is not practical, for example, for a dawn patrol session, you'll want to eat a smaller, more easily digestible meal containing foods with high glycemic indices, such as a muffin, bagel, or yogurt with honey. With these foods, sugars are more immediately available for your body to utilize. The downside of relying solely on these types of carbohydrates is that the spike in blood sugar lasts for less than an hour and may be followed by a blood sugar crash. To avoid this crash, particularly for longer surf sessions, add a bit of dried fruit or oatmeal, which fall under the category of foods with low glycemic indices.

Immediately after surfing, as with all your workouts, carbohydrates should be ingested with protein with an optimal ratio of 4:1. Most of the body's beneficial adaptations to exercise don't actually occur during exercise, but afterward, as the body repairs, rebuilds, and strengthens itself during periods of rest—which is why this is such an important time to eat. Carbohydrates are needed to replenish stores of the muscle-fuel glycogen (stored in the muscles and liver), which can get depleted after prolonged periods of physical activity, and proteins are needed to repair and build muscle. Chocolate milk is one of the most readily available and nutritious post-workout snacks as it contains simple sugars, which are easily converted to glycogen as well as the milk proteins casein and whey. Ideally, your most substantial meal should be eaten within an hour or so of surfing to capitalize on the body's recovery systems and to build lean muscle. Try to make this a well-balanced meal with high-quality protein (tofu, poultry, or fish), carbohydrates (whole grains), clean and fresh vegetables prepared with olive oil, and fruit for dessert. Drink plenty of liquids with this meal to rehydrate, particularly if you have been surfing in a tropical climate.

*"It seems that high-quality, nutrient-dense, fresh, organic, plant-based foods like vegetables, fruits, grains, and beans are just easier for us to process and are what our bodies crave. Eating them regularly will improve how you perform, feel and recover (from surfing and even injury). After a short period of time of improving your nutritional choices, you'll even see an upgrade in how you look (skin, hair, eyes, waistline). When you eat processed foods for example, foods that are in a box, can, or from a fast food place, you are eating 'food' produced and heavily marketed by companies that are economically driven. They are profit driven—not health driven. You might be saving money in the short term, but every time you eat it you're making it really tough on your body's digestive system to break it all down and put it to use. These foods make it much, much tougher and take the body much longer to break*

down and absorb the nutrients, vitamins and minerals it needs in order to do important things like provide you with energy, perform bodily functions and build a healthy immune system. Most of your immune system is in your lower intestine—the better your digestion, the stronger your immunity." —Dr. Tim Brown and Dr. Doug Andersen, (Surfline.com Health and Fitness Column)

## Surfer's Reflux: Chumming and Bumming

It is not uncommon for surfers to get heartburn (indigestion) while they surf, and many a surfer has had the unpleasant experience of getting reacquainted with his or her recently eaten breakfast during a dawn patrol paddle out. The combination of strenuous exertion while lying in a prone paddling position puts significant upward pressure on your stomach, which often leads to reflux (backward flow) of stomach contents into the esophagus (swallowing tube). Though a valve (the lower esophageal sphincter) ordinarily prevents food and stomach acid from burbling back into the esophagus, this valve can be overcome by excessive pressure on the stomach, particularly if you are prone to reflux to begin with. The simplest solution to this problem is to avoid any significant meals at least two hours before surfing. If you must eat just before a surf, make it just a small snack of easily digested food (that won't taste so bad on the way up) like a banana or non-fat yogurt, and avoid foods that are slowly digested such as solid foods rich in fats or protein. Avoid foods that relax lower esophageal sphincter tone (fatty foods, chocolate, and alcohol) and don't drink highly acidic liquids such as orange juice and colas before a surf. If you continue to suffer from symptoms of reflux despite steering clear of pre-surf meals, try using over-the-counter antacids such as Maalox, Mylanta, or Pepto-Bismol to neutralize stomach acids. Other medications such as Pepcid or Zantac work by decreasing acid production but need to be taken regularly because it takes a few hours for their effects to kick in.

If you still suffer from heartburn despite following the measures above, it is time to see a doctor and you may need a type of acid-reducing medication known as a proton pump inhibitor. With repeated episodes of reflux, stomach acids can cause damage to the poorly protected lining of the esophagus, leading to esophagitis (inflammation of the esophagus). If this process continues unchecked, digestive juices can actually burn a hole in the esophagus and, in the worst-case scenario, result in a bleeding ulcer.

# Wetting the Whistle

Fluids are lost from the human body via so-called insensible losses such as exhaled water vapor and sweat, as well as from urine and stool. The average inactive male in a temperate climate requires about 3.7 liters of water from food and drink daily to replace those losses, and the average female about 2.7 liters. However, unlike most sports where there is always a water bottle on the sidelines, liquids are not readily available when you are out in the lineup, so it is a good idea to start hydrating well before entering the water. For every hour of surfing, drink approximately one liter of water or juice thirty to sixty minutes before surfing. Fluids pass through the stomach most rapidly if taken a cup at a time, as opposed to a full guzzle, so drink slowly to avoid that bloated feeling when you paddle out. In tropical climates, fluid requirements are even greater, and there can be significant losses of electrolytes (salts) through your sweat. In hot and humid conditions, fluids should contain salt and a small amount of simple sugars as well, as is found in most sports drinks. You can easily make your own sports drink by diluting fruit juice 1:1 with water and adding half a teaspoon of salt.

If salt and fluids are not replaced during extended exercise in hot weather, you will tire more quickly, become irritable, and run the risk of muscle cramps and dehydration. Even when surfing in cold water, proper hydration remains important. Cold water is a diuretic (makes you pee), so even though you are not sweating off fluids in cold conditions, you lose them in your wet suit (toasty!). In chilly climates, your metabolism is in high gear in an attempt to produce heat, and warm sugary fluids like hot chocolate or tea with honey are an excellent way to fuel your fire and ward off hypothermia.

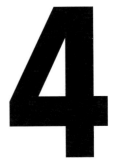

# Surfing Injuries and Injury Prevention

Almost everything worth doing in life involves an element of risk, and surfing is no exception. For many surfers, some of the sport's allure lies in the challenge of safely negotiating the powerful natural forces found in the surf zone—an area long feared by mariners for its hazardous waves, reefs, and strong currents. Indeed, the rush that comes from sticking a late drop or charging big surf is fueled in part by fear—fear that errors in judgment or technique could result in a serious thrashing (or worse). Sensationalism in the media would lead us to believe that surfing is a highly dangerous sport where close brushes with death from underwater hold-downs and man-eating sharks are commonplace. The surf industry also goes a long way to perpetuate the notion that surfing is a risky "extreme" sport ('cause it helps sell board shorts in Ohio), and most surfers seem happy to bask in the macho aura that has come to be associated with the sport.

## HOW DANGEROUS IS SURFING?

 But, ego stroke and media hype aside, just how dangerous is surfing anyway? Contrary to popular belief, a number of studies suggest that, overall, surfing is a relatively safe sport. Nathanson's worldwide study of competitive surfing found it to be less risky than other competitive sports like college-level football, soccer, and basketball, but more risky than college baseball. Brian Lowden, a researcher from Australia, surveyed 360 recreational surfers and found that the risk of "moderate to severe" injuries—the kind of injury that would keep you out of the water a day or more—was 3.5 per 1,000 days of surfing, which is roughly in keeping with injury rates reported for recreational alpine skiing and somewhat safer than snowboarding. Compared with other sports in which violent collisions frequently occur between players or with the ground, injury rates in surfing are tempered by the cushioning effects of water and the relatively low speeds usually attained by surfers. In all likelihood, the most dangerous thing about surfing is the drive to the beach—particularly when the driver is a stoked surfer who's got an eye on the swell, an ear on the cell phone, and the pedal to the metal. Probably the most effective way to avoid a surfing-related death is to keep your eyes (and ears) on the road and wear your seatbelt.

| Sport | Injury Rate per 1,000 Hours |
|---|---|
| Professional Rugby | 69 |
| College Football | 33* |
| Men's College Soccer | 18.8* |
| Men's College Basketball | 9* |
| **Competitive Surfing** | **6.6** |
| College Baseball | 5.8* |
| Snowboarding | 5.4 |
| Skiing (Recreational) | 4–5 |
| Softball (Recreational) | 2.3* |

*Injury rate per 1,000 games
Nathanson, Bird, Dao, & Tam-Sing, "Competitive Surfing Injuries: A Prospective Study of Surfing-Related Injuries among Contest Surfers." *American Journal of Sports Medicine* 35, no.1 (2007): 113–17.

But how about Mavericks or Pipeline, you ask? Surely many of us would feel safer playing soccer than dropping into a bomb at Pipeline. In fact, your fears are well founded. While on average surfing is pretty safe, researchers at Brown University found that the risk of severe injuries increases in big surf and when surfing over a reef or rocky bottom. The risk of injury among competitive surfers in big surf (overhead or higher) is 2.4 times that of smaller surf (head high or smaller). This is probably due the fact that large waves travel faster than small waves and carry more energy. The energy of a wave increases as the square of its height, so other factors being equal, a ten-foot wave isn't just twice as powerful as a five-foot wave, but it's actually four times as powerful. Similarly, the risk of injury has been found to be more than doubled when surfing a reef break as compared to a beach break. These risks are cumulative, so overhead Pipeline works out to be about six times as dangerous as your hometown beach break on a small day. These facts are borne out by an analysis of contests held at Pipeline, Hawaii, which showed that an hour of surfing at that ultraheavy wave spot carries slightly more risk of significant injury than an hour of college football. So while on average, surfing is a comparatively safe sport, it will come as no great surprise to those who have braved the likes of sketchy spots like the Box in Western Oz or Temples in Bali that surfing in big, powerful waves, which break over shallow reefs, can indeed be dangerous.

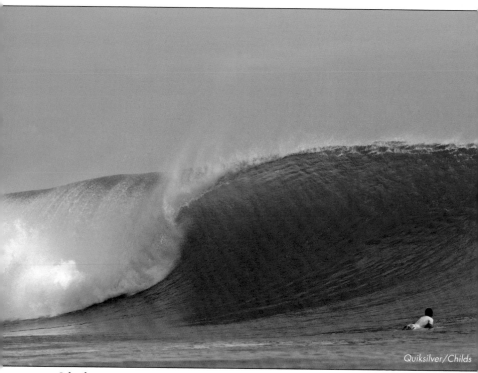

Quiksilver/Childs

**G-land monster.**

Paradoxically, being an expert surfer is also a risk factor for injury. Expert surfers have been found to have higher rates of injury than intermediates—even when wave height is accounted for, probably because they surf more dangerous spots and surf more aggressively, pulling into more barrels and attempting more aerials, steep drops, etc., than their less-experienced counterparts. Rank beginners are also prone to injuries, but for a completely different set of reasons: they tend to surf in more gentle waves but are less familiar with the marine environment and have little wave sense, board control, or board awareness. Those of us who learned how to surf the old-fashioned way—from the school of hard knocks—know that injuries during one's first year of surfing are not uncommon. An oft-repeating scene is one in which a beginner surfer is pushing his board out through the shore break and unwittingly allows the board to come broadside between himself and a breaking wave—and then, in classic kook style, proceeds to get mowed down by his own stick.

## How Do Most Injuries Occur?

Hint: The biggest teeth in the water are the fins on the bottom of your board.

## Surfboard-Related Injuries

While sharks grab all the headlines, by far the biggest danger lurking in the water is your very own surfboard. Most studies have found that fully two-thirds of all surfing injuries are board related, with the majority of those injuries being caused by the fins, rail, and nose of the rider's own board.

Most surfboard-related injuries are variations on the following sequence:

1. Surfer botches takeoff and gets pitched forward, or otherwise wipes out.

2. Surfer proceeds to get worked in the impact zone.

3. During the ensuing chaos, collides with fins, nose, or rail of own or other surfer's board.

### Causes of Surfing-Related Injuries

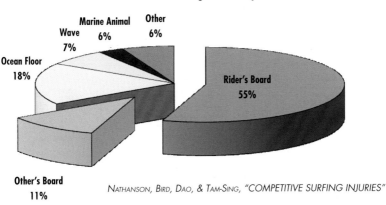

Ocean Floor 18%
Wave 7%
Marine Animal 6%
Other 6%
Rider's Board 55%
Other's Board 11%

NATHANSON, BIRD, DAO, & TAM-SING, "COMPETITIVE SURFING INJURIES"

## Parts of a Surfboard Resulting in Injury

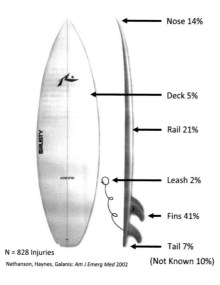

Nose 14%

Deck 5%

Rail 21%

Leash 2%

Fins 41%

Tail 7%

(Not Known 10%)

N = 828 Injuries

Nathanson, Haynes, Galanis: *Am J Emerg Med* 2002

If the surfer happens to hit a fin with significant force, chances are pretty good that the encounter will result in a laceration (cut). Surfboard fins have sharp trailing edges, which are capable of causing lacerations through even the most leathery skin (and wet suits) and are undoubtedly the most common type of surfing injury, accounting for nearly a quarter of all significant surfing injuries in some studies.

While most fin cuts are superficial, be aware that what may appear to be a relatively modest surface laceration may actually be a much deeper stab wound that has damaged underlying structures or other vital pieces of anatomy (yes—even *that* vital piece has seen damage). For this reason, most any fin cut that is bleeding warrants a trip back to shore for closer inspection. There are a couple of well-documented reports of surfers who took a fin to the head—and despite a bit of bleeding, kept on surfing, only to find out later that the fin had actually penetrated through their skulls and into their brains!

Collisions with rounded surfaces of the board can also cause a variety of injuries. Light blows to well-padded parts of the body cause little more than bumps and bruises, but hard blows to poorly padded parts of the body, such as the scalp, lip, and ribs, can split open skin, break bones, knock out teeth, and cause concussions. Clearly, heavily glassed long boards and guns

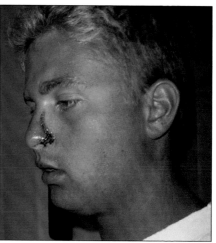

**Nose job courtesy of fin.**

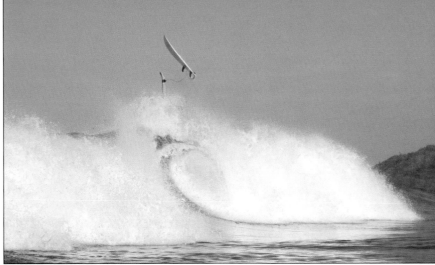

**What goes up must come down.**

are more likely to cause significant injuries in this way than are smaller lighter short boards. After a wipeout, head injuries from surfboards (yours or someone else's) are relatively common because a board's buoyancy tends to keep it tumbling near the surface—aimed right at the head of any surfer who happens to be in its path. When surfing in offshore winds, be wary of the heightened risk of injury from your board. The updraft of wind on the wave's face can launch your board like a pinwheel after a wipeout, and if you are unlucky, it will come down on your head just as you come up for air.

Although bodyboards are relatively soft, they, too, can cause blunt force injuries. There have been a series of reports of bodyboarders who have suffered from internal (abdominal) bleeding after pearling in the shallow waters of a shore break. This occurs when the nose of the bodyboard jams into the sand and the tail of the board is thrust forcefully under the rider's ribs and into his or her abdomen (like a sucker punch to the solar plexus), which can cause damage to the liver or the spleen.

## Seafloor

While water is a forgiving surface on which to fall, the same cannot be said of the seafloor. In fact, injuries from the seafloor are the second leading cause of injury after injuries from one's own surfboard and can be some of the most severe. A large percentage of these injuries occur when surfing hollow reef breaks where a powerful swell jacks up out of deep water and pitches over a shallow reef or ledge.

While tube riding is a pinnacle of the sport and there is perhaps no experience (surfing or otherwise) more intense and rewarding than

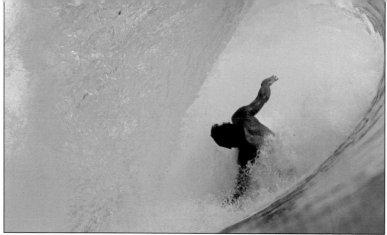

**Paying the piper.**

scoring a great barrel, sometimes you've got to pay to play. Even the most skillful surfers occasionally get sucked over the falls and bounced unceremoniously off the bottom in their quest for a few epic moments in the green room. Depending on the force of the impact, the composition of the seafloor, and the orientation of the rider, the resultant injuries can vary from minor to catastrophic. Though "reef rash" (from getting dragged across coral reef) is a common badge of honor when tube riding reef breaks, more serious injuries like fractures and head injuries are not unheard-of.

## SURF SURVIVAL LESSON

Chris McAleer, a hard-core surfer, moved to the beach at age nineteen so he could surf every day. At age twenty-three, he was surfing two- to three-foot waves at 48th Street in Newport Beach, California, and fell forward off his board, striking his head on a shallow sandbar. He felt a click in his neck, a tingling sensation throughout his body, and found himself conscious but facedown in the water, unable to move his legs or flip himself over. Through the quick action of an off-duty lifeguard and other bystanders, he did not drown, but remains paralyzed and wheelchair-bound. Though Chris lives an active and productive life as a spokesman for Hoag Memorial Hospital's Project Wipeout — teaching kids about water safety — and is a school educator, his days of standing on a surfboard ended in an instant on that fateful day.

Injuries from hitting the seafloor are not just a problem when surfing big hollow barrels but are also a risk when surfing small waves anywhere, because small waves invariably break in shallow water (remember—waves begin to break at a depth that is 1.3 times their height). In fact, some of the most tragic injuries in surfing take place not in giant surf, but on small days, when a surfer dives off his board in shallow

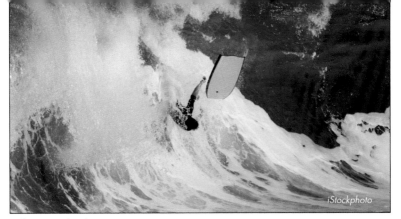

**A dangerous header.**

water and hits the bottom headfirst, resulting in a broken neck or head injury. Surfers share a common misperception that they are immune from significant injury from the seafloor when surfing over a soft sandy bottom in small waves—but as evidenced by Chris McAleer, and others, this could not be further from the truth. Wet sand has the consistency of concrete when struck with sudden impact—and countless neck injuries (particularly among bodyboarders and bodysurfers who ride headfirst) have occurred at sand-bottomed breaks such as Sandy Beach, Hawaii, which has been dubbed by lifeguards as the Break-Neck Capital of the World. The Wedge, a pitching sand-bottom beach break in Newport Beach, California, shares a similar distinction, and one summer, the local hospital (Hoag Memorial) had five of its eight intensive care unit beds occupied by young watermen who lay paralyzed from spinal cord injuries sustained in the surf.

A Hawaiian study showed that those at highest risk for neck fractures from wave-riding accidents were inexperienced tourists in their forties of heavy build that were bodysurfing or bodyboarding at beaches with a hollow, heavy shore break. Learning how (and when) to bail off your board is a critically important surfing skill that needs to be mastered in order to minimize the risk of injury from the seafloor and is discussed in detail in the section below on injury prevention.

## Wave-Force Injuries

The power that is carried by a ground swell and then dissipated as kinetic energy when its waves break in shallow water can be considerable. It has been estimated that a mere three-foot-wide slice of a nine-foot, twelve-second-period swell has the equivalent of seventy-four horsepower—enough to power a motorcycle. Most of the power of a breaking wave is concentrated in its cascading lip, and in heavy top-to-bottom waves, the breaking lip should be respected, and avoided if possible, because it has sufficient force to blow out your eardrum, force you deep underwater, yank your shoulder out of its socket, and in rare cases even break bones. That being said, injuries resulting purely from the hydraulic force of a breaking wave are surprisingly rare, even in big surf. With the exception of injuries to one's eardrums (which are paper-thin), it is pretty unusual to get injured solely from the force of a wave.

Of course, every surfer's nightmare in big waves is an underwater hold-down that exceeds their breath-holding capacity. Fortunately this is exceedingly uncommon. Although time seems to slow down when getting "rag-dolled" underwater, the reality is that it is rare for a surfer to be held underwater for more than thirty seconds, even in enormous surf. While those who venture into big surf should be seasoned surfers and need to be incredibly fit, the overwhelming majority of big-wave riders have never even experienced a dreaded two-wave hold-down.

Though holding one's breath while at rest for well over a minute is not a problem for most people, breath-holding capacity is significantly reduced with even moderate exertion. Those most likely to be at risk for drowning are surfers who push their limits to excess and frequently cross the double yellow line. (See "Surviving Big Surf.") They go out in conditions far beyond their level of expertise, may be under the influence of alcohol or drugs, or surf until near exhaustion, get held under—and then waste oxygen trying to fight the turbulence in a panicked attempt to surface.

## Falls

Ever walked down a particularly steep and slippery access path to a break at the bottom of a bluff and started sliding downhill, clinging to small shrubs thinking, *Maybe this isn't such a good idea?* Many surf breaks (e.g., Indicators, Palos Verdes, California) are located at the bases of cliffs with approach trails that would give mountain goats pause, yet surfers seem to think nothing of heading down (or up) these precipitous trails, board under arm, shod in perhaps the worst hiking shoes known to mankind—a beaten-up pair of neoprene booties. Some of these paths are notorious for having claimed the lives of surfers and should be approached with extreme caution if at all and only when wearing high-traction footwear. After heavy rains, avoid the hairiest of these trails altogether and either use an alternate route to access the break, paddle from somewhere farther away but easier to get to, or surf somewhere else.

# What Are the Most Common Types of Surfing Injuries?

## Lacerations

In reviewing the literature on surfing trauma, a few common patterns of injury emerge; lacerations (cuts) have consistently been found to be the most common type of surfing injury accounting for as many as half of all injuries, followed by bruises, sprains, and fractures. Lacerations to the scalp, face, feet, and legs are all very common and often require stitches or some other form of wound closure (see "Wound Care" in Chapter 10). Most of these are the result of collisions with surfboard fins or contact with the seafloor. As mentioned above, some fin lacerations can be very deep and it is not unusual for them to cause damage to arteries, nerves, and tendons.

**Distribution of Surfing-Related Lacerations**

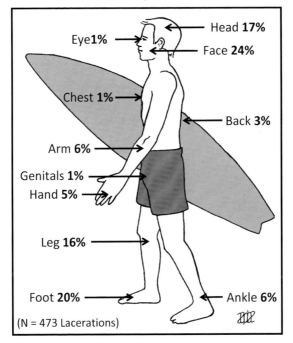

Eye **1%**

Head **17%**

Face **24%**

Chest **1%**

Back **3%**

Arm **6%**

Genitals **1%**

Hand **5%**

Leg **16%**

Foot **20%**

Ankle **6%**

(N = 473 Lacerations)

SURFING INJURIES AND INJURY PREVENTION

**81**

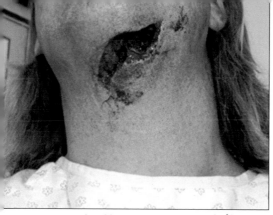

**Fin-induced laceration.**  *SurfCo Hawaii*

Foot lacerations from sharp objects on the seafloor, the beach, or access trails nearly top the list of surfing-related injuries, especially among those with tender "haole feet." In many parts of the world, the seafloor is strewn with sharp objects—from sea urchins, barnacles, and coral reef, to rusty cans and broken bottles—any one of which can inflict a nasty gouge on the bottom of your foot, putting an abrupt end to even the best-planned surf trip. Even seemingly minor lacerations and abrasions to the foot and ankle can be problematic because they are painful, slow to heal, and prone to infection. With continued daily saltwater exposure, some of these wounds may stubbornly refuse to heal and can go on to become what are known as *sea ulcers*. Proper attention to wound care is crucial, particularly in hot, humid environments where *Staphylococcus* and other bacteria flourish, and can make the difference between a speedy return to surfing or being dry-docked for weeks by an infected wound or ulcer.

## Sprains and Strains

As surfing maneuvers become more radical, knee and ankle injuries traditionally associated with land-based sports like football, soccer, and skiing are becoming more commonplace, particularly at the elite levels of the sport. Dynamic maneuvers that score

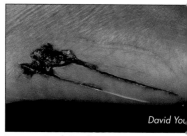

*David You*

**Foot vs. Reef. Reef won.**

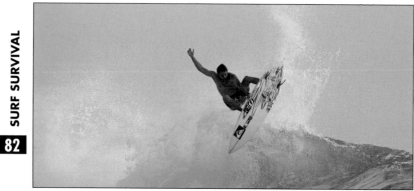

**Preparing for re-entry.**

*Quiksilver/Childs*

highly in competitive surfing—like radical snaps, cutbacks, and especially aerials—put high stress loads on knees and ankles. If these forces are poorly distributed due to improper technique, insufficient flexibility, or inadequate leg strength, the ligaments holding the joint together can be sprained (partially torn) or ruptured (completely torn), and the cartilage that forms the smooth weight-bearing surface of these joints can be damaged. Structures that are particularly vulnerable to these dynamic force injuries include the anterior cruciate ligaments (ACL), medial collateral ligaments (MCL), and medial meniscus (cartilage) of the knee, as well as the ligaments (on the inside) of the ankle. Warning signs that a knee or ankle injury is more than just a minor sprain include instability (it gives way when you walk on it), immediate swelling, and persistent pain, which has not improved after a few days of rest, ice, compression, and elevation (RICE). If *any* of these warning signs are present, it's best to seek medical care because some joint injuries will require extensive rehabilitation, and occasionally surgery, before a return to normal activities is possible. (See Chapter 5 on rehabilitation.)

**Distribution of Surfing-Related Fractures**

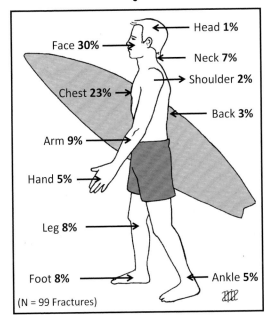

Head **1%**
Face **30%**
Neck **7%**
Shoulder **2%**
Chest **23%**
Back **3%**
Arm **9%**
Hand **5%**
Leg **8%**
Foot **8%**
Ankle **5%**
(N = 99 Fractures)

## Fractures and Dislocations

While fractures are common in land- or snow-based sports, they account for fewer than 10 percent of all surfing injuries. The fractures most often associated with surfing involve the face (nose, jaw, facial bones) or ribs and are typically the result of getting slammed in the face or chest from one's own board after a poorly executed duck-dive or during a wipeout. Fractures to the arms and legs are rare and are usually caused by hitting bottom or from board-related impact to thinly padded parts of the shin and forearm. Fortunately fractures to the spine, discussed above, are rare, though they can have disastrous consequences.

Shoulder dislocations are relatively common among surfers, body-surfers, and bodyboarders. Prone wave riders can dislocate a shoulder by hitting bottom with an outstretched arm, and surfers suffer these injuries when they fall under the lip of a big wave with an arm extended overhead or simply by exuberant paddling if they have a history of prior shoulder dislocations. On land, this injury is painful and somewhat debilitating, but in the water, it can be a major emergency, because getting back to shore with one arm completely out of commission is difficult. If you ever do dislocate a shoulder, be sure to put serious effort into your rehab program before returning to the water. Surfing is an overhead sport, and without properly strengthening the muscles that stabilize your shoulder, you run the risk of recurrent dislocations, which could jeopardize your surfing career.

Over the years we've seen a number of surfers dislocate fingers in strange ways. In the leash-wrapped-around-a-finger scenario, the surfer is in the water, tugging on his leash in an attempt to pull his board toward him when a wave jerks the loop in the leash taut, either dislocating or fracturing the finger. The same injury can happen to SUP'ers when they wipeout with a one-finger (or two) death grip on their paddle. and the shaft of the paddle gets forcefully torqued by wave action, twisting fingers beyond their normal range of motion.

## How Can You Minimize the Risk of Injury?

Though surfing is a relatively safe sport, like many outdoor activities, it carries a small risk of catastrophic injury and even death. While most of us have our guards up when surfing in conditions that test our limits, most injuries occur in mundane, everyday surf (because that is where we do the vast majority of our surfing). By making minor modifications to your equipment, following some of the recommendations below, and surfing in conditions that match your abilities, you should be able to lower your risk of of getting seriously dinged.

## Surfboards

If you want to reduce your risk of injury, look no further than your own board. While the reef and sea urchins are there to stay, chances are you could be riding a less-dangerous stick. Remember that 55 percent of all surfing injuries are caused by your surfboard, and more than half of those are caused by the board's fins and nose.

Do the trailing edges of your fins really need to be as sharp as samurai swords? And does the nose of your board really need to be shaped

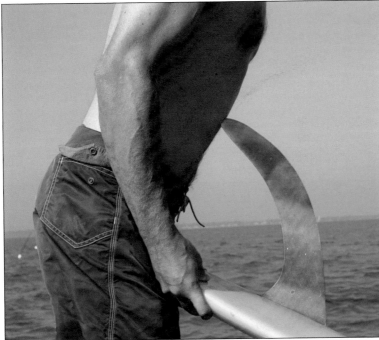

*Nainoa Nathanson*

Just say no to surf seppuku ('68 Greg Noll glass-on).

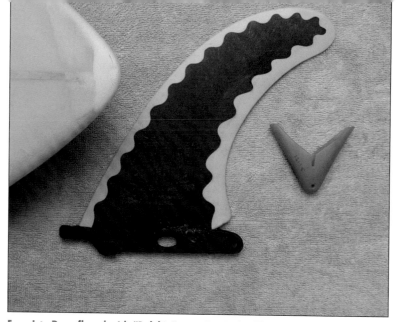

From L to R, surfboard with "Dolphin" nose, Pro Teck rubber-edged fin, "Noseguard."

like the tip of a harpoon? These sharp board appendages are perfectly set up to inflict major bodily harm and are just plain bad design from a safety perspective. Perhaps it's time to reconsider the current fashions in board construction. While the trailing edge of a fin does need to be thinner than its leading edge for a proper foil, a razor-sharp trailing edge is completely unnecessary. We recommend dulling the tips and edges of your fins with fine-grit sandpaper to a thickness of just over one-sixteenth of an inch (two millimeters), which could make the difference between your fin causing a superficial nick in your leg or causing a deep gash that severs a major artery. Fin lacerations are so commonplace that a few manufacturers have gone to great lengths to develop fins that are less likely to fillet you open. Some are made with break-away tabs so as to snap off in the event that they are struck with significant force, others have flexible rubberized edges, and those on many beginner boards are completely flexible. SurfCo Hawaii makes a variety of Pro Teck Fins with rubberized edges that are also equipped with breakaway tabs. These seem to provide the best compromise between performance and safety. Long, glassed-on single fins with pointy tips and sharp edges are the most hazardous.

Surfboards, particularly short boards, have a tendency to recoil on their outstretched leashes after a wipeout, and the sharp nose or tail of the board may spring back and hit its rider, often in the face. As you can imagine, the results of this scenario aren't pretty. Wet suit pioneer

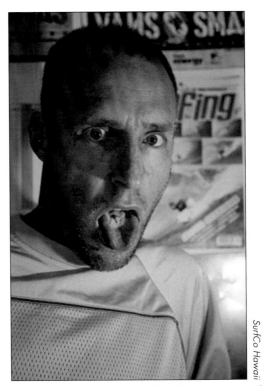

SurfCo Hawaii

**Took the tip of his board through the cheek and into his tongue — now *that's* gnarly.**

Jack O'Neill (founder of O'Neill wet suits and early adopter of the surf-board leash) lost an eye in such an injury, and he is not alone in this regard. Many of these injuries could be prevented by rounding the nose (and tail) of surfboards to a minimum radius of one and a half inches (37 mm). Promoted as a safety measure by the Surfrider Foundation (Australia), and coined the "dolphin nose," this design feature has not gained wide popularity probably because it bucks the current fashion trend of short boards with sharp pointy tips. However, next time you have a custom board shaped, insist on a dolphin nose; it won't noticeably change the performance of your board, yet it could prevent a life-altering injury. Covering the tips of boards you already own with rubber nose-guards is helpful in protecting you and others from penetrating injuries but may not provide complete protection from eye trauma.

It is not just the sharp fins and tips of surfboards that cause injuries, but also the deck and particularly rails can cause major trauma if they strike their rider (or someone else) in the face or head. To minimize this risk, many beginner soft boards are made out of closed-cell foam whose impact-absorbing properties significantly soften the blow should a surfer be hit by his or her board. Due to their excellent safety characteristics, these boards have become very popular with surfing schools, and we highly recommend them for young children, beginners, and those surfing in close proximity to swimmers. So-called soft-top boards have a rigid epoxy core whose rails and deck are wrapped in a thin layer of nonskid foam to provide a bit of padding. They are a good compromise between the performance characteristics of traditional rigid fiberglass (or epoxy) boards and the safety afforded by the all-foam varieties.

## Leashes

Your leash serves as your lifeline because it keeps your board close at hand, and your board can serve as an excellent flotation device should you become exhausted. Surfing without a leash puts you at risk for a potentially long and dangerous swim and puts others in the water at risk of getting clobbered by your loose board. That being said, don't get accustomed to being overly dependent on your leash. When conditions allow (i.e., uncrowded days), try surfing old-school, without a leash, which will force you to get in the habit of maintaining control of your board and make you more proficient at locating and retrieving your board when you lose it.

Unfortunately, leashes tend to break when you need them most (in big surf), so show this oft-neglected piece of equipment a little love; take care of it, and it will usually take care of you. Remember, a leash is only as strong as its weakest link, so periodically check the cord, swivels, ankle, leg or biceps strap, and most importantly check that little string that keeps the whole thing attached to your board. Buy quality leashes, and use one that is appropriate for the conditions and for your board; bigger boards and bigger days call for longer and thicker leashes.

### SURF-SURVIVAL TIP

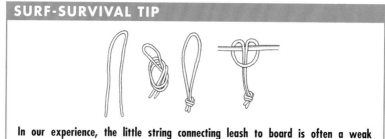

In our experience, the little string connecting leash to board is often a weak point—either it breaks or gets untied. Attach the string to your board correctly by first tying an overhand loop and then using a girth hitch to secure it to the bar in your leash plug.

In certain circumstances, your leash can prove to be a serious liability. Some of the most tragic and preventable surfing deaths occur when a surfer snags his or her leash on an object on the seafloor, gets tethered to the bottom, and drowns. Coral heads, rocks, kelp, and crab traps have all been implicated as culprits in these needless drownings. Should you ever get held down by your own leash, you'll only have seconds to free yourself, so make sure you know how to pull it off quickly. Make it a habit to always put your leash on the same way (clockwise or counterclockwise), with the pull tab always located in the same place. Every now and again while you are waiting for waves in the lineup, roll off your board and (like Houdini) practice taking your leash off underwater without looking. If you are cold-water surfing with gloves on, make sure to increase the size of that little bitty pull tab with a piece of duct tape so you'll have something you can get a grip on. Better yet, buy a leash equipped with a quick-release pin, which allows the leash to separate from the Velcro ankle strap with a simple upward pull. (See page 246.) Using a quick-release leash could save your life and is especially important when surfing in areas with underwater structures or overhangs around which your leash could snag. Large SUP boards should also be equipped with these leashes because there are some conditions in which you could get dragged by your own board, ankle first, into a dangerous (e.g., rocky) shoreline. In such situations, and as a last resort, you may want to rapidly disengage yourself from your board so you can swim to safety, and a quick-release pin makes it that much easier.

## Personal Protective Gear

While a wet suit's primary function is to keep you warm, it also shields you from the sun, provides some positive flotation, and may save you a little skin should you get dragged across the shallows. Even a rash guard provides some protection from the sun, from the abrasive action of your deck, and from jellyfish stings. For these reasons, we recommend wearing a rash guard as a bare minimum every time you go out for a surf. (For more on wet suits, see "Hypothermia" in wilderness first-aid chapter.)

Similarly, though booties are typically used to keep your feet warm in cold water, they can provide considerable protection from the seafloor. Ideally, you never touch bottom when surfing on coral reef—it is bad for the reef and bad for your feet, but if you are surfing over live coral and happen to get caught inside, booties can help prevent your feet from getting torn to shreds on the reef and may prevent injuries from sea urchins, barnacles, and other critters. If you are surfing a reef break for the first time or anticipate that getting pushed into the shallows is a possibility, it is prudent to wear some form of foot protection.

Although head injuries account for between 20 and 40 percent of all surfing injuries and are responsible for a significant percentage of surfing fatalities, few surfers don protective headgear. However, it is safe to say that given the relatively modest speeds involved while surfing (as opposed to, say, skiing), helmet use can prevent most surfing-related head trauma. The hard shell of a helmet provides significant protection against penetrating injuries caused by contact with sharp parts of your surfboard or the seafloor and should also prevent loss of consciousness in the vast majority of situations. Remember, even a brief loss of consciousness while in the water (a blow to the head from your nine-foot gun is all

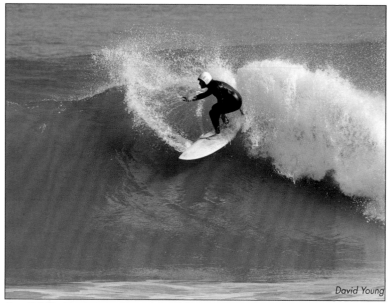

David Young

A stylish Kiwi surfer wearing a stylish lid.

it takes) can have dire consequences, and novice as well as elite surfers have been pulled out of the water unconscious after such incidents, both dead and alive. At Pipeline alone, pro surfers Tamayo Perry and Jack Johnson sustained horrific head injuries, barely making it back to shore, while Moto Watanabe and Malik Joyeux were not so lucky and drowned there likely as a result of head trauma. None were wearing helmets.

Surf-specific helmets (Gath) have been available for quite some time now, but surfers have been slow to adopt them for a variety of reasons. Unlike sports such as white-water kayaking and mountain biking where helmets have gained widespread popularity and are considered de rigueur, by and large, helmets aren't considered cool by most surfers. There are also some legitimate concerns about helmet use. Helmets can make duck-diving slightly more difficult because they add to the surface area of a surfer's head, and if not snug fitting, can fill up like a bucket, pulling the surfer's head back when passing through a wave. For the most part, this can be overcome by purchasing a close-fitting helmet and keeping your chin slightly tucked when duck-diving. Lastly, most surfers are minimalists, preferring to wear less gear in the water rather than more.

However, the safety benefits of helmets clearly outweigh the risks in the vast majority of situations, and we particularly recommend wearing one when surfing hollow waves breaking over shallow or exposed reefs (e.g., Teahupoo), when surfing in very crowded conditions (where collisions between surfers are a distinct possibility), when surfing alone, or if you're a beginner, learning on a heavy glass board. Aside from preventing head injury, helmets have the added benefits of protecting your ears from surfer's ear and eardrum blowouts and keep sun off your head.

## Exit Strategies: The Art and Science of Bailing

All surfers wipeout. If you don't wipeout, you aren't pushing your limits, and if you don't push your limits, you can't progress as a surfer. But just like wave riding, wiping out is a skill, and to be a good surfer, you need to know how (and when) to wipeout so as to minimize your risk of injury.

Though the best wipeout strategy often depends on the specific situation, a few general principles apply. Just prior to a wipeout, attempt to take in a big gulp of air. If you have any control of the situation, make an effort to direct your board shoreward so you fall behind it, or try to fall to either side of your board, but not in front of it. While going through the rinse cycle, protect your head and face with your arms and relax the rest of your body (and your mind), which will keep your heart rate low and conserve oxygen. Struggling against the turbulence in an attempt to reach the surface quickly is generally futile and needlessly burns more oxygen. Your best bet is just to go with the flow, enjoy the ride, and wait for the turbulence to subside before swimming to the surface. (For more on breath-holding technique, see Chapter 12.)

Because some of the most catastrophic surfing injuries involve the

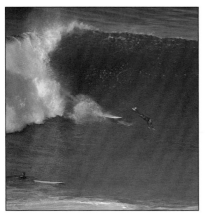

"9.5" for style.

head and neck, under the majority of circumstances, it makes sense to fall with your arms crossed over your head and to keep them there until you surface and locate your board. Predicting where your board will be as you surface from a wipeout is often impossible, so as a precaution, keep your head covered as you break through the surface. It is not uncommon to find that your board is directly above you, zinging back at you from the elastic recoil of your leash, or airborne and ready to land squarely on your head. Maintaining this defensive posture (arms crossed overhead) will serve you well by protecting your head, face, and neck should you hit the seafloor, collide with your own board, or be struck by another surfer's board.

Immediately upon surfacing from a fall, quickly look around to assess your surroundings. Where is your board? Is there a surfer, set wave, or loose board bearing down on you? Are there any exposed rocks or sketchy-looking boils in the near vicinity? How about other surfers nearby? Do you really want to be right behind that guy wearing nose plugs on a rental board when the next set rolls through? Once you have scoped out your situation, reel in your board and paddle hard out of the impact zone, angling toward the channel (if there is one) to avoid subsequent drubbings.

## Specific Wipeout Situations

### 1. Shallow-Water Wipeouts

When surfing in shallow water, your greatest risk is striking bottom, so make every effort to fall flat like a starfish so you can maximize the cushioning effect of the water. Try to fall parallel to the seafloor (belly flop or back flop) and avoid diving in headfirst at all costs. If you can, try to fall back into the soup (white water), which puts you in deeper water and keeps you away from your board. Cover your head as described above.

## 2. Tube-Riding Wipeouts

The trick here is to avoid getting sucked over the falls and driven onto shallow reef. You also want to avoid getting axed by the lip. There are two schools of thought on how this is best accomplished. The most common tactic when the door slams shut in front of you is to dive head-first and horizontally penetrating through the base of the wave, popping out the back. Another less-common move is to fall backward, behind your board, and into the partially collapsed tube, the theory being that the lip of the wave behind you has already lost much of its juice. If your wipeout is completely uncontrolled in a hollow reef break, cover your head, tuck into a crouch, and try to orient your feet toward the seafloor so if you strike bottom, you'll hit feet first. Good luck! Wiping out in the tube is technically the most difficult of all wipeouts.

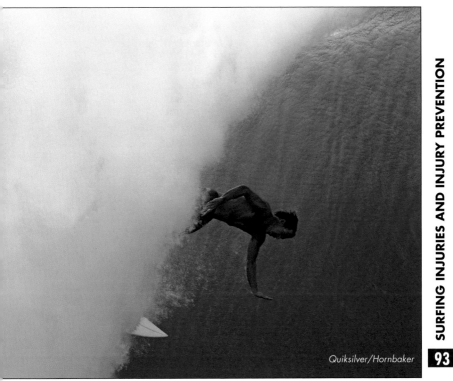

*Quiksilver/Hornbaker*

**SURFING INJURIES AND INJURY PREVENTION**

**Diving through the face?**

### 3. Shore Break

Shore break is primarily the haunt of bodysurfers and bodyboarders (and should generally be avoided by stand-up surfers). Prone wave riders have a disproportionately high rate of neck injuries undoubtedly due to the fact that the waves are being ridden in a headfirst position, often in very shallow, hollow conditions. Inexperienced bodysurfers and bodyboarders tend to ride straight toward the beach and can go over the falls and get pile-driven head first into the sand. To avoid the pile-driver routine, always angle off along the wave face and ride waves with at least one arm out in front of you, leading the way to fend off the bottom if needed. Use good judgment regarding wave selection and don't bodyboard/bodysurf in hollow dumping shore break unless you are an expert—and willing to take the risk. The over-fifty crowd or those with a history of spinal stenosis are at significantly increased risk for neck fractures and may want to consider retreating from the front lines.

### 4. Crowds

As surf breaks become ever more crowded, injuries from other surfers and their boards have become a significant risk, particularly at breaks that are crowded with beginners (e.g., Waikiki and Malibu) who are apt to lose control of their boards. When surfing in a crowded lineup and getting caught inside by a cleanup set, make a quick assessment of those around you and try finding a bit of open space so you can avoid getting clobbered if someone loses their board. If a surfer or loose surfboard is bearing down on you and a collision appears imminent, use your board as a shield to protect yourself from the impact.

### 5. Rocks and Logs

If riding a wave and a rock or exposed reef appears in front of you, you have a couple of options. If the rock is just above the surface, sometimes you can have the wave take you over it by riding higher up the face. If that is not an option, or you encounter a large floating object such as a log, try to jump over it, feet first, landing on the far side. Should you encounter a number of low rocks right in front of you, quickly ask yourself the question, "Who do I like more—my board or myself?" If the answer is "myself," you can prone out, steer clear of the bigger ones, and let your board take the brunt of the damage taking care to keep your fingers on the deck of your board so they don't get smashed. As a last resort, you can bail off your board diving horizontally through the base of the wave you are riding and relying on good karma that when you surface your situation will have improved.

### 6. Big Waves

Read the section on wipeouts, beginning on page 240, in Chapter 12, "Learning How to Survive Big Surf."

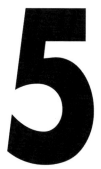

**5**

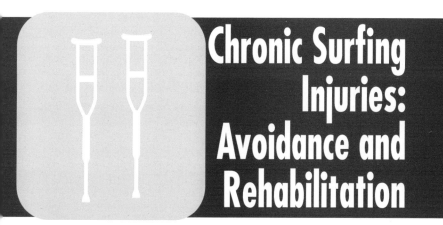

# Chronic Surfing Injuries: Avoidance and Rehabilitation

All athletes look for effective methods of dealing with injury. Some of the most frustrating of these injuries come from overuse. Some surfers may try to work through their injuries and avoid medical attention for fear that doctors will say they need time away from surfing.

Others who do seek medical attention may receive less-than-optimal care because the vast majority of physicians and other health-care providers are unfamiliar with the sport and some of the unique types of overuse injuries it can lead to. A surfer who is well versed in the diagnosis and treatment options for surfing-specific injuries should be able to provide self-care for many of these aches and pains and will be a more informed consumer when it comes time to seek the advice of a specialist.

## Sprains and Strains

### Strains in Surfing

The shoulder, elbow, neck, back, and hip are the areas of the body that are predominantly vulnerable to strains in surfing. Strains are partial to complete muscle tears caused when a muscle is overstressed, and for the most part, these injuries can be avoided with a proper dynamic warm-up prior to surfing and by stretching out on a routine basis as described in Chapter 2, Fitness for Surfers. They are graded on a scale of 1–3, with grade 1 strains being microscopic tears within the muscle fibers. Overuse-type strains are generally grade 1 and have a distinct pain pattern; the pain is absent while surfing, but soreness sets in one to two hours after getting out of the water. The best treatment is to take a break from surfing for a week or two. Ignoring the pain and failure to listen to your body can lead to chronic injury, scar tissue deposition, and further damage. There is no loss of strength with these minor strains, and with adequate rest, the muscle itself should heal with minimal intervention.

Unlike grade 1 injuries, grade 2 strains hurt right away—like when you slip on your board into a split and strain your groin. Because a large number of muscle fibers have been torn, those suffering from grade 2 strains will notice weakness of the injured part and may develop swelling and even bruising a couple of days post injury. These types of injuries often require physical therapy and may take up to four weeks to heal.

Grade 3 strains are a complete muscle rupture and are distinctive because the muscle is torn in half and no longer works. The pain is immediate and severe, the muscle may appear to be balled up, and bruising is common. These injuries will require a month or more to heal and, depending upon which muscle is involved, may require surgical repair. A classic example of this type of injury is a torn hamstring muscle that leaves a nasty bruise in the back of the leg and will have you limping around for at least a month.

The initial rehabilitation of muscle strains involves rest, ice, elevation, and compression with an elastic wrap. After a week or more of rest, depending on the extent of your injury, you can begin gentle controlled stretching of the muscle to prevent shortening by scar tissue. This stretching should follow the general principles of modern sports medicine that (1) early mobilization leads to quicker recovery, and (2) pain should be used as the rate-limiting factor in the pace of rehabilitation. In other words, listen to your body. Minor discomfort is to be expected with any rehab, but significant pain means that you are advancing your rehab too quickly. Gentle stretching should be accompanied by isometric exercise, which should then be followed by isokinetic exercise. Isometric exercises involve contracting a muscle without changing its length (like putting your hands in a prayer position and pushing them together to contract your chest muscle), whereas with isokinetic exercise, the length of the muscle does change—like doing a push-up to contract your chest muscle. Rehab of specific injuries is described later in this chapter.

## Sprains in Surfing

Ligaments are tough fibrous tissues that hold bones together across a joint. Sprains are injuries to a ligament that can occur if the joint is stressed and the ligament gets stretched beyond its functional length. Docs aren't overly creative, and just like strains, these too are graded on a scale of 1–3. Grade 1 sprains are associated with microscopic tears within the ligament, but the basic integrity of the ligament remains intact. While these injuries are accompanied by pain and swelling, the injuries usually heal with rest, ice, compression wraps, and elevation, best remembered by the acronym RICE. Most grade 1 sprains are caused by excessive twisting of a joint beyond its normal range, as when landing awkwardly from an aerial and twisting an ankle, but some like "surfer's elbow" and multidirectional shoulder instability are simply caused by overuse and muscular imbalances. Grade 1 sprains may progress to grade 2 when surfers ignore early symptoms, neglect to ice and elevate the injured part, and surf through the pain.

Grade 2 sprains are partial ligament tears that stretch out a ligament and weaken it. They cause considerable pain and swelling and, unlike grade 1 strains, may cause some instability (laxity) within the joint. These types of injuries may require physical therapy and a splint or brace along with prolonged rest, ice, elevation, and compression. Functional bracing, like an air cast for an ankle sprain, allows for early mobilization which reduces stiffness, yet protects the ligaments from further damage.

Grade 3 sprains are complete ruptures of the ligament and paradoxically may be less painful than grade 2 sprains but usually involve more swelling and cause joint instability. Magnetic resonance imaging (MRI) may be useful to determine the need for surgical repair versus bracing. These injuries are typified by rupture of anterior cruciate ligament (ACL) in the knee, an injury that has become increasingly common among pro surfers.

## Healing and Rehabilitation

There are three phases of healing from a sprain or strain: an inflammatory phase, a phase where scar tissue forms, and a maturation phase where scar tissue shrinks while functional capacity recovers. Once functional capacity recovers, you are ready to return to surfing. Several modalities can be used to accelerate this process, including icing the area for twenty minutes up to four times daily, massage, steroid injections, and either electrical stimulation with corticosteroid cream (iontophoresis) or electrical stimulation alone (TENS). Ibuprophen (Motrin, Advil) 400–800 mg every 8 hours (with food) is often prescribed by physicians to treat the pain associated with sprains and strains and may also help to decrease inflammation. While these medications may delay the healing of fractures, there is no firm evidence that they delay healing of sprains and strains.

Heat, contrary to popular opinion, will actually increase inflammation and swelling within the first three days of an injury and should be avoided unless you are certain you have a muscle spasm (knot) and not sprain or strain. Osteopathic manipulation has been safely and effectively used in treating surfing injuries but should be done only within a normal physiologic joint range of motion.

Physical therapy (PT) is probably the most important factor in rehabilitating an injury. The main purpose of a PT program is to regain strength, endurance, and flexibility and integrate that back into surfing-specific activity. Another important facet of physical therapy is to improve balance and proprioception (one's sense of body position), which can be significantly impaired after a sprain or strain. Tendons (connecting muscle to bone) and ligaments aren't just lifeless ropes. Inside these structures lie nerves that feed information to your brain about how hard and fast they are being stretched, which helps coordinate balance, and these nerves are damaged right along with the connective tissue during a sprain or strain. After recovering from an ankle sprain, for example, you will find that your ability to balance yourself on the ball of that foot is significantly impaired. Fortunately this skill can be retrained with dedicated physical therapy.

Don't be discouraged about gains lost or setbacks resulting from injury. Consistency, focus, and a positive attitude are the most important factors in successful rehabilitation.

## Neck Strains

All acute traumatic injuries of the neck warrant formal evaluation! Any numbness, tingling, or weakness in the arms or legs after a neck injury are major red flags. If you really tweaked your neck after a wipeout, your neck should be immobilized right away, and you should be examined in a hospital or clinic where X-rays or CT scans can be obtained if necessary. (See "Spine Injuries," Chapter 10.)

Surfing can be a pain in the neck, and that's not only when you get skunked after having driven 350 miles overnight to chase a swell. The prone paddling posture requires constant contractions of the muscles in the back of the neck, upper back, and lower back, causing tension and muscular shortening of the trapezius and other muscles in the neck. This causes muscle soreness in the back of the neck, which is a common complaint among surfers, particularly weekend warrior types who often overdo it by surfing for hours despite the fact that they are out of shape. Low-grade muscle strain may not be evident until a few hours after getting out of the water, when the neck muscles go into spasm, and you feel hard, tight muscles in your neck that are tender to the touch. The pain is worsened by moving your head to either side to side or up or down. Five minutes of warm-up, particularly before entering cold water, will go a long way toward preventing this stiffness. Attention to core strength and proper paddling form is also important. When paddling from a prone position, the back should be slightly arched to raise the shoulders and chest up off the board's deck. This chest-forward posture puts your neck in a more neutral position, taking some burden off the muscles in the back of your neck and placing your shoulders in position to add leverage to your paddling stroke. Be sure to actively engage your abdominal musculature to create a firm paddling platform and to take stress off the low back. For minor neck strains, massage and gentle stretching should improve discomfort and aid in the healing process. As well as pain, trapezius muscle spasms can also cause headaches in the back of the head, as this muscle originates at the base of the skull. Other symptoms may include neck stiffness, dizziness, or unusual sensations, such as burning or a pins-and-needles feeling. Stingers are electric-shock-type pain running down the arm and may occur from sternocleidomastoid muscle or trapezius muscle strain but need a doctor's formal evaluation to rule out the possibility of a pinched nerve in the neck.

These five exercises are meant to help your neck remain flexible:

*Neck flexion.* Touch your chin to your chest and hold for twenty seconds, and then relax. This stretch can be done out on the water and will stretch out the muscles in the back of your neck that can get tight after a long paddle.

*Chin tucks.* Place your fingertips on your chin and gently push your head straight back as if you are trying to make a double chin. Keep looking forward as your head moves back. Hold five seconds. Do a number of these throughout the day.

*Upper trapezius stretch.* The upper trapezius muscle connects your shoulder to your head. Gently grasp the right side of your head with your left hand to help tilt your head toward the left. You will feel a gentle stretch on your right side. Hold for twenty to thirty seconds. Repeat often.

*Scapular squeezes.* While sitting or standing with your arms relaxed, squeeze your shoulder blades down "into your back pockets" and hold for five seconds. This should activate the lower trapezius heads, which stabilize the scapulae. Do as many as possible during the day.

*Thoracic extension.* Clasp both arms behind your head. Gently arch backward and look up toward the sky. Repeat ten times. Do this several times per day.

# Shoulder Strains and Rotator Cuff Injuries

The shoulder is the most frequently injured joint in surfing, so it is worth spending some time discussing its anatomy, injury patterns, and rehabilitation. Surfers depend on their shoulders as a principal means of locomotion and are overhead athletes, predisposing them to two surfing overuse injuries known as rotator cuff strain and multidirectional instability. Postural problems with rounded shoulders and a forward head posture (think Neanderthal man) known as the upper-crossed syndrome are also common among surfers and can lead to rotator cuff strains, biceps tendon-itis, and the neurologic symptoms of thoracic outlet syndrome (TOS).

## Anatomy

The shoulder has the widest range of motion of any joint in the body, and to allow for this movement, it is kept in place primarily by ten-dons (muscle-to-bone attachments) as opposed to the stronger, but less flexible ligaments (bone-to-bone attachments) found in other major joints. The structure most vulnerable to strains in the shoulder is the rotator cuff, a series of four muscles that serve to keep the shoulder from popping out of its shallow socket in the scapula (shoulder blade). These four muscles originate on the scapula, and their tendons come together to form a fibrous capsule or "cuff" that surround and stabilize the golf ball–like humeral head (upper arm bone), while allowing the arm to rotate freely. If you want to get extra credit on the quiz that follows, those four muscles are the supra- and infra-spinatus muscles, teres minor, and subscapularis. Forming the roof of the shoulder joint and stabilizing it is the relatively immobile acromio-clavicular joint where the scapula and clavicle (collarbone) come together. Running through the front of the shoulder joint is the biceps tendon, and lub-ing up the joint is a fluid-filled sack known as the subacromial bursa. The scapula, in turn, is held on to the rear rib cage by the muscles of serratus anterior.

### Frontal View of the Shoulder

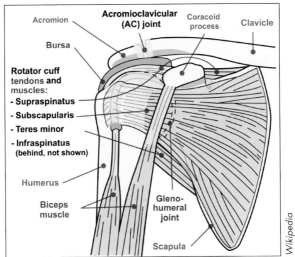

*Wikipedia*

# Rotator Cuff Injuries

Shoulder problems most commonly occur when the tough but thin rotator cuff is overstretched or torn. Occasionally this happens from an acute injury, like getting smashed by a wave, but more typically it's just the result of simple wear and tear from paddling. This should come as no surprise when you consider the fact that over half of one's time in the water is spent paddling, amounting to hundreds of paddle strokes per session, and that the shoulders are also called into action when duck-diving and taking off.

The area of the rotator cuff most prone to injury is the supraspinatus tendon, which can get impinged (pinched) as it slides though a narrow gap between the acromio-clavicular joint and the humeral head. It turns out that this bony gap is narrowest when the arm is overhead, as happens when paddling a surfboard (or throwing a baseball), which is one of the reasons us surfers so often suffer from shoulder pain. Impingement of the supraspinatus tendon can lead to inflammation and tendinitis. The now fatter, swollen tendon gets even more irritated and chafed as it attempts to squeeze under the acromium, setting up a vicious cycle. If you continue to surf through the pain and allow this process to remain unchecked, the inflamed tendon will start to fray and eventually break down, causing a tear right through the rotator cuff.

The most common symptoms of a rotator cuff injury are pain in the top and front of the shoulder and restricted movement of the arm. To test for this injury, stand with the affected arm out to your side, thumb up and raised slightly above shoulder level, as if hitchhiking. Have someone push down on your hand as you try to keep your outstretched arm up. If this reproduces the pain you get while surfing, chances are good that you have rotator tendinitis or a rotator cuff tear. If symptoms don't improve after a couple of weeks of rest and some ibuprofen, it may be time to visit a sports medicine doctor. Small rotator cuff tears are often treated successfully with physical therapy, but larger tears may require surgery.

Another chronic shoulder problem common to overhead athletes such as swimmers and surfers can occur with the gradual stretching out of the rotator cuff. This results in laxity of the shoulder joint, rendering it prone to dislocation or a near dislocation known as subluxation, in which the shoulder partially pops out of its socket, but then pops right back in. This condition referred to by sports docs as multidirectional instability can be overcome by exercises directed at strengthening the muscles that form the cuff, which in turn help to tighten up and stabilize the joint.

# Upper-Crossed Syndrome and Thoracic Outlet Syndrome

Overdeveloped paddling muscles can contribute to the rotator cuff impingement and strain described above. Muscle-bound surfers who have thick chest and shoulder musculature, but poorly developed muscles in the upper back can develop chronic postural issues in which their shoulders and neck get rolled forward. This is due to a muscular imbalance wherein the pectoralis muscles in the chest get tight and shortened, while the weaker rhomboid muscles and other scapular stabilizers allow the shoulder blades to get pulled forward, creating a hunched-over carriage. Similar problems can occur to those with desk jobs who spend hours on end leaning over a computer, with their necks craned forward. This so called upper-crossed syndrome causes movement of the humerus high into the shoulder socket, resulting in compression of the rotator cuff tendons or the subacromial bursa leading to strain or bursitis, respectively.

The upper-crossed syndrome is also a risk factor for the rare condition known as thoracic outlet syndrome (TOS), whereby nerves and blood vessels can get compressed between the clavicle and upper ribs. The symptoms of TOS vary depending upon whether it is the bundle of nerves of the brachial plexus, passing from the neck to the arms, or the subclavian artery passing from the chest to the arm that are most affected. Neurologic symptoms are most common and cause pain in the neck, arm, and hand. The pain is usually described shock-like, but may also be a burning type of pain and radiates from the inner aspect arm to the last three fingers or may involve the entire hand. Eventually weakness and/or changes in temperature of the hands can occur if the condition goes untreated.

The upper-crossed syndrome and TOS can be treated by having a friend, therapist, or athletic trainer help you assume a supine position (lying on back) on a table and placing a rolled towel under the midline of your back. Having the trainer gently push your shoulders toward the table will help the contracted pectoralis minor relax and stretch. Many athletes report this stretch to be not only painless but also comfortable. Specialized shirts designed to pull the shoulders back and improve posture, such as IntelliSkin from Dr. Tim Brown, can also assist in correcting this dysfunction. If the symptoms of TOS are not improved by stretching exercises and correcting posture, occasionally surgery may be needed to remove part of the uppermost rib and relieve pressure on the brachial plexus.

Prevent and rehabilitate shoulder and biceps overuse injuries with the following exercises. Those who have suffered prior dislocations, instability, pain shooting down the arm or into the neck, limited range of motion, or who have had prior surgery may need to be evaluated by a sports physician.

***Isometric shoulder rotations.*** If shoulder pain is severe, start with this gentle exercise. Standing near a tree (or door frame) with your elbow bent 90 degrees and the back of your wrist pressing against the tree, try to press your hand outward into the tree. Hold for five seconds. Alternate by trying to press the palm of your hand into the tree, holding that for five seconds.

Do two sets of fifteen repetitions every other day.

***Isokinetic shoulder rotations.*** Attach an elastic cord to a fixed object like a doorknob at waist height. Stand a few feet away, right shoulder toward the door, and grasp the elastic with your right hand. With your elbow bent at 90 degrees and held against your side, rotate your lower arm 180 degrees toward your left hip, pulling the elastic cord taught. This moves your shoulder in *internal* rotation.

Do two sets of fifteen repetitions every other day.

***Now turn facing the opposite direction.*** Again grasp the cord with your right hand starting at your left hip and move your shoulder in *external* rotation 180 degrees.

Do two sets of fifteen repetitions every other day.

***Side-lying external rotation.*** Lie on the floor sideways with your arm flexed 90 degrees at the elbow. Rotate your upper arm until it is pointed at 45 degrees toward the ceiling, while keeping your lower arm next to your body. Hold for two seconds and then lower it slowly. Start this exercise with no weight. As you get stronger, add a light weight.

Do two sets of fifteen repetitions every other day.

***Horizontal abduction.*** Lie on a table or the edge of a bed facedown with one arm hanging down straight to the floor. Raise your arm out to the side, with your thumb pointed toward the ceiling until your arm is parallel to the floor. Hold for two seconds and then lower it slowly. Start this exercise with no weight. As you get stronger, add a light weight or a bungee cord for resistance.

Do two sets of fifteen repetitions every other day.

***Scapular squeeze.*** Just like the neck rehabilitation sequence. While sitting or standing, squeeze your shoulder blades down.

Do two sets of fifteen repetitions daily.

***Thoracic extension.*** Just like the neck rehabilitation sequence, contract shoulder blades back and look up toward the sky several times per day.

Do two sets of fifteen repetitions daily.

***Mid-trap exercise.*** Lie on your stomach with your elbows straight, fingers pointing toward feet and thumbs toward the ceiling. Slowly raise your arms toward the ceiling while squeezing your shoulder blades together. Lower slowly.

Do two sets of fifteen repetitions every other day.

***Biceps stretch.*** Stand holding your surfboard with both hands behind your back like the vintage Hawaiian photos for twenty to thirty seconds several times after your surf session. You should feel a stretch in your biceps muscles.

***Biceps curls.*** Stand and hold some kind of weight that does not cause discomfort when lifting. Bring your hand up toward your shoulder.

Do as many as possible every other day but stop if it becomes painful.

***Push-up plus.*** Begin on the floor on your hands and knees. Keep your arms a shoulder width apart and lift your feet off the floor. Arch your back as high as possible and round your shoulders forward to activate the anterior serratus muscles (this is the plus part or the exercise). Bend your elbows and lower your body to the floor. Return to the starting position and arch your back again. Push-up–type exercises with an Indo board promote shoulder stability by training the shoulder muscles on an unstable surface, much like duck-diving a surfboard on the water.

Do as many as possible every other day, but stop if pain develops.

## Low-Back Pain: The Bane of Two-Legged Mammals

Like many other athletes and the population at large, surfers often suffer from chronic low-back pain. Back pain is so common among humans that some people are beginning to think of it as a normal part of the human condition, rather than as a disease process. In fact, the vast majority of adults, over 80 percent, will eventually suffer a bout of back pain severe enough to keep them out of work, or otherwise out of commission. Perhaps this is because we humans are the only mammals truly capable of standing upright, which places our spines in a constant state of compression. But, hey, it is a small price to pay for

## Lumbar Spine (Highlighted)

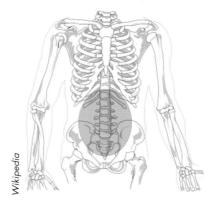

*Wikipedia*

being able to score a stand-up barrel (can't really do that on all fours). But enough speculation. The good news is that in the vast majority of cases (over 90 percent), low-back pain will resolve within six to eight weeks—with little more than tincture of time. The section that follows lays out some exercises to help you rehab a bad back and, if you stick with the program, help prevent future flare-ups.

Surfers spend prolonged periods of time in spinal hyperextension (arched back and neck) while paddling, which can gradually lead to neck and low-back muscular strain. This is particularly common if you haven't been out surfing for a while or partake in an exceptionally long session. Muscle strain is generally a self-limited process and is thought to account for the majority of back problems among surfers.

The discs between the bones in the spine (vertebrae) can also be the source of back problems. These intervertebral discs that serve as padding between the vertebrae are composed of a tough fibrous outer layer, the annulus fibrosus, surrounding a softer gelatinous inner core, known as the nucleosis pulposus. With wear and tear, or subject to enough pressure, the outer layer of the disc can tear, allowing the nucleosis pulposus to bulge out, causing what is commonly known as a herniated disc. The material that bulges outward can press against local structures like the spinal cord, or more commonly the nearby spinal nerve roots that exit both sides of the spinal cord. If a nerve root is compressed or even irritated due to inflammation from herniated material, it can often cause pain that radiates down the leg and, in severe cases, will also cause leg weakness. Sounds pretty grim, eh? But even those with disc herniation have a favorable prognosis. In fact, more than half will be better in six weeks, and nearly three-quarters will be healed up in twelve weeks, without any surgery.

Chronic injuries to the bones in the spine (vertebrae) are far less common causes of back pain, but athletes whose sports rely on spinal hyperextension such as football players, gymnasts, and surfers are at increased risk for a category of vertebral injuries in which the bridge-like facet joints that connect each vertebra to its neighbors break down. In a process called spondylolysis, the support structure for these facets joints breaks, which can lead to slippage of one vertebra over another (spondylolisthesis). Despite the ominous-sounding nature of this condition, treatment is rarely surgical, and symptoms generally improve with physical therapy.

### Disc and Spinal Cord

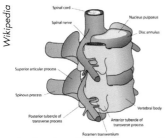

Wikipedia

So when *should* you see the doctor for back pain? Cases in which pain is shooting down the legs or into the groin imply involvement of nerves, often the sciatic nerve. Though sciatica is generally treated conservatively, that is to say, nonsurgically, it is wise to consult a physician. In most cases, sciatica will flare up for a few weeks and then resolve for months to years before becoming symptomatic again. Back pain associated with numbness or weakness in a leg (or legs) or back pain associated with difficulty urinating or controlling one's bowels also implies nerve damage and is worrisome; see a doctor right away for any of these symptoms. Lastly, acute trauma to the spine should always be evaluated by a physician.

With the exception of leg weakness or problems involving the bowels or bladder, be wary of any surgeon who wants to operate on you without a three-month trial period of rest and physical therapy. Know that even those with herniated discs usually improve without going under the knife. In fact, the significance of a herniated disc is becoming less and less clear. Recent studies done on healthy volunteers without any back pain whatsoever show that 30 percent of *them* have a herniated disc on MRI! The bottom line here is that back pain is very common and mostly goes away on its own. Maintaining strong core musculature, attention to proper posture in the workplace, and working on flexibility will go a long way toward avoiding back problems.

To stay clear of back pain, perform these exercises most days of the week:

***Back flush.*** Stand with your back to a wall. Tighten your abdominal muscles and push your lower back into the wall until the lower back is flush with the surface. Hold this position for ten to fifteen seconds, then relax.

*Piriformis and gluteal stretch.* Lying on your back, grab one ankle with the opposite hand and pull out until you feel a stretch along the buttocks and possibly along the outside of your hip. Hold this for twenty to thirty seconds. Switch legs and repeat.

*Bird dogs.* Get down on your hands and knees. Tighten your abdominal muscles to stiffen your spine. While keeping your abdominals tight, raise one arm and the opposite leg away from you. Hold this position for five seconds. Lower your arm and leg slowly and alternate sides. Do this ten times on each side.

## Case Study: The Unusual Case of a Surfer's Myelopathy

Renee, a twenty-five-year-old accountant from New York, went to Hawaii on vacation and, like most twenty-five-year-old accountants from New York, wanted nothing more than to learn how to surf. After a two-hour surf lesson in Waikiki, she noticed that her legs felt weak, and her midback hurt quite a bit. Figuring that she was just out of shape, she thought nothing of it until upon returning to her hotel an hour later, she found that she had trouble walking. An MRI at a local hospital revealed that her spinal cord lacked blood flow (like a stroke). She was suffering from a rare and recently described condition known as surfer's myelopathy, curiously seen only among first-time surfers. Renee was fortunate in that she regained a full recovery, but others have been less fortunate. The cause remains shrouded in mystery—but probably has something to do with a kinking of tiny arteries supplying blood to the spinal cord, which occurs when a beginner is paddling with an arched back. First-time surfers should probably limit their intro session to an hour and return to the beach at the first hint of back pain.

## Hip

The hip flexor and extensor muscles are heavily used during surfing pop-ups and turns, respectively. It is common for a lower-crossed syndrome that causes back pain to overlay into tight but weak hip flexor muscles. These muscles are commonly strained during surfing and could predispose to further injury in the hip socket leading to impingement, functional limitations, and ultimately, arthritis. Preventative and rehabilitative stretching and isokinetic and isometric exercises are important and can include Indo board variations to add more of a challenge.

You can begin stretching your strained hip muscles right away by doing the first two exercises. Make sure you only feel a mild discomfort when stretching and not a sharp pain. You may do the last exercise when the pain is gone.

**Scorpion stretches.** Lay facedown on a towel and kick one heel over and across your back like a scorpion's tail. There should be a gentle stretch in the hip flexor area just lateral to the groin. Hold for twenty to thirty seconds for each hip.

**Straight leg raise.** Lie on your back with your legs straight out in front of you. Bend the knee on your uninjured side and place the foot flat on the floor. Tighten the thigh muscle of the other leg and lift it about a foot off the ground, keeping the thigh muscle contracted. Slowly lower your leg back down to the floor. Do until the muscle feels fatigued.

**Kicks.** Hold arms out and gently kick out, aiming to hit each hand with the opposite foot. This activates the hip flexors. Do as often as possible.

# Knee

Certain exercises intended to strengthen leg muscles are counterproductive to athletic performance yet are still recommended by the pros. These exercises, such as treadmill running, deep squats, and leg extensions, have been popular over the years and will likely be difficult to quash. They are also the most common cause of worsening knee arthritis and anterior knee pain (runner's knee).

Anterior (front) knee pain syndrome can be relieved by avoiding activities that make symptoms worse like knee paddling and sitting or kneeling in the bent-knee position for long periods of time. Biking is one of the best aerobic replacements for treadmill running and is excellent rehabilitation for anterior knee pain and osteoarthritis (wear and tear arthritis) of the knee. Adjust a bicycle or exercise bike so that the resistance is not too great and the seat is at an appropriate height. The rider should be able to spin the pedals of an exercise bike without shifting weight from side to side, and the legs should not be fully extended at the lowest part of the pedal stroke. Avoid bent-knee exercises, such as squats, deep-knee bends, or leg extensions, where the knee is bent greater than 90 degrees.

Sometimes overly bent knees cannot be avoided. For example, when riding a fast tube back side in the "pig-dog" stance, you will compress the patella (kneecap) of the bent knee against the thigh bone. Landing airs causes immense stress on the knee joint and ligaments. Even if the ligaments and cartilage are not torn, a small amount of swelling or minor muscle strain can cause pain at the back of the knee. This needs

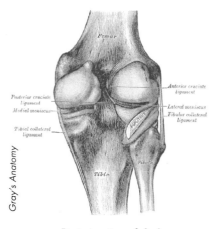

Posterior view of the knee.

simple rest, ice, compression, and rehabilitation exercises unless the knee is grossly swollen or unstable, in which case it should be seen by a doctor.

When associated with plantar fasciitis (heel pain), shin splints, and low-back pain, the knee alignment may need to be evaluated by a sports physician to rule out flat feet, patellar malalignment, or a combination called pronator distortion syndrome. Rehabilitation exercises help the body find a way to adjust from knee hyperflexion to hip flexion and abduction. Remember, any instability, catching, or locking of knee should be evaluated by a sports physician.

Strong yet limber quadriceps and hamstring muscles buttress the knee and hip joints. Try the following prevention and rehabilitation program:

**Hamstring tree stretch.** Lying on the ground, place the heel of each leg on a tree or lifeguard tower until you feel a gentle stretch. Stretch twenty to thirty seconds for each leg.

**Side-lying leg lift.** Lying on your uninjured side, tighten the front thigh muscles on your top leg and lift that leg about a foot away from the other leg. Keep the leg relatively straight and the tempo slow. Do as many as possible, focusing on the gluteal muscles.

**Quad sets.** Done by tightening the muscles on the top of your thigh. Hold this position ten to twenty seconds. Relax. Do as often as possible.

**Straight leg raise.** Lie on your back with your legs straight out in front of you. Bend the knee and place the foot flat on the floor. Tighten the thigh muscle

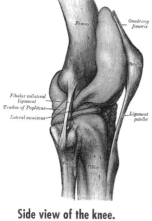

Side view of the knee.

of the other leg and lift it about 6 inches off the floor, keeping the thigh muscles tight throughout. Slowly lower your leg back down to the floor. Repeat for the other knee and perform as often as possible.

## Ankle

With the progression of aerial surfing and recent adoption of foil surfing, ankle sprains and even fractures among surfers are on the rise. Most injuries are to the back "power foot" and occur when a surfer lands awkwardly on their board, forcing the front of the foot up and out, placing stress on the inside of the ankle. This can result in a sprain of the inside (medial) "deltoid" ligament as opposed to most other sports where the foot rolls inward spraining the outside (lateral) part of the ankle. In contrast to the far more common lateral ankle injury, medial ankle injuries from surfing are associated with "high ankle sprains" (stretching the intraosseous ligaments between the two bones in the lower leg), and even "Maisonneuve" fractures of the upper, outer leg (fibula).

Medial ligament sprains can be easily diagnosed because they cause swelling and tenderness to the inside of the ankle. Those with more serious high ankle sprains have tenderness extending high up the front of the ankle and lower leg and experience increased pain and instability when attempting to push off the toes or pivot inward with the foot planted. These types of ankle injuries take extended periods (four to six weeks or more) to heal and occasionally require surgery. Those that continue to have pain after initial conservative therapy may require an MRI.

A phased rehabilitation program is described below. The acute phase is aimed at protecting the joint while minimizing pain, inflammation, muscle weakness, and loss of motion. Those with severe pain and swelling will initially require a boot, or "functional" ankle brace at the onset of injury before progressing to gentle range of motion exercises. For the exercises below, only move the ankle to the point of mild discomfort.

*In a standing position* trace the alphabet with your toe which encourages ankle movement in all directions. Trace the alphabet one to three times.

*From a seated position* slowly move your knee side to side while keeping your foot pressed flat. Continue for two to three minutes. Raise the front of the foot up with the heel on the floor and hold for a count of ten. Do this slowly, while feeling a stretch in your calf. Repeat ten times. Raise your foot just off the ground and point the toes toward the other leg for a count of ten. Repeat ten times. Again, with the foot slightly raised move the front of your foot up and out. Hold this everted position for a count of ten. Repeat ten times. From the starting position, point your toes down and hold this position for a count of ten. Repeat ten times. From the starting position, wave toes up, then down. Repeat ten times.

Once ankle range of motion has been almost or completely restored, you must strengthen your ankle. Along with strengthening, you should work toward a feeling of stability and fine motor control, which we sports medicine specialists call "proprioception."

Consider these home exercises when recuperating from an ankle sprain. Perform them twice per day. Start this program only when the pain from your ankle sprain has significantly subsided:

*Stand 12 inches from a wall* with your toes pointing toward the wall, arms in front horizontal. Squat down and hold this position for a count of ten. Repeat ten times.

*Balance on one leg* with the affected leg on a pillow or bosu ball. Hold this position for a count of ten. Repeat ten times. Try standing tiptoe on the floor while balancing on one leg. Lift up and down ten times. For additional challenge close your eyes. For a more sports-specific rehab, get on an balance board and roll side-to-side, or preform lightweight squats on a bosu ball. Progress to surfing aggressively when able to jog and perform a series of hops without pain.

## Elbow

Chronic elbow pain is relatively common among surfers. A condition commonly known as golfer's elbow that causes pain at the inside of the elbow (medial epicondyle) is related to repetitive paddling. Pain at the very back of your elbow (where the triceps attaches) can occur from repetitive pop-ups on the unstable surfboard. This is called surfer's elbow. Anterior (front) elbow pain is caused by overuse of the biceps or brachioradialis muscles. These muscles are stressed with sustained or repetitive flexion of the elbow, particularly during long stalls in heavy or barreling surf, or during layback snaps. This type of repetitive stress may result in tendonitis of these muscles and may be considered another unique surfing injury. The ulnar nerve can also be inflamed from irritation or injury, causing the same burning pain shooting into the tips of the ring and small finger as when you hit your "funny bone."

Rehabilitation exercises for these elbow injuries involve stretching and strengthening the flexor, extensor, pronator, and supinator muscles of the wrist and forearm. Do these stretching exercises at the first sign of pain and continue doing them throughout your surfing career. Begin the strengthening exercises when stretching is nearly painless.

Supination of the forearm involves bending the elbow to ninety degrees, turning your palm upward and holding for five seconds. Slowly turn your palm downward for pronation and hold for five seconds. Make sure you keep your elbow at your side and bent 90 degrees throughout this exercise. Do five sets of ten. Include wrist flexion and extension as well as forearm internal and external rotation. Wrist flexion exercise involves grasping a weight in your hand with your palm facing up. Bend your wrist upward. Slowly lower the weight and return to the starting position. Do five sets of ten. Gradually increase the weight you are holding.

Wrist extension exercise involves holding a comfortable weight in your hand with your palm facing down. Slowly bend your wrist upward. Slowly lower the weight down into the starting position. Do five sets of ten. Gradually increase the weight of the object you are holding.

Elastic tubing or bungee exercises for external rotation involve resting the hand of your injured side against your stomach. With that hand, grasp elastic rubber or bungee cords connected to a doorknob or tree at waist level. Keeping your elbow in at your side, rotate your arm outward and away from your waist. Make sure you keep your elbow bent 90 degrees and your forearm parallel to the floor. Repeat ten times. Build up to five sets of ten.

# Ribs

The twelve ribs on each side of your chest may be bruised, strained, broken, or separated during surfing. Women and thin men commonly develop lower rib soreness a few days into a good swell, particularly if they haven't been out on the water for a while. With little natural padding between themselves and their boards, any bony prominences in the ribs (and even hip bones) become pressure points when paddling. Constant irritation at these contact points between rider and board causes bruising and irritation. This type of soreness to the front lower part of the rib cage can be minimized by wearing a thicker wet suit, using a full deck pad, or trying a recently developed wet suit (paddleair.com), which incorporates air bladder in the chest for optimum

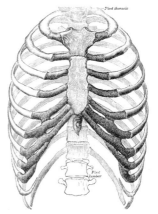

*Gray's Anatomy*

**Human rib cage. Note cartilage (dark area) connecting ribs to sternum.**

padding. Occasionally the pain can continue for weeks after the cessation of surfing, which is a sure sign that you've developed inflammation of the cartilage connecting ribs to sternum (chest plate), a condition known as costochondritis. The best treatment for this is to take ibuprofen (Motrin) and abstain from surfing for a week or so. Adopting a slightly more arched paddling posture will transfer weight off your ribs and onto your abdomen, and may provide a long-term fix. If you develop painless bumps at the contact point between chest and board, you probably have a benign condition known as surfer's knots—for more on those, see the chapter "Skin Problems of Surfers."

With overuse or trauma, ribs may tear away from the cartilage that attaches them to the breastbone in front, causing what is commonly known as a popped rib, but we doctors call a costochondral separation. This may occur when you land hard from a wipeout, hit your board, or even when you pop-up on your board. With a separated rib, you may feel a popping sensation or even movement of the front part of a rib when you take a deep breath or cough. If you have severe pain when you take a deep breath, cough, or sneeze, you might have broken a rib and should be seen by a doctor and get an X-ray to rule out the possibility of an underlying injury such as a collapsed lung or injury to your spleen. Separated ribs and broken ribs usually heal on their own without any specific treatment, though the pain will probably prevent you from surfing.

To help a rib injury heal, rest and put an ice pack over the injured rib for twenty to thirty minutes every three to four hours for two to three days or until the pain goes away. Do not surf if it hurts to breathe or paddle. Actively seek medical attention if you cannot breathe comfortably at rest. Take an anti-inflammatory or other pain medicine. Adults aged sixty-five years and older should not take nonsteroidal anti-inflammatory medicine for more than seven days without their health-care provider's approval. Bruised ribs and a costochondral separation usually take three to four weeks to heal. Broken ribs take six to eight weeks to heal and should be evaluated by a physician.

Surfer's rib is an isolated first-rib stress fracture that occurs in surfers who perform the lay-back maneuver excessively. It may also be associated with thoracic outlet syndrome described in the section on shoulder injuries.

*Scalene stretch.* This stretches the neck muscles that attach to your ribs. Clasp both hands behind your back, lower your left shoulder, and tilt your head toward the right. Hold this position for 15–30 seconds and then come back to the starting position. Lower your right shoulder and tilt your head toward the left until you feel a stretch. Hold for fifteen to thirty seconds. Repeat three times on each side.

*Pectoralis stretch.* Stand holding your surfboard behind your back like the vintage Hawaiian photos for twenty to thirty seconds several times after your surf session. You should feel a stretch in your chest muscles.

*Scapular squeeze.* Just like the neck and shoulder rehabilitation sequences. While sitting or standing, squeeze your shoulder blades down as many times as possible.

*Thoracic extension.* Just like the neck and shoulder rehabilitation sequences, contract shoulder blades down and look up toward the sky several times per day.

*Mid-trap exercise.* Just like neck and shoulder rehabilitation sequences. Lie on your stomach with your elbows straight, fingers pointing toward feet and thumbs toward the ceiling. Slowly raise your arms toward the ceiling while squeezing your shoulder blades together. Lower slowly. Do as many as possible.

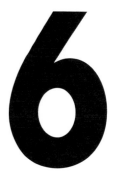

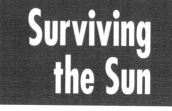

# Surviving
# the Sun

The sun is a surfer's best and worst friend. Were it not for the sun—heating the atmosphere and creating wind that caresses the seas—the ocean would not make waves. And were it not for the sun—bombarding the DNA in our skin and eyes with harmful radiation—we would not have to worry about skin cancer and premature aging of our skin and eyes.

Even though the sun is increasingly seen in a negative light, in truth it is also a powerful contributor to our health, particularly by triggering vitamin D production in our skin. Sun exposure is linked to better immune function, healthier bones, less cancer, and lower incidence of high blood pressure and diabetes. And in general, it reduces the risk of seasonal affective disorder (SAD) and increases our ability to experience feelings of happiness (the sun boosts our endorphin levels). In fact, there is even a field of health called heliotherapy—the use of the sun to heal. We surfers all know that to be true.

This chapter will examine our present understanding of the dark side of the sun for surfers and what can be done to survive it.

## Case Study

As a young man, Robert began surfing at Zuma in the late '50s, and before long he had a garden-variety skin cancer cut off his forehead. The doctor told him that if he wanted to stay alive, he should stop surfing. So he did, for years and years, until he finally realized the doctor didn't know what he was talking about, that most skin cancers do not threaten your life.

Most surfers, even back then, would not have fallen for their doctor's admonitions, as Zuma Robert did—they'd have found some way to keep surfing. Check out Christopher Snow, a surfer in *Fear Nothing*, the 1998 mystery novel by Dean Koontz. Snow had xeroderma pigmentosa, a rare but devastating skin condition for which all sunlight must be avoided, so he only night-surfed, at a place named Midnight Bay. Fictional, hard-core, real!

# The Texas Surfers Skin Study

 No one had studied the relationship between surfers and sun-damaged skin compared to the general public, until 1992, when a group of dermatologists screened forty-nine surfers competing in an amateur surfing contest in Galveston and compared them to sixty nonsurfing locals. Although this was not a large study, the results were startling.

The surfer group had a median age of just thirty years, but 41 percent of them were found on skin examination to already have pre–skin cancers—called actinic keratoses—and that keratoses' group was only slightly older, by two years. And eight of the forty-nine surfers (16 percent) were found to have actual skin cancers, of the basal cell type, with that group, again, being just a bit older still, with thirty-eight years as their median age. There were no squamous cell cancers or melanomas found, but eighteen of the forty-nine (37 percent) had the kinds of moles that are considered worrisome, as per the ABCD rule: Asymmetrical and irregular Borders, variations in Color, and Diameter larger than six millimeters (the width of a pencil eraser). So, all told, almost 75 percent of surfers who had a median age of only thirty were well on their way to having skin cancer, or already had one!

And ominously, their development of pre- or actual skin cancers was occurring with only a slight laddering upward of their quite-young-to-begin-with ages. Not surprisingly, there was a statistically significant difference as to both the incidence and the age of onset of skin cancer in the surfers compared to nonsurfers. Unfortunately, these findings would have not surprised many surfers, especially those over forty, because by that age most surfers already have had something cut, frozen, or burned off by a dermatologist, or at least one of their buddies has, and exclaimed to all, "I'm not even that old!"

Sun product marketing surveys report that about two-thirds of Americans never or rarely use sunscreen, and, those who do, don't use enough. The authors of the Texas study also reported that most of the surfers expressed reluctance to wear sunscreen. There has never been a true study of sunscreen use among surfers, but it would be safe to say that a large percentage of surfers do not regularly use them, particularly young surfers, whose lifelong risks of skin cancer are greatest.

## Sun Damage 101

The science of solar radiation isn't complicated. The earth's outer atmosphere, especially the ozone in it, filters out the most damaging sunrays, which are the shorter wavelengths in the violet-and-blue spectrum (that's why the sky is blue!). What makes it through and comes invisibly hurtling down upon us is a slightly longer wavelength of light called ultraviolet, or UV for short.

The UV spectrum is divided into A, B, and C, but most of the UVC is also filtered out by the atmosphere. That leaves us with A and B. UVA is the more powerful, with longer wavelengths, at 320–400 nanometers. UVB are weaker and of shorter wavelengths, at 290–320 nanometers. UVB can't penetrate very deeply and concentrates in the outer skin (the epidermis, the skin you can see). UVA goes into both the outer skin and the deeper tissues under the skin (the dermis).

UVB is associated with sunburn—redness and burning in the skin—which is what sunscreens have traditionally targeted. Until recently, UVB was thought to be the main cause of skin cancers. But the less-visible damage from UVA is more insidious and is now understood to be more destructive, causing extensive photoaging of the skin—wrinkles, premature aging, and cancers. UVA is also harder to screen out, whether with sunscreens, hats, and clothes, even car or house windows!

Visible light is of a longer wavelength than UV, in the 400–700 nanometer range, and isn't thought to have much downside, healthwise. Infrared is the next longer wavelength (greater than 700 nanometers), is invisible (except to night-vision goggles), and is of emerging health concern. Infrared slowly cooks even the deepest skin tissues and is also now thought to contribute to photodamage and skin cancer causation. Infrared radiation is not easy to block.

## A Life in the Sun: Photodamaged Skin

Some surfers imagine that if they just maintain a nice tan, their skin will be protected from sunburn and sun damage. Wrong. In fact, the regular sun/UV exposure needed to maintain a tan will set them up for even earlier premature skin changes. All but the most dark-skinned surfers wear their sun-exposure history on their faces, literally.

# The Face of a Surfer

Surfers' faces show sun-damaged skin about ten to twenty years earlier than nonsurfers. Realize that before they get into the line of lemmings on their way to a conventional world of life indoors, the average person receives 80 percent of their lifetime sun exposure by age eighteen, the age when hard-core surfers are just getting started!

### Age 20–30

- Minimal wrinkling
- Mild pigment changes (age/sunspots)
- Early pre–skin cancers

### Age 30–40

- Smile lines and faint crow's-feet by eyes
- More obvious age/sunspots
- Pre–skin cancers and basal cell skin cancers

### Age 40–50

- Wrinkles more widespread over face
- Obvious age spots
- Multiple keratoses and pre–skin cancers
- Basal and squamous cell cancers
- Some baggy skin

### Over 50

- Furrowing of wrinkles
- Broken blood vessels (telangiectasia)
- Yellow grayish color to skin
- Multiple skin cancers
- More and more baggy, loose skin

Notes: 1. Melanomas can occur at any age, but peak in the forties.
2. Cigarette smoking will exaggerate photodamaged skin.

3. A similar chronology could be constructed for eye-specific sun damage (pinguecula, pterygium, corneal and macular degeneration, see "Eye and Vision Problems" chapter).

## Sunburn—Ouch!

Sunburn can occur in less than fifteen minutes of UVB sun exposure at midday in a fair-skinned individual, but in surfers the usual scenario is either to have forgotten to put on any sunscreen, to have found the surf so ridiculously good that they just couldn't bring themselves to come in, or to be on their first day of a surf trip to the tropics. Sunburn has two phases. The first phase is a faint redness that develops shortly after exposure but then fades within thirty minutes. If you are observant and notice the first phase reaction and get yourself out of the sun, and, best of all, actively cool your skin (cold water), you may reduce the degree of phase 2 reaction (but there is scant research on this). The phase 2 full-bummer

**"This is how I tan!"**

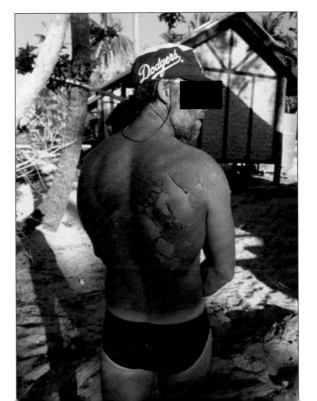

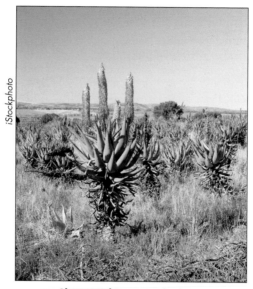

**Aloe vera plants in South Africa.**

reaction begins two to six hours after overexposure and peaks at sixteen to twenty-four hours, but can last up to forty-eight hours. There is the characteristic redness, but often warmth, tenderness, and swelling. If severe, there will be immediate blisters (or they may come after one to three days), and there may be fever, chills, nausea, and even delirium.

The treatment for acute sunburn is (1) get indoors, (2) immerse in cold freshwater (not ice-cold) or cool compresses for up to two hours or longer, and (3) begin nonsteroidal anti-inflammatories such as ibuprofen (e.g., Advil, Motrin). Note: you may need larger doses than over-the-counter products indicate, which for ibuprofen usually is 200 mg every four to six hours, but if it looks severe, you may want to start with 400 mg every four hours. Ibuprofen peaks at about one hour, so if the pain is still severe then, think nothing of taking another 400 mg right then. Aspirin will also work well while acetaminophen/Tylenol less so.

Severe sunburn may require prescription pain medications, such as codeine or Vicodin (a combination of hydrocodone and acetaminophen). Sometimes, oral steroids are needed, but applying steroid creams to the sunburn hasn't been shown to do much. There is some research that proves what surfers have always known, that aloe vera can help with sunburn. You can buy aloe in most health food stores as a gel or liquid, but there may be aloe plants available for use right where you surf: aloes are those spiky succulents that are often red or orange, which grow in many parts of coastal California, Hawaii, and South Africa. Surfers just tear off a leaf and smear the juicy pulp right on to their skin. Iced milk compresses applied to sunburned skin can also be soothing, as can tea compresses to blistering sunburn.

First-degree (nonblistering) sunburn usually resolves in about three days, but some skin may peel off days later. Second-degree (blistering) sunburn may take longer to resolve, with larger portions of the skin still sloughing off for many days. Post-sunburned skin often remains darker, with a different pigment pattern.

## Sunscreens and Sunblocks

The United States sunscreen product industry is estimated at about 11 billion dollars per year, and like most multibillion-dollar health-product industries, it is hard to discern fact from promotion, and hard to regulate. To their credit, the sunscreen industry has seized upon and made use of most every scientific discovery, even minor ones, so driven are they by the heat of competition.

For instance, a study in the late '80s found that PABA (para-aminobenzoic acid) nicely blocked UVB protection so PABA was immediately added to sunscreens and PABA sunscreens became all the rage. But soon PABA was found to cause allergic reactions and stain clothes yellow, so the next big advance was to promote—you guessed it—PABA-free sunscreens. Now it is all but absent from sunscreens.

And so it goes. Know that what sunscreens mainly do is prevent sunburn (and sunburn is mainly caused by UVB). More recently, when the industry was criticized for only targeting UVB and all but ignoring UVA radiation, so called "Broad Spectrum" suncreens were developed which provide at least some UVA protection. This followed a period when the industry seized upon a combined UVA/UVB blocker called oxybenzone (and its chemical cousins such as oxinoxate) and soon it became the big tag for promotion. But then it was found that oxybenzone was systemically absorbed through the skin, may promote cancer and disrupt your endocrine system, and was harmful to coral reefs and marine life. In 2018, Hawaii passed a law (to go into effect January 1, 2021) banning any sunscreen containing oxybenzone or octinoxate. While there are still a number of sunscreens containing these chemicals, the Hawaii model should be how all surfers approach this, no matter where they surf: best not to use them!

The same thing happened as to the strategy of adding in an antioxidant, specifically, a type of vitamin A (retinyl palmitate), with the thought that it would help prevent skin cancer. But a recent study showed it causes more skin cancers than it prevents. Oops. A goodly number of sunscreens still contain retinyl palmitate, but, again, their days are numbered. Steer clear of sunscreens with vitamin A added in.

Same with sunscreens trying to sound oh-so-modern by advertising they contain "nanoparticles" and are therefore more effective. Same deal, reefs don't like nano-containing sunscreens, and neither should you.

The type of sunscreens we are recommending are those that contain minerals such as zinc oxide and/or titanium dioxide, without nanoparticles, and no additional chemicals such as PABA, oxybenzone, or vitamin A, even if they are advertised as "organic" chemical sunscreens. Added "inert" or "inactive" organic products such as beeswax, honey, calendula, coffee, hemp, and a multitude of oils and scents are okay, if you are not allergic to them.

Keep in mind that there is no such thing as a sunblock—at least some portion of the sun's radiation gets through everything. In fact, the FDA has essentially banned the use of the term "sunblock." But most of us have a pretty good idea of what a sunblock is versus a sunscreen: a sunblock is something that physically blocks out the sun, such as zinc oxide or titanium oxide, versus sunscreens, which, by chemical wizardry, somehow neutralize or absorb the sunrays. Part of the chemical wizardry of sunscreens is why they keep backfiring—to chemically weaken the sunrays leaves a byproduct of oxidative chemicals, called reactive oxygen species, which are more, not less, likely to cause DNA mutations and cancer. Furthermore, the blocking of the sun's natural effects in the skin dramatically hinders the body's normal production of vitamin D, and vitamin D deficiency is now being seen as epidemic in the United States and tied to an increase in not just melanoma but also many other cancers, including breast, lung, and colon.

So what sunscreens to use and who to trust as to their recommendations? Well, it turns out the American Cancer Society and Skin Cancer Foundation have effectively sold their logos to endorse certain sunscreen products, so scratch them off the list. Many health-minded organizations began calling foul on the sunscreen industry back in the early '90s and even filed various false-advertising, class-action suits. The FDA has dragged its heels, which may have been why President Obama finally signed a bill in 2014 called The Sunscreen Innovation Act. We have listed some of the top-rated products by the United States–based Environmental Working Group (EWG) below that surfers may want to consider using.

At this point, the most comprehensive and precautionary-minded information is coming from the EWG. Each year, the EWG puts out an updated informative report (readily available online, just type in "Environmental Working Group Sunscreens") and over five hundred sunscreen products will appear for which they have given detailed ratings. We have listed some of the top-rated products below that surfers may want to consider using.

| Best Sunscreens for Surfers (adapted from the Environmental Working Group's 2018 Sunscreen Guide). | |
| --- | --- |
| Note: what each of the following have in common is that they are sunscreens which contain both zinc and titanium, and do not, in general, contain oxybenzone or vitamin A. Since most surf shops or drugstores will not have many of these brands, you probably will need to order online. Beware: most of the tried-and-true sunscreens we surfers have been buying for years in surf shops aren't so "true," and we canaries in the coal mine shouldn't even be trying them. | |
| All Terrain | 8 lotion and stick products, all zinc-based |
| Badger Sunscreens | 12 adult and kids' lotion and stick products, all zinc-based |
| California Baby | All products titanium-based |
| Coral Safe | Lotion, stick, and spray products, all titanium-based |
| Maui Natural Organics | Zinc and titanium products |
| Raw Elements | Lotions, sticks, and tins, zinc-based and titanium-based |
| Tropical Sands | Lotions and sticks, zinc-based and titanium-based |
| Zeb's Organics | Zinc lotions |

Because it will be on the midterm, you are all expected to know a few basic things about SPF (sun protection factor). SPF is a laboratory measurement of sunscreen protection. If, in the laboratory, your unprotected skin burns in one hour, an SPF 5 product would help you not burn until five hours; an SPF of 30, for thirty hours, etc. Know that any SPF rating beyond 30 is probably bogus outside of laboratory conditions, since sunscreen products won't be active or adhere to the skin for much longer than two hours, no matter how high the SPF. In open acknowledgment of the falsity of high SPF ratings, Australia won't even allow an SPF rating above 50! A while back, the FDA banned the term "Water Proof" for all sunscreen products, since they are never completely water proof. The present term is "Water Resistant," either forty or eighty minutes. And the more active you have been—sweating, smashing through lips, rubbing your face—the quicker you will lose protection. Under real-life conditions, we've found that the "velvety, clear" products never last eighty minutes, no matter how they are labeled, and that heavier, whiter zink products work best.

The bottom line is that surfers will do well to get SPF 30+, eighty-minute water-resistant sunscreens and reapply them at least every eighty minutes. Short of going in early to the beach (no one wants to do that), you would do well to bring a sunscreen product out with you. The thin stick types will slide under a wet suit sleeve or leg, or if you are in warm water and have no wet suit, aim to use trunks with a back pocket that snaps shut.

How much sunscreen to smear on? The majority of people put on too little sunscreen, probably by a factor of one-half. Figure one-fourth to one-third of a teaspoon for your face and two tablespoons (about one ounce or a jigger full) for your whole body if you're going to surf nude. Sunscreen is less likely to wash off and will work best if you put it on at least thirty minutes before you paddle out—and that kind of foresight is rare among surfers, who usually want to go to the beach to check it out before deciding if they'll even go out, but once they've decided to go out, they'll scramble and get out there fast. There has never in the history of surfing been a surfer who announced that he or she was delaying their paddle out to give their sunscreen a full thirty minutes to fully bond to the skin! The best strategy is to apply your sunscreen in the morning at home before heading out to look for surf. Plus, that may give you more incentive to go out if the surf looks marginal, if only not to waste your already-applied sunscreen!

Sun-protective clothing is by far the best sun protection, beginning with wet suits. De rigueur ocean sports clothing may carry a UPF rating (ultraviolet protection factor). UPF is roughly equivalent to the SPF rating for sunscreens, so aim for a UPF of 30 or higher, though higher UPF clothing gives far better protection from the sun than any high SPF sunscreen. By comparison, a regular T-shirt has a UPF of about 6. Caps, hats, and visors can help immensely in reducing sun exposure to the upper face and eyes. If the surf is small and you're not having to punch through many waves (i.e., point breaks), wearing a cap or hooded rash guard in the surf is a good idea—especially in the tropics. Various surf wear companies make hats or visors with strong straps that go around the neck and under the chin.

## SURF-SURVIVAL TIP

You will always underestimate how much sun protection you need.

# Know Your Skin Type

Far more people know their blood type than their skin type, probably because skin-type classification wasn't thought up until the mid-'70s by a Dr. Thomas Fitzpatrick, who sought to explain why darker-skinned people don't get much melanoma. He divided all of humanity into six skin types (see table), and in a glance you'll be able to see which type you are. He and others extrapolated upon his work and made recommendations as to rational approaches to sun protection. Then we surf docs adapted those recommendations to surfers.

| Skin Type | Tanning | Hair and Eye Color |
| --- | --- | --- |
| 1—Very light, freckly | Always burns easily | Red, blond, light brown hair |
| Celtic/Nordic descent | Doesn't tan | Blue/green/gray, light eyes |
| 2—Light skin | Easily burns | Light to darker hair |
| N. European | Tans minimally | Any eye color, but not dark |
| 3—Intermediate colored skin | Seldom burns | Brown hair |
| Middle-European | Tans gradually/ uniformly | Any eye color, rarely dark brown |
| 4—Darker, olive colored skin | Burns minimally | Dark to black hair |
| Mediterranean | Tans well | Any eye color, can be dark brown |
| 5—Dark, brown skin | Rarely burns Tans profusely | Black hair Brown or hazel eyes |
| 6—Very dark, "black" skin | Never burns Already deeply pigmented | Black hair Dark brown eyes |

## Skin Type 1 Surfers

You've got your work cut out for you. Yes, you can be a full-time surfer, but you have to be calculating if you want to avoid fully nuking your skin. For instance, skin type 1 surfers really shouldn't surf in the midday (oh, okay, except for the best day of the year) and should ardently seek to avoid surfing between 10:00 AM to 3:00 PM in the winter and 9:00 AM to 4:00 PM in the summer.

And then there are the things you should do even when not surfing, for instance, on days you're just going to school or work. Really, truly, even if you are young, you need to apply sunscreen *every day* to your face and head, with special attention to your nose, lower lip, tops of your ears, back of your neck, and exposed areas of scalp, as well as to the sun-exposed parts of your arms, wrists, and hands. Do this when you get up in the morning, ideally after showering. Use SPF 30 or higher products and be sure it protects both for UVA and UVB. Keep in mind that if you initiate this daily habit, it will let you stretch things a bit when it comes to water time.

When you go surfing, reapply sunscreen and be sure to use more sunscreen than you think you need. Take it out with you in the water and reapply it after each hour to your face. A Vaseline–based high-SPF chap/lipstick may be useful for your lips and nose, given that you can feel with your finger to know if any is still on you and reapply accordingly. Except at dawn and sunset, when the sun is all but gone, don't even think of surfing without a wet suit or some kind of body covering, such as a 30+ UPF rash guard. Wet suits are your friends; use legged and sleeved suits even in warmer water (you can get one to two millimeter suits). If the water is above eighty degrees, use a full-body, light-colored, thicker-fabric Lycra suit. Surf type or size permitting, wear a hat or visor in the water. If in the tropics, type 1s readily fry their eyes, so use sunglasses even when in the water or specially tinted contact lens. Don't linger in the sun before and after you go out.

## Skin Type 2 Surfers

Think of yourself as a slightly less vulnerable type 1. If your skin is already showing signs of being ravaged, then you really should put on a sunscreen lotion every morning, regardless of whether you're planning to surf. You should also try to avoid midday sessions, but if tides and swell call for it, you can feel reasonably safe surfing for about ninety minutes. Again, use at least an SPF 30 sunscreen, with both chemical and physical blocking agents. As with type 1s, the most vulnerable time may be when you get out of the water and your sunscreen is all but worn-out, but who can resist standing around for a few minutes chatting with your surf buddies? Danger, Will Robinson!

## Skin Type 3 Surfers

Feel free to stay out a lot longer in the midday but still use broad spectrum SPF 30 or higher, with an emphasis on UVA protection. Just remember to reapply sunscreen at least every two hours. You don't have a green card to just hang out on the beach—photodamaged skin is still a problem for type 3s.

## Skin Type 4 Surfers

Yes, you still need sunscreen, but you can use a lower SPF, keeping in mind that UVA can still make you look leathery before your time. However, midday sessions on the North Shore, no problem.

## Skin Type 5 Surfers

You can still get sunburned, so you'll want to use some kind of sunscreen for midday sessions, but the rest of the time you're probably okay. Three months in Indo, you're on it.

## Skin Type 6 Surfers

Born to be a surfer. Sunburn and skin cancers extremely rare, even without sunscreen, though the sun can prematurely age the skin. Overall, though, live and surf anywhere, anytime.

# 7

## Skin Problems of Surfers

Just as the outer skin of one's surfboard is easily dinged (and often needing repair), so, too, does our actual skin receive the brunt of physical damage from surfing. Scrapes, cuts, scars, sunburns, strange discolorations and growths, infections, irritations from surf trunks and wet suits, weird lumps—we surf docs always find a surfer's skin interesting to examine! In fact,

**rare would be the hard-core surfer who doesn't have at least one abnormal skin condition purely as a result of being a surfer.**

## Keratoses and Pre–Skin Cancers

 Keratoses are the general name for various skin changes that are slightly raised and more often initially felt by your finger rather than being seen. They can feel rough to touch, like fine-grit sandpaper. They commonly appear in fair-skinned people in sun-exposed areas, especially the face and the tops of the ears. Most often these are not actual skin cancers, but are pre–skin cancers—what are technically called actinic keratoses (actinic = sun-caused). It takes years of sun exposure to develop an actinic keratosis, and once present, only a small percentage, usually after many years, go on to develop into an actual skin cancer, most often of the squamous cell type. However low the risk of an actinic keratosis turning into a skin cancer, if you don't do something about them, they'll eventually make your skin look pretty ragged and considerably aged. Dermatologists usually can easily recognize actinic keratoses (no biopsy needed) and remove them with liquid nitrogen (said to have been "burned" off, though, really, they are frozen off). Know that with sun avoidance and rigorous daily use of sunscreen, actinic keratoses can slowly get better. Actinic keratoses can be made to shrink and then disappear by daily use of various prescription cream/gels, such as tretinoin/Retin A, which is a vitamin A derivative most often used to lessen wrinkles, or a skin preparation of the cancer chemotherapy drug fluorouracil.

There is a more common type of keratosis that isn't a pre–skin cancer, but once noticed by a surfer, invariably freaks them out, because it is often pigmented and may be growing fairly quickly, so they think they must have a malignant melanoma-type of cancer. These usually turn out to be what is called a seborrheic keratosis (seborrheic = oil-producing). They are painless, sometimes black or brownish, can feel rough and a bit greasy or oily, and are usually flat, as if they'd been stuck on, like an old piece of chewing gum. If picked at or peeled off, they may bleed and usually regrow. Again, a dermatologist can usually diagnose one without a biopsy and can freeze it off.

There is increasing evidence that a high intake of antioxidants—vitamins A, C, E, pomegranate, and especially green tea—helps protect against or reverse sun damage to the skin. Applying these antioxidants to the skin as creams or lotions may seem like a logical approach, but oftentimes a product's claims have little justification, their antioxidants being of such low concentration or of such poor quality that they are already oxidized and useless. More worrisome is that multiple recent studies show that adding vitamin A (retinyl palmitate) to sunscreens and skin products may actually *increase* the rate of skin cancer development. Increasing oral intake of antioxidant-containing foods and beverages is the safest and best strategy.

# Skin Cancers

At close to three million cases per year (and still rising fast) in the United States, skin cancer is by far the most common type of cancer. Fortunately, it is also, overall, the least-dangerous cancer type, particularly the nonmelanoma skin cancers. The three most common types of skin cancers (named for the type of skin cell they arise from) are as

## ABCDs of Malignant Melanoma

| Normal Mole | Melanoma | Sign | Characteristic |
|---|---|---|---|
| | | Asymmetry | when half of the mole does not match the other half |
| | | Border | when the border (edges) of the mole are ragged or irregular |
| | | Color | when the color of the mole varies throughout |
| | | Diameter | if the mole's diameter is larger than a pencil's eraser |

Photographs Used By Permission: National Cancer Institute

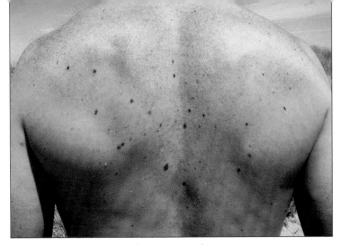

**Dysplastic nevi syndrome.**

follows: basal cell, squamous cell, and melanoma. Basal cell far outnumbers squamous cell cancers, and both far outnumber melanoma, which accounts for "only" about 180,000 cases per year in the United States. Even so, melanoma is the number one cancer in ages twenty-five to twenty-nine. Basal and squamous cell skin cancers tend to occur in older people, but melanomas can occur in all ages. There can be an inherited predisposition to develop melanoma, and individuals with large numbers of moles (dysplastic nevi syndrome) are more at risk. Melanoma is also, as is more widely known, an often deadly cancer, more prone to be truly malignant and spread throughout the body (metastasize).

While it has been heavily promoted that skin cancers, including melanomas, are caused by sun exposure, there is the strange fact that both basal cell skin cancer and melanoma often turn up in nonsun-exposed parts of the body. So, to be clear and evidence-based, one would only be able to say that squamous cell skin cancers are purely caused by the sun (but rarely they, too, turn up in nonsun-exposed areas of the body). While sun exposure is well established as a risk factor for melanoma—the highest rate of melanoma in the world is among those of English descent living in sunny Australia—there is a still emerging story in the field of melanoma-causation research pointing less at ultraviolet radiation as the biggest culprit and more at the interrelationship between genetics and epigenetics (gene-affecting exposures, such as hormone-disrupting chemicals). Though you can't control your genetic risks, recent long-term studies have shown that you can decrease your risk of melanoma, particularly the invasive type, as well as basal cell cancers, by about 50 percent with regular use of sunscreens.

# Skin Lesions

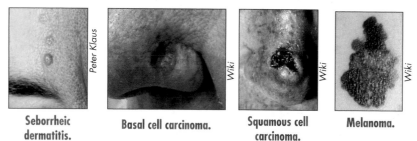

Seborrheic dermatitis. | Basal cell carcinoma. | Squamous cell carcinoma. | Melanoma.

Peter Klaus

Wiki

Wiki

Wiki

The rule of thumb with any skin growth is that if it has gotten bigger or worse after a month, it's time to go into your doctor and have it checked out. Your local primary care practitioner would be fine for that and more often will be able to accurately tell you if it is a skin cancer and can biopsy it themselves or send you on to a dermatologist. Treatment for nonmelanomas can be as simple as a simple removal by shaving or cutting it off with a scalpel, usually not requiring stitches (unless it is larger). With rare exceptions, anything resembling melanoma should not be shaved off (don't let your GP do that!), but needs more careful wider surgical removal.

## Case Study

Beginning at a young age, Kevvy diligently applied sunscreen to his face each time before he surfed, but somehow, in his carefree manner, he'd usually miss getting the sunscreen onto a small triangle of skin, just below his right eye. And that's exactly where the skin cancer appeared, at age forty-six, when, after getting a skeg into that part of his face, the plastic surgeon who sewed him up noticed a small basal cell cancer. Because removing skin cancers on that part of the face can be disfiguring, the minimum of normal tissue is removed if a stepwise technique called Mohs surgery is pursued, which is what Kevvy had done. Now Kevvy has a happy face, and generously and thoroughly slathers sunscreen on his face.

# Wet Suit–Related Skin Problems

## Underarm and Neck Rashes

Underarm and neck rashes are common among surfers, caused by repeated friction from an imperfectly fitting wet suit. It is such a common problem that a protective undergarment came into being: the rash guard, which is a thin, skin-tight Lycra or polypropylene under-shirt that can also be useful if worn without a wet suit to prevent sun-burn in the tropics. Although bodyboarders and kneeboarders and div-ers also wear wet suits, they seldom get such rashes, mainly because they aren't continuously windmilling their arms, but they do get rashes behind their knees from swim fin use. The main cause of wet suit rashes are from tight-fitting wet suits, especially if snug in the armpits and neck, and if the rubber has become stiff. The other common variable is being out of shape (more fat, less muscle) and having put on a few pounds, as is frequently the case for weekend warriors and Fiji–and Indo–bound surf vacationers. Don't assume the wet suit that fit you per-fectly the last time you wore it, say, six months ago, still will fit you well. Try it on before you head off, and if it feels too snug, realize that (1) put-ting a rash guard under it may be too constricting, (2) that it might be time for a different-sized wet suit, or to try a different brand. Using gobs of petroleum jelly (Vaseline) is the tried-and-true remedy for preventing a rash, or for keeping a rash from getting a whole lot worse. Most experi-enced surfers always travel with something that can help in that way, if not a tube of petroleum jelly, at least a tube of lip balm or vitamin A and D ointment. In a pinch, if there is any seaweed or algae floating nearby and it is slippery to touch (kelp is often covered with a sleek biological substance called surfactant), then rubbing that piece of kelp on a wet suit rash area can be a wonderful preventive remedy.

## Wet Suit Acne

Wet suit acne (acne mechanica) is also extremely common among surf-ers, and can look just like acne on the face, all red and angry and zitty, and this most often occurs in the oily skin in the upper and midcentral back. It appears to be from both the occlusive properties of the wet suit causing sweat retention and not letting the skin breathe, and the some-what rough inner surface of most wet suits rubbing across oily skin, with the resultant irritation and inflammation causing skin pores to plug. This can even happen when wearing wet suits in more tropical waters (for example, from short-sleeved, thigh-length "spring suits," worn in Hawaii year-round). To prevent wet suit acne, keep your wet suit clean, and try not to have it on when not in the water. For instance, leave your wet suit down to your waist when walking to and from the surf, and afterward don't stand around gabbing with your friends with your wet suit zipped up. If particularly red and zitty, take care to use soap and scrub the area when showering, and even consider daily use of benzoyl peroxide (5 percent should be enough), as used for facial acne.

Beware, though, of benzoyl peroxide on the body bleaching color from fabrics and clothes.

## Wet Suit Dermatitis

Wet suit dermatitis (contact dermatitis) is less obvious than wet suit acne, without all the redness and flare, but instead there will be a sense of thickened skin with subtle, itchy bumps, occurring more often on the wrists, underside of your lower arms, and over the shoulders. There won't be such a temporal relationship with wet suit dermatitis—its onset and persistence may not be in direct relationship to your having just used your wet suit. Wet suit dermatitis can be both from what is called an irritant contact dermatitis (being in contact with the abrasive wet suit material or some noxious physical agent or scum caught up in it), or less commonly from what is called an allergic contact dermatitis (having an actual allergy to the wet suit material, most often the thiourea chemicals used in rubber manufacturing). The best test for whether it is an actual chemical allergy is to firmly tape a small square of the wet suit material onto a sensitive skin area, like the inside of your forearm, and see if leaving it on at least overnight makes the skin under it break out. In general, wet suit dermatitis is best approached preventatively. For many surfers, it is simply a matter of carefully rinsing or actually washing their wet suits after each use, particularly if surfing was done during a red tide (phytoplankton blooms) or in polluted water. Wet suits do fine with gentle detergents in a washing machine set on "Delicate." If itching is a problem, over-the-counter hydrocortisone 1 percent or diphenhydramine (Benadryl) 1–2 percent cream, gel, or spray should take care of it. Note: occasionally someone can be allergic to Benadryl applied to the skin.

## Water and Sun Problems

## Heat Rash

Heat rash (also called prickly rash and miliaria rubra), while not unique to surfing, is frequent in hot climates. It's not a sun rash and in fact occurs most often under clothing or a wet suit, so it can be confused with a wet suit rash. Heat rash is a scattering of tiny reddish spots, sometimes bumpy, sometimes tiny blisters, and is experienced most often as a prickliness rather than pain or itching. Getting into cool air or a cool water environment will relieve it within an hour, as can an over-the-counter hydrocortisone 1 percent cream or gel.

## Sun Rash

Sun rash (also called solar urticaria) is quite different from heat rash, if only that it itches intensely, occurs within minutes of sun exposure (and ends within an hour of being out of the sun), occurs on sun-exposed skin and looks altogether different, with actual hives, which are rounded, freaky-looking raised skin spots, that can be red or white, quite small or quite large, and may lead to more generalized problems such as wheezing and dizziness. Oral antihistamines can help (such as diphenhydramine/Benadryl).

## Water Itch

Water itch (aquagenic pruritus) is an uncommon condition in the general population but, for some reason, more common in surfers, probably related to how much time surfers spend in water of varying temperatures. It is caused by exposure to either warm or cold water, with intense itching and a prickly skin discomfort without any visible skin changes that can last up to two hours then disappear, making you wonder, "What the hell was that?!" A red pepper cream (capsaicin) can help, as can a paste of baking soda. Rarely, water itch can lead to hives, called aquagenic urticaria (use oral antihistamines to treat).

## Cold Water Hives

Cold water hives (cold urticaria) is also generally uncommon, but, again, surfers turn up with it fairly often, probably due to the extremes of water temperature to which they subject themselves. Often it is when going from quite cold to quite warm water. It can happen while in the water, soon after leaving, or upon rewarming (jumping into a hot shower). There can be strange color changes in the skin (reddish, blue, purplish), swelling, and always itching, sometimes with actual hives. Again, there can be a whole-body reaction, with trouble breathing, dizziness, even unconsciousness! Sometimes there is a family history for it, but most often it just starts happening sometime between eighteen to twenty-five years of age, and tends to lessen and then stop happening over a handful of years. It is largely a histamine reaction, so antihistamines (even over-the-counter ones, such as chlorpheniramine, or diphenhydramine/Benadryl) tend to prevent it. There is a continuum of severity, with many surfers getting some degree of itching in their hands on cold-water exposure or on rewarming, but very few surfers getting full-blown cold urticaria. The crudest way to determine if you have it is to hold an ice cube to your skin for about five minutes and look for a local reaction such as welts or hives. If that is positive and you are wondering if it is safe to surf, stick a thermometer in a sink filled with water and get it to about the temperature of the water you surf in, and see if that, too, triggers the reaction. If so, then try taking oral antihistamines to see if you can block the reaction at that same (or lower) immersion reaction. If so, you may want to preventatively take antihistamines before going surfing in cold water. If you have had a whole-body reaction, see an allergist.

## White Fingers and Toes (Raynaud's Phenomenon)

White fingers and toes (Raynaud's phenomenon) are quite common in surfers, and can be spooky because single or multiple fingers or toes can suddenly become bone white, as if there isn't a drop of blood in them. This is due to local vasoconstriction, a selective shutting down of the blood vessels, and is most often caused by exposure to cold, and sometimes by an extreme change in water or air temperature, most often when going from very cold to very hot water (as in going into a hot shower after winter cold-water/cold-air surfing). There will be numbness and sometimes pain, but not usually itching; there will not be permanent damage. If it occurs, after a few minutes of keeping the digits immersed in warm (not too hot) water, they will suddenly pink up and come back to normal. Or, if you don't have warm water, just get your whole body warmer with heavier clothes, and drink a hot beverage. Tell a doctor about this and use the word "Raynaud's" and they will suspect you of having an underlying autoimmune disease, but that will almost never be the case.

## Surfer's Lip

Surfer's lip is a condition of the lower lip usually triggered by intense overexposure to the sun (a sunburn reaction), but with exaggerated swelling and discomfort, and not uncommonly a subsequent breakout of herpes labialis (from a herpes virus that lies in wait in the nerves of the lip). The way you'll know it is a herpes infection is if it crops up in exactly the same place over and over again. And in case you were wondering (but were too scared to ask), no, this is not (usually) the sexually transmitted type of herpes. Applying acyclovir/Zovirax cream (a prescription drug in most countries) every four hours can help, especially at the first sign of the herpes outbreak, but sometimes five times a day oral acyclovir or the more expensive but only twice a day valacyclovir is needed (again, by prescription). The best strategy is to avoid sunburning your lip and, if you are a person prone to this problem, plastering zinc oxide cream on your lip (and bringing some out in the water to reapply).

## *Staph* and Other Skin Infections

For varying reasons, surfers, especially those frequenting or living in the tropics, suffer from an inordinate number of skin infections, such as cellulitis (red, hot, spreading infections of the skin, commonly in the ankles) and abscesses (pockets of pus under the skin). These infections can occur while in the tropics, usually from a coral or skin scrape that wasn't thoroughly cleaned, or upon returning home. Sitting for hours in a plane with reef-ravaged feet is a perfect storm for developing a raging infection. Plus, there can be subtle differences in the types of *Staphylococcus* bacteria from place to place in the world, some to which we have little to no resistance (probably from overuse of antibiotics), and those *Staph* can displace the *Staph* that normally live on our skin and start causing recurrent cellulitis or abscesses. As always, the best possible approach is preventative, with frequent inspection, rigorous cleansing and care of any cuts or scrapes. If a hand or foot starts feeling or looking infected (redness, swelling, heat, discomfort), elevate that body part above the level of your heart for as much of the time as possible (to improve drainage) and generously use warm compresses, at least four times per day. Over-the-counter antibiotic ointments can sometimes be quite helpful, such as Bacitracin or Polysporin, and if those aren't working, try a Staph–specific prescription ointment called mupirocin/Bactroban (though increasingly, even that may not work). Sometimes an oral antibiotic like cefalexin/Keflex will be needed. If red streaks up the arm or leg have appeared, which means the infection is moving up through your lymphatic vessels, that may even call for intravenous antibiotics! If Staph infections keep recurring or just won't heal, there may be some foreign material in there (e.g., a splinter of coral or wood). Many surfers swear by use of oral homeopathic arnica (a "30c" dose, four tablets under the tongue up to four times per day) for traumatized tissues, particularly if foreign objects may be embedded under the skin; arnica is thought to help the body expel such objects and to better recover from blunt trauma.

## Trauma-Related Skin Conditions

### Sea Ulcers

Sea ulcers are seen almost exclusively among hard-core oceangoers (not weekenders), especially devoted surfers, fisherman, and sailors—those with prolonged daily exposure to saltwater. Most common in warm climates, they begin innocently enough as small scratches or cuts (often from rocks) on the hands, legs, or feet that don't get the cleaning and early attention they deserve. So, instead of healing up like most cuts will,

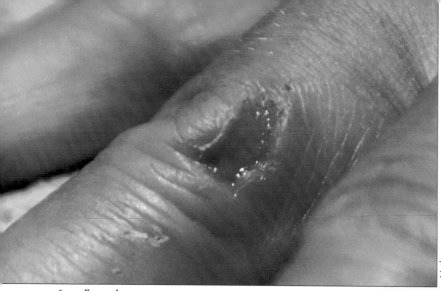

*Nathanson*

**A small sea ulcer.**

they actually get bigger, more painful, and deeper over time, stubbornly refusing to heal. The problem is that each surf session is interfering with the normal scabbing process, particularly if the wound is repeatedly rubbed or chafed by your board, wet suit, or paddling motions. You may be able to avoid having to stay out of the water for the week or so needed to let healing take hold if you pay special attention to (1) freshwater rinse and clean the sea ulcer after each ocean immersion, getting out any sand particles or debris, (2) dry the wound with a clean towel and twice daily dab it with an antibiotic ointment (Bacitracin, or Bactroban), and then cover it with loose gauze and tape so it can breathe, trying to leave it as uncovered as possible when sleeping, and (3) before each surf session, apply a waterproof dressing (such as Opsite or Tegaderm) to keep the ocean water out, and put duct tape over it all to hold things down better and to provide protection from the ulcer area being bashed while you surf. If it is not healing with these extra steps, it may be that a splinter or sliver of ocean material is still stuck deep in the ulcer, so you may need to visit a surgeon. Or it may be that you have an underlying condition associated with nonhealing skin ulcers, such as diabetes.

## Talon Noire

Talon noire is a lovely name for a pseudo-condition quite common in surfers and other athletes who pound their feet on hard surfaces (such as the deck of a surfboard), causing a small hemorrhage under a callused area of the foot, especially the heel, which can result in a dark-pigmented area within the callus that you or a doctor may think is a melanoma. It very likely isn't. Stick a needle into it and a drop or two of black blood may come out, or scrape down to it through the callous with the edge of a razor blade and you may find it is just a blackened callus.

## Wax Folliculitis

Wet suit-less, warm-water surfers who repeatedly rub their skin on the waxed portions of their surfboards, for instance, on the lower part of their rib cage when paddling or their inner thigh surfaces when sitting on their boards, quite often get plugged, irritated hair follicles. A rash guard can protect your chest area, and not applying your wax so far to the edge of the board can help with the legs. Or you can give up on wax altogether, and just use traction materials on your deck.

## Surfer's Knots or Knobbies

Surfer's knots or knobbies are also surprisingly common; famously sung about by the Beach Boys, these are the bumps that form on a surfer's feet or knees from knee-paddling a long board without the padding afforded by a wet suit or booties. They can also occur just below the breasts, on the edge of one or both sides of the rib cage, and can be soft and look like small boobs. Also, surfers can get them just under their chin, from riding boards too thin or short and needing to push down on the front of their board with their chins in order to catch a wave. They shouldn't hurt, even if you press on them. They are not zits or an infection, just an adaptive response of your body by adding a fat/fibrous pad under your skin to keep you from bashing the underlying bone. If you add some padding (wet suit or booties, or add some padding to the deck of your surfboard), you can get these lumps to slowly shrink and go away. No matter where such chronic friction and pressure lumps or bumps occur on surfers, if you make the mistake of going to a doctor or surgeon who knows nothing about surfing, they will tell you it may well be cancer and that it should be surgically removed. Beware—you may want to get a second opinion, ideally from a surf doc!

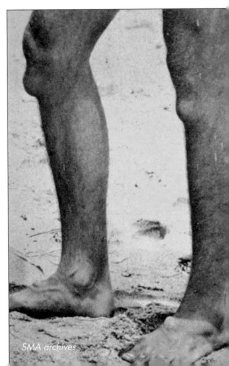

**"Oh my! What large knots you have."**

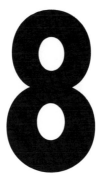

# 8

## Surfer's Ear, Nasal, and Sinus Problems

For every sport, there are unique and repeated traumas of a particular weak link body part: the elbow in tennis, knees in skiing, hands in rock climbing. Surprisingly, in surfing, it is the ears. Huh? Yep, the bane of surfers—affecting an absurdly high

percentage of us, close to 100 percent if you surf long enough—
is a condition called surfer's ear. (Note: this is not the same as
swimmer's ear—we'll get to that later.)

## SURFER'S EAR

 Mention surfer's ear to a nonsurfer—most importantly, to a
nonsurfing physician—and watch their face go blank: they
almost certainly won't know what you are talking about,
even though "surfer's ear" is an actual medical term. Surfer's
ear is just not covered in most medical schools, so unless a doctor lives
on a surfed coastline, they likely will have never seen a case of it. Out of
self-protection, it is incumbent upon all surfers to know as much as they
can about surfer's ear, since they will almost certainly be afflicted by it.

Surfer's ear is a bizarre bone-growth condition of the outer ear
canals. Although it may affect other water sportsmen, such as swimmers, divers, kayakers, and sailors (in fresh- and saltwater), it is most
common among surfers, particularly in those who have surfed cold-water
places for many years. The more precise medical term for surfer's ear is
"exostoses," but calling it surfer's ear is more fun, if only to get a rise.

You can't see surfer's ear by looking at someone who has it—from
the outside, there is nothing wrong with their ear. When a doctor looks
into a person's ear with an otoscope or speculum, they are peering down
an inch-long, slightly S-curved canal to the eardrum, the drumheadlike

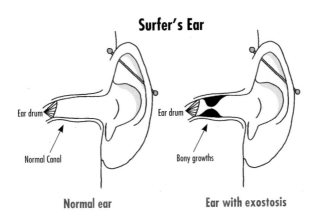

**Surfer's Ear**

Ear drum     Ear drum

Normal Canal     Bony growths

**Normal ear**      **Ear with exostosis**

membrane that completely closes off the inner parts of the ear from the outside. In surfers, though, it can be hard to even see the eardrum, because at different points along the canal can be one, two, or commonly, three rounded skin-covered bony bumps growing in from the bottom, sides, and top of the canal. Not too many years ago, and even today, unknowing physicians have thought they were looking at cancerous growths! To be fair, surfer's ear can look like cancerous growths.

## Case Study: The Dixon Family (As Told by Mother Sarah)

"I took my children in for their annual checkups, but this time we had a new pediatrician—I think he was from back East. He had a grim and puzzled look on his face after he finished examining the ears of my eight-year-old daughter. But he didn't say anything until he had checked the ears of my eleven-year-old son. Now he looked real worried. Then, as if he'd suddenly thought of something, he asked to also examine my ears. He looked oddly contented when he'd finished. 'Just as I thought,' he said reassuringly, 'there appears to be some kind of a genetic ear problem in your family—you each have peculiar little bumps in your ear canals.' He had neglected to obtain the most pertinent part of our family history: we all surf!"

For half of surfers with exostoses, the case is only mild—defined as less than one-third closure. Then there are a quarter who have moderate surfer's ear, with between one-third and two-thirds closure. And about one-quarter of surfers have severe surfer's ear, in which the bumps have grown so large that they block off over two-thirds of the canal. Mild and moderate surfer's ear doesn't cause much in the way of problems, but

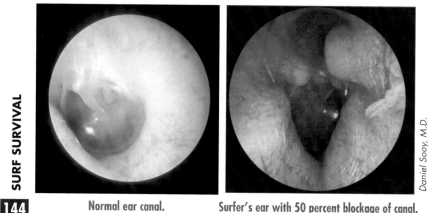

Daniel Sooy, M.D.

Normal ear canal.          Surfer's ear with 50 percent blockage of canal.

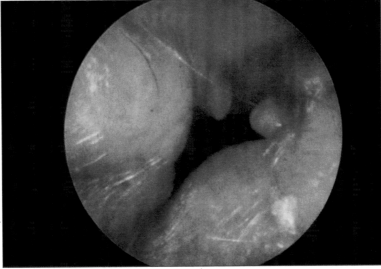

**Surfer's ear with 75 percent blockage of canal.**

severe surfer's ear is full of troubles. That amount of closure leaves only a tiny opening for air and sounds to reach the eardrum, and worse, it is harder for water, sand, and earwax to slide out of the ear canal, leading to a chronically wet mass of debris trapped amid the growths (and sometimes pushing up against the eardrum)—all contributing to a vicious cycle that even further blocks the ear canal.

Surfer's ear itself causes few symptoms: the bumps produce no pain, no bleeding, no discharge, and rarely do they fully close the canal and block hearing. But if debris builds up, and the canal never has a chance to dry out from session to session or shower to shower, then you can develop what is called swimmer's ear or, more precisely, external otitis or otitis externa (same thing).

## SWIMMER'S EAR

Swimmer's ear is caused by inflammation and possibly infection of the external ear canal. The symptoms include the following: itching, pressure, pain, discharge, pus, maybe a little bleeding, ringing in the ear (tinnitus), and even trouble hearing. If you pull upward on the top of your ear and it causes pain, you are likely to have swimmer's ear.

Swimmer's ear is more common among those with surfer's ear because those bony bumps in the ear prevent sloughed off earwax and other debris from naturally falling out of the ear canal, and it takes a long time to dry after being in the water. In other words, it is a set up for inflammation and swelling, and frank infection. Once there are symptoms, resist the temptation to stick something in to try to itch or remove gunk. Q-tips/cotton buds, matchsticks, keys, and bobby pins being the most common offenders, you may get some debris out, but at the same time, you'll be pushing some farther in, making things worse. And if you aren't careful, you'll scratch open the skin covering the surfer's ear bumps (the skin is stretched extremely thin over the knobs and has no fat under it—just bone), and that will be a setup for an even deeper-seated infection. Bring on the antibiotics!

## SURFER'S EAR SURVIVAL TIP No. 1:

**Never try to clean or scratch an itch in your ear canals with pointy objects.**

# Medical Treatment of Swimmer's Ear

Broad-spectrum antibiotic ear drops are the most immediate treatment. In most countries, that requires a prescription. The usual ingredients in prescription ear drops are glycerol or glycol (the thick, slippery fluid), an antibiotic, and some steroid. Of the antibiotic ingredients, polymyxin or ciprofloxacin is preferred over neomycin, because a small percentage of people are allergic to neomycin. The steroid is usually hydrocortisone, of varying strengths (if bad swelling/ear closure, go for the higher steroid concentration). Sometimes an antifungal is thrown in, but that isn't necessary. And sometimes there is some anesthetic, such as benzocaine or lidocaine, which can ease pain quickly. Antibiotic eardrops come as a solution or a suspension, of which the suspension is preferred, because it has a pH more favorable to an irritated ear canal (and to the delicate middle ear, if you have a hole in your eardrum). Note: if the infection has spread outside the ear canal, oral antibiotics may be necessary. Most surfers with more than mild ear closure from surfer's ear keep a stash of antibiotic drops nearby and won't leave home without it. Primary care doctors are usually quite willing to prescribe a stash of ear drops to their surfing patients. Usually you put in about four drops, three to four times per day, for as little as one to three days (but may be needed for longer). Make sure you are lying on your side when you do it, with your bad ear up—and once you've put the drops in, try to stay in that position for about ten minutes (good time to read a surf magazine). This will let the drops seep into your ear canal. Undoubtedly, one of the main reason ear drops work is that the glycerol or glycol softens up the debris, allowing the body to more easily discharge it. Keeping that in mind, realize that painful ear canals are more likely to be impacted (stuffed) than infected. So, following the ear-flushing methods described further on in this chapter may be all you need. Ear candles are a more naturopathic treatment for otitis externa: long hollow cones lit on the noninserted end, the idea being that heat will draw the infection out. Some surfers, mostly in or from Oregon, swear by them, but ear candles have little published support, and can not be recommended. Some surfers, mostly from the Big Island, report good success with tea tree oil eardrops.

A number of recent studies of surfer's ears have finally increased our understanding of this peculiar malady. Here is a summary of what is known:

## Surfer's Ear/Exostoses Index

- Coastal Chilean mummy skulls with exostoses: 30 percent
- Highland Chilean mummy skulls with exostoses: 0 percent
- Arctic hooded seals at birth with exostoses: 100 percent
- Surfers at birth with exostoses: zero
- Started surfing before age ten, years until operation: twice as long as if started after ten
- Youngest surfer needing a surfer's ear operation: seventeen
- Years surfing on average before first exostoses: five years
- North and South New Zealand surfing for more than ten years: 90 percent with exostoses
- North Island (warmer water): less-severe exostoses
- Reddened (irritated) ear canal from fifteen seconds of 104-degree water: one minute
- If 60-degree water: forty-five minutes of reddening
- If 60-degree water and also have exostoses: eighty minutes of reddening
- Regularly surf in water less than 60 degrees: 2.6 times more likely to have severe exostoses
- Exostoses on prevailing coastal wind side of head: twice as likely to be severe
- Osteomas (a nonskin-covered, single bony knob) in surfer's ears: 20 percent
- Male to female Australian surfers with exostoses: 78 percent versus 69 percent
- First surgical treatment for exostoses: 1763 (the patient died!)

- First use of chisels for removing exostoses: 1845
- First use of a dental drill for exostoses: 1873 (no anesthesia)
- First use of leeches to heal a broken eardrum after exostoses surgery: 1877
- Operating microscope, power drills, burrs, curettes: after 1969
- Use of posterior flap-ear approach (cut open ear from behind): 90+ percent (to this day)
- Average time to get back into the water with flap ear and drills: eight weeks
- Use of one-millimeter chisels for transcanal approach (no flap): 1999
- Average time to get back into the water after transcanal approach: three and a half weeks
- Painless Partridge's ears operated on: five times each side
- Use of earplugs to prevent exostoses or recurrence: recommended by all
- Evidence for earplugs preventing exostoses or recurrence: minimal
- Also using wet suit hood to warm ears and prevent exostoses: makes sense
- Doc Scott's idea of keeping ears warm 24/7 to reverse exostoses: well, maybe . . .
- Sight of Doc Scott in a Fijian village wearing wool earmuffs: priceless

## SURFER'S EAR SURVIVAL TIP No. 2:

**If you are a hard-core cold-water surfer and have been at it for at least five years and particularly if you already are having ear problems, find and go to an ear, nose, and throat doctor (ask around for which ENT other surfers go to) to get some idea of how severe your exostoses are and for guidance in caring for the problem.**

## Prevention

The obvious goal is to try to prevent the development of exostoses, but short of never taking up surfing or only surfing in the warmest of water and getting out of the water if it gets windy, if you become a lifelong surfer, you are going to get some degree of exostoses. Despite there being no published studies on preventing exostoses by wearing earplugs and/or using a wet suit hood, that doesn't mean that it doesn't work—most every surf doc and ENT professionals recommend it. And for surfers who take those precautions, they truly do seem to stave off worsening of their exostoses and the need for an operation. The most affordable earplugs made specifically for surfing are called Doc's Proplugs. They are silicon and have a patented pinhole opening feature that lets some sound get in, but not water. Doc's Proplugs are in most every surf shop worldwide. You can also have custom earplugs made, through an ear, nose, and throat doctor's office. Most every surfer who has an operation will use custom earplugs until they lose them and realize it's almost as good—and far cheaper—to buy ear putty (also in many surf shops), which can be similarly fashioned to fit their ears. The biggest problem with all earplugs except Doc Scott's is that they tend to push too far into the canal, which then pushes wax and debris still farther in (stethoscopes and some cell phone earbuds can cause the same problem). And for the cheapo putty and compressible plastic plugs, pieces can break off and add to the logjam in your ear. Some surfers find they can't hear well enough in the water with earplugs in or that the plugs disturb their balance. However, these problems can be improved, and they may still be able to have significant protection by just wearing an earplug in their worse ear (usually the upwind side). Many surfers use alcohol eardrops after surfing, as a way of helping dry their ear canals, and this may help prevent swimmer's ear (but won't improve surfer's ear). Hydrogen peroxide drops are not a great idea after surfing—it will just remove earwax, and you actually don't want it all removed, since it helps control infections. Some surfers swear by use of a hair dryer to dry their ear canals after surfing and showering—these are usually the folks with severe exostoses, approaching 90 percent closure. Again, *never* try to dry your ear canals with Q-tips or a wisp of tissue—you'll just wreak havoc. Lastly, although the research hasn't gone so deeply as to look at genetic risk of surfer's ear, it seems clear that some people are genetically programmed to have more exuberant bone and tissue response to trauma. They are probably the ones who develop severe surfer's ear more rapidly and, even if they take every precaution after being operated on, have rapid regrowth.

## Aural Toilet

You gotta love ear doctors. Aural toilet is what they call it when they clean your ears out. Under direct magnification, they can use tiny suction, washing, and forceps devices to clear your ear canals. This is highly recommended for any surfer with severe exostoses who is plagued by recurrent infections and their ears getting plugged up. For some, it may need to be done every six months, but most could get by doing it once a year or less. It's particularly useful before long surf trips where there wouldn't be good ear medical care available. For some reason, cold-water surfers with bad surfer's ear fare poorly when traveling to ultrawarm water spots—perhaps the warmer water melts and solidifies their wax debris even more deeply, or it may have to do with the entirely different water bacteria leading to infections.

Self-aural toilet can usually be accomplished, however crudely, by one of the following two methods:

1. Place your ear directly in the path of a warm jet of shower water—you'll have to carefully cant and twist your head to the exact position that results in the most direct and loudest effect on the eardrum (but not causing discomfort). This will, at a minimum, melt and mobilize wax and debris, which may flop out right then, or within the next day or so. If it doesn't work outright, each night put a few drops of olive oil in your ear (while lying down, with your ear up—and stay in that position for five to ten minutes). This will help soften the wax debris so that the shower approach will help dislodge it.

2. Buy an ear bulb syringe (a fig-shaped plastic squirter often used for baby care), which most every drugstore sells. Use it to shoot into your ear a solution of 1:1 warm water and hydrogen peroxide. Make up a batch of about one cup and shoot it in three to five times. Again, you'll have to experiment with what angle to place the teat to your canal to hit the target. And again, you'll know you're hitting home if you hear and feel it on your eardrum. If it's painful, back off. If you do this over a plugged sink, you'll find that all kinds of waxy brown debris comes out. Using olive oil for two to three days before will also help make it come out easier.

Note that store-bought earwax-removal solutions are *not* recommended for those with surfer's ear. Yes, they can melt wax, but more often the exostoses causes the wax to flow farther down the canal and harden on the eardrum. Only use an earwax remover if right afterward you can use a bulb syringe or shower jet to wash the stuff out. And remember, those little wax-producing glands in your ear canal are producing that wax for a reason: it helps prevent infections. Only remove wax if it has built up excessively or is trapping water.

## If You Need an Operation

Oh, if it were only as simple as going to your local coastal ENT and having an operation. It turns out that each of these surgeons have their own special ways of doing the operation and are utterly convinced they have the best results. Very few are willing to go straight into the ear canal (the transcanal approach), saying they can't see well enough. Most want to cut the ear from behind (the posterior auricular approach) and flap the ear forward, more fully exposing the whole ear canal. At the end of the operation, they sew the ear back down again (which is your chance to ask for Spockian ears). Some want to place special protective devices in front of the eardrum. Some leave bone exposed. Some want to use skin grafts. Some want to use power drills. Some will go to great lengths to make you understand they could hurt your facial nerve, which runs inside nearby bone, within millimeters of the exostoses. Some will do both ears in one day; others won't. And on and on. They mostly all fail to realize that surfers mainly want to know one thing: "How long do I have to be out of the water after the operation?"

If it were strictly on the basis of published evidence, all surfers would have their operations done by Douglas Hetzler, MD, a Santa Cruz ENT doctor. He clearly threw down the gauntlet for other ENT surgeons with his 2007 paper, "Osteotome Technique for Removal of Symptomatic Ear Canal Exostoses," published in the ENT journal named *The Laryngoscope*. He reported on his use of one-millimeter-wide straight and curved chisels (osteotomes) by a direct, incremental trans-canal approach (straight down the ear canal, from the outside in, not using a posterior ear-flap approach). He analyzed his own consecutive series from 1999 to 2005, of operating on 221 cases of ear canal exostoses (in 140 patients, 96 percent of which were surfers; note: he often did both ears). His success and complication rates were as good or better than all other published work using other operative methods. But most importantly, in his series, healing was achieved on average at three and a half weeks (range of two to eight weeks)—meaning that's when you could go back in the water. That is a lot earlier than other papers describe (the few that even looked at that key variable), or what most ENT surgeons would tell you to hope for with their method (you'll hear things like, "Some of my surfers get back into the water in less than a month, but you should figure on six to eight weeks"). Hetzler more recently reports that between 1998 and December 2010, he operated on 878 ears in 512 patients, and that only 7 ears needed reoperation. It is likely that by now other ENT doctors are using similar techniques, so they presumably would be getting equally good results. Be sure to ask, though, before you sign up: Do you go from behind the ear, or down the canal? Do you use a drill or chisels? How long on average do your patients have to stay out of the water after the operation?

# Eardrum Injuries

It is really quite surprising how seldom surfer's rupture or break their eardrums, given how hard they may splat against the water in a wipeout or when trying to blast through a lip when paddling or pulling out, or even from sudden shifts in water pressure (barotrauma) while diving under a huge wave. There aren't any studies on eardrum injuries in surfers, but they appear to happen a lot more frequently in advanced rather than beginning surfers (i.e., those going faster and in bigger, heavier waves) and in those with more advanced surfer's ear. It may be that surfer's ear alters the recoil elasticity of the ear canal, allowing more force to directly impact the eardrum.

When you've even slightly injured your eardrum, you'll usually know it immediately: it will hurt. The eardrum is rich with nerve endings, so it hurts if it is only minimally buffeted by sudden shifts in air or water pressure or temperature. Besides pain, there can be a reflexive sudden flooding of thick mucus into the back of your throat. All such symptoms are more likely if your eardrum is already compromised, perhaps from a recent cold or viral infection or if the ear can't equalize pressure normally due to a blocked eustachian tube (see below). The symptoms of a fully blown-out eardrum may also include dizziness or vertigo and decreased hearing.

## Case Study: Greg Long and His Ear at Mavericks

Greg is one of the most talented Mavericks surfers, but Mavericks eventually takes its toll on everyone who surfs it. On a notably powerful and bigger day than usual, in 2009, Greg had made it through all the normally hard parts of the wave—the takeoff and first section—but then the usually makeable second section took him down, and down he stayed, for two waves! So Mavericks legend Jeff Clark powered over on his Jet Ski™ and found Greg on the surface but trying to swim back down like a floppy fish, thinking that down was "up." Jeff dragged him onto the ski and buzzed back to the safety of the channel, where it became evident Greg had probably broken his eardrum: he couldn't hear worth a damn out of that ear and was still having vertigo.

If you are having any such traumatic eardrum symptoms, paddle out of the lineup, sit up, and take stock. If you feel it was only a zinger, and the symptoms back off within a handful of minutes, well then, you're probably okay to stay out. To double-check that there isn't a rupture or perforation, try to click your ears, as you would to equalize pressure in an airplane (shift your lower jaw forward or blow against closed nostrils). If the injured ear won't click, that may mean there is more of a problem than you realize. Worse would be if, on blowing against a closed nose, you feel air being blown out your ear canal: that means you broke your eardrum! So if that is the case, or there is persistent pain or decreased hearing, then you should paddle in, trying to keep your head from being dunked. Most physicians you enlist to look into your ear will be able to tell if it is broken or if there is an obvious perforation (hole). If so, antibiotic drops may be prescribed (to prevent infection), your ear canal may be packed with gauze, and you'll likely be referred to an ENT doc or simply told to keep the ear dry for six to eight weeks, which means keeping it covered while showering and staying out of the water. Most surfers will try going out sooner than that, say, at about four weeks, and, yes, there have been several who then rebroke it. If you do try to shortcut things, surf preventively for the first couple weeks: no falls, no blasting through the lip, wear earplugs and, wear a hood (to dampen direct water or air pressure).

If a broken eardrum doesn't heal, which happens only rarely, there may need to be a tethering-down or eardrum-reconstruction type of operation, called a tympanoplasty (may only be a three- to four-week recovery time). Sometimes, if there is a small residual hole in the middle of the eardrum, a patch can be placed over the hole by an ENT (the favored patch among ENTers, believe it or not, is a piece of Zig-Zag home-rolling paper!).

The other important thing to take note of is that immediate surgical closure of a ruptured eardrum will almost certainly have you in the water sooner—as early as two weeks, versus waiting the usual six to eight weeks, depending on the degree and type of rupture.

## Plugged-Up Ears and Sinus Problems

These two problems tend to go together and are usually due to inflammation and irritation of the entire nose, sinus, throat, and eustachian tube system. Connections between all these parts of the head are through narrow, mostly mucous membrane–lined passages that may normally be only a few millimeters wide (especially in the eustachian tube, which goes from the back of the throat to the middle ear) but when inflamed and full of thick snot can plug up easily. Some surfers are luckier than others when it comes to how reactive they are to all the stuff in ocean water—bizillions of bacteria and viruses, algae, sand, dirt blown in from the shore, pollution, and chemicals. For those surfers who are more reactive, with a history of asthma, allergies, or hay fever, when they punch through a lip or wipeout and have seawater forced up into the sinus and ear passages, they are far more likely to get symptoms: a runny nose, heat and pressure and sometimes pain in the sinuses, feeling plugged up in the nose or ear(s), perhaps low energy, sometimes fever, and even pus coming from your nose. All surfers after a particularly long and good session will occasionally have the unique problem of, sometimes hours after surfing, bending forward and having a sudden large saltwater discharge from their nose. Surf docs listening over a patient with their stethoscope have been known to let loose mightily. It ain't pretty.

Preventing seawater being pushed up your nose is the obvious solution, which means not being so cavalier on junky days when the ocean seems particularly dirty. If there is an algae bloom (red tide), a lot of sewer drainage during or after rainstorms, or just a lot of scum on the sea surface, paddle and surf defensively as to your orifices. For instance, when duck-diving or punching through, consciously exhale through your nose (with mouth shut, obviously). Also, before going out, about fifteen to twenty minutes beforehand, try taking a 30 mg tablet of pseudoephedrine (over the counter as Sudafed—but you may need to ask the pharmacist for it, since it is a prime meth lab ingredient). If you know you are an allergic type, you might also beforehand take a 4 mg tab of the over-the-counter antihistamine, chlorpheneramine, and also give a squirt into each nostril with oxymetazoline hydrochloride (Afrin, also over the counter). Then when you get out of the water, don't stand around and gab, but go straight to a freshwater source and rinse your face, eyes, and nasal passages as best you can. Best is to snort some fresh- or saltwater into your nasal passages and then blow it out—but that can take some practice to not choke. You can also use a neti pot, which you can buy in health food stores and some drugstores, which lets you pour freshwater into your nose on one side and have it come out the other nostril, cleansing as it goes.

If your ear is so plugged that it can't equalize pressure (when you try to "click" your ears or try to blow air out of your nostrils when they are pinched shut), the tried-and-true home remedy is to take pseudoephedrine 30 mg and, then an hour or so later, follow up with oxymetazoline (Afrin) nasal spray, but *not* to inhale it or let it go so far in that you taste or feel it going down your throat. Then wait about five minutes and pinch your nostrils shut and blow out hard five times in a row—which has the effect of forcing the oxymetazoline up into your eustachian tubes. You may need to repeat this twice daily for up to four days before the ear opens. It rarely fails.

If you appear to have more than just inflammation of your sinus passages, you may have an actual infection—though this is not as common as most surfers might think, based on how miserable their inflamed sinuses feel. Before begging for antibiotics, you may find that hot compresses over the uncomfortable area helps a lot. Remember, you have sinuses above and below each eye, and up against each side of the nose all the way down to near the upper lip. If any of those areas are specifically tender, put heat on it as much as you want—the longer and more frequently the better. Even just to stand in a shower with hot water beating down on the area for a minute can help, but try for longer, up to five minutes (you may need to cover your upper mouth so you can breathe). Again, keep it up for several days if needed. Don't be surprised if things improve quickly. Acupuncture can often help with such throat/nasal passage rising heat conditions. So can osteopathic manipulation to help the sinuses drain. Finally, if nothing else is working, a broad-spectrum antibiotic can be quite effective. Each physician has their favorite for sinusitis, but for surfers, the best may be doxycycline, given the range of marine organisms that can get up there. If an initial course of antibiotics doesn't work, it may be useful to have a physician culture your discharge to see what might best kill your unique bugs. Surfers rarely have fungal sinus infections, so there usually isn't need for antifungal drugs. Traveling surfers with recurrent antibiotic-requiring sinusitis should carry the antibiotic that usually works best for them.

Enterprising surfers who may wish to examine and document their own and other's ear canals can now easily purchase optical devices that plug into their iPhones or laptops. The cheapest device is about $16, consisting of a pencil-thin flexible fiberoptic device that can be placed just inside your ear canal and which transmits what it is seeing to your computer. Probably safer and niftier is a $50 iPhone attachment that uses a doctor's ear speculum on the end of a digital camera. The images can be sent to a doctor for review, and, importantly, can be stored to document one's surfer's ear growths over time. Markus Emerich, MD, a German ENT and member of the Surfer's Medical Association, has done a pioneering field study of surfer's ears around the world with just such an iPhone device.

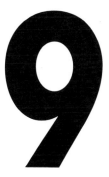

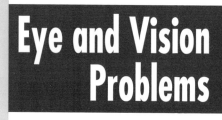

# Eye and Vision Problems

**S**urfing is hard on the eyes—not as a result of blunt trauma, but from the surfing environment: the wind, water, and sun. Surfing is often done in windy conditions—in fact we regale in offshore winds—but while straining to look for incoming waves or while taking off and riding, powerful blasts of wind often buffet the surfaces of our eyes, and those winds often carry sand

and soil particles from land causing further irritation. Although we usually close our eyes when wiping out or punching through a wave face, it is critical to keep our eyes wide open when taking off and riding. The glare from the sun also becomes problematic after even an hour or two of surfing, especially in early morning or late afternoon when the water's surface is smoother and more reflective.

## SURFER'S RED EYE (CONJUNCTIVITIS)

 Having chronic red eyes from surfing's environmental exposure to wind, sun, and sand only adds to the surfers' reputation as being druggies—our dripping noses after surfing only make that perception worse (oh well, their problem, not ours). Surfer's red eye is a result of physical irritation to the outer surfaces of our eyeballs. Usually the irritation affects the conjunctiva (the blood vessel–rich tissue covering the whites of our eyes and the inner eyelid linings) rather than the corneas (the clear tissue in the center of our eyes). With wind and water irritation comes swelling of the conjunctival tissues, which includes dilation of the eye's many blood vessels (ergo, red eye). Your eyes might begin to feel gritty and uncomfortable while out in the water, and the irritation can be enough to drive you back to shore to seek relief from the wind, spray, and sun. As soon as you can, rinse your eyes with cool freshwater and put on sunglasses or go into a dark or shady place. Use of lubricating eye drops (such as artificial tears) can help. Cucumber slices or used tea bags placed over the eyes can give some relief (and will amuse your friends). Eye drops that promise to "get the red out" aren't helpful symptom-wise, but they will make your eyes less red, since most contain adrenaline-like chemicals that cause the eye's surface blood vessels to constrict (but daily use will lead to tolerance and they won't work as well—best to only use occasionally). Use of sunglasses or goggles in the water will help prevent red eye, but contact lenses don't cover enough of the eyeball to make much difference. Thankfully, surfer's red eye won't usually affect vision.

# Corneal Sunburn

This is particularly common when surfing for several hours in the midday tropical sun when there is a lot of reflected sunlight. It is a plain-and-simple sunburn of the corneas, and as with sunburn of the skin, you may not realize it is happening until it is too late, sometimes hours after you've come in. There can be considerable pain, especially in bright light, as well as blurred vision from a swelling of the corneas. Rinsing your eyes with cool water won't help. Oral aspirin (650 mg) or ibuprofen (400–800 mg) every four hours can bring effective relief, as can avoiding light. The symptoms usually resolve in twenty-four to thirty-six hours. Wearing sunglasses in the water and/or use of tinted contact lens can prevent corneal sunburn. Repeated corneal sunburns take their toll on the cornea, causing subtle but progressive scarring resulting in vision that becomes progressively worse and may necessitate a corneal transplant. Lifelong surfers who are also lifelong sailors are high-risk. Surfers who have had corneal laser vision correction procedures (e.g., Lasik surgery) sometimes complain about having greater corneal sensitivity to the sun and wind.

# Pinguecula and Pterygium

Repeated microtrauma to the eyes leads to an adaptive response in the conjunctivae resulting in a small yellowish, fibrous triangular or sail-shaped area of tissue that begins to build up on the white of the eye, most often on the inner corners. This is a common condition in surfers, especially among tropical surfers, and is called a pinguecula (in

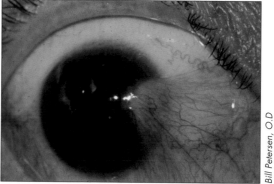

Bill Petersen, O.D

**Pterygium.**

the beginning stages) or a pterygium (larger and encroaching on the cornea). They are often in both eyes, but usually one will be a lot worse than the other. In any hard-core surfer, a good ophthalmologist should be able to find some degree of pinguecula in one or both eyes. Pinguecula are usually painless, but pterygia can become more easily irritated (e.g., just stepping outside into the wind or sun) and can be a chronic source of foreign body–like discomfort, particularly when using contact lenses. In addition, this discoloration and buildup can look really bizarre. Pinguecula require no treatment, but pterygium, if affecting vision, may need to be surgically scraped off by an eye surgeon (which can be expensive). Obviously, the best strategy is prevention (avoiding extreme wind, water, sun, and the use of sunglasses or goggles), but even after damage has been inflicted, careful management of causative factors can lead to improvement. The less often you have surfer's red eye, the less likely you are going to develop a progressive pinguecula or pterygium. As with surfer's red eye, eye drops don't help reverse the condition.

## Eye Cancer

Eye cancer is extremely rare and is only mentioned here because most surfers, on first noticing they have a pterygium, will think they have an eye cancer (see above condition). But it is worth knowing that, given our years of sun exposure, surfers are at risk for eye cancers—the most frequent being a precancerous condition on the outer eye surface called Bowen's disease, or an actual squamous cell cancer. Visit your doctor or ophthalmologist if you're concerned about any changes in your vision or the appearance of your eye. Prevention is to wear sunglasses and not sunburn your eyes!

## In-Water Vision Correction

Contact lens technology is now so advanced that most any surfer who needs vision correction can be successfully fit by an eye doctor with a pair of contact lenses that can be worn both on land and when surfing. Numerous studies have shown surfers only rarely lose a lens (just keep your eyes closed when underwater). Surfers who wear glasses on land but find contact lens irritating usually do fine just putting on contacts before going surfing, then taking them off when they get in. Sunglasses or goggles with custom prescription lenses can be used, but are easily lost while surfing, so a strong tether around the neck is needed as well as a frame material that floats. In small surf, if one doesn't have to punch through many waves, one's regular glasses can be used, but again, a tether is essential. For an uncorrectable, near-blind, or low-vision surfer, an innovative surfing "telescope" lens was developed in Sydney, Australia, which is worn like a diving mask.

## Sudden Vision Loss: Retinal Detachment

Surfers have a higher-than-normal incidence of retinal detachment (a lifting away of the "seeing" tissue in the back of the eye). It is most common in surfers who are nearsighted (have trouble seeing in the distance). When it does occur, it often follows a face-plant kind of wipeout—an acceleration-deceleration injury that causes the retina to pull away from the back of the eye, resulting in varying degrees of lost vision. It may manifest as a dark spot in your vision (a small area of detachment), or as if a windowshade just went down (complete detachment). Retinal detachments are painless, but this is serious stuff: go straight to shore and head to the emergency room. You will almost certainly need eye surgery, but know that the sooner you receive it, the better the chance of successfully reattaching the retina.

## Sunglasses and In-Water Eyewear

It makes sense that various sunglass companies developed along with the surfing culture, not because surfers are concerned about fashion, but rather that most surfers know to protect their eyes from the sun, at least on land. It is surprising, then, how few surfers wear eye protection while surfing (for protection against the sun's rays as well as blunt trauma from a fall). In the tropics, eye protection can be essential, particularly for those with light-colored eyes that are more susceptible to damage. With a strong string tethering the eyewear to the neck, loss can be minimized. Even surfers who don't need vision correction can use a nonprescription, darkly tinted contact lens, especially in the tropics. Most surfing helmets will compress and anchor the arms of glasses at the ears, so it takes a lot to lose them. Some surfing helmets even have a plastic visor that can be lowered to give protection from the sun. Custom-made hats or visors for surfing or even baseball caps with a tether can easily be worn while surfing. A strip of darkly tinted zinc oxide under each eye will help reduce reflected light. Every surfer needing vision correction, and all surfers by age forty, should get a thorough eye exam at least once every two years—the better you can see in the water, the better you'll see incoming waves, surfers, and other hazards.

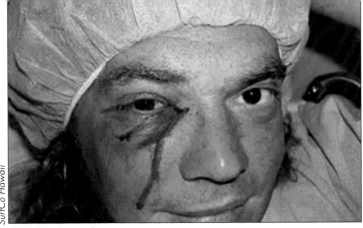

SurfCo Hawaii

**Too close for comfort.**

# Trauma to the Eye

While a rare occurrence, sometimes a surfer will be struck in the eye while surfing, most commonly by the tip, tail, or fins of their surfboard, but occasionally by something floating or airborne, like a kelp bud. A surfboard that is loose in the wind or on recoil from the leash is dangerous—keep your hands over your face and head whenever you come back up to the surface and until you know your board is not rocketing back at your face. Take care to order or purchase surfboards with blunted "dolphin" noses and tails. Round sharp fin tips with a file or sandpaper. Soft plastic fins are less dangerous but they don't perform as well in good surf. Fins with softer rubber on the tip and trailing edge are a good compromise. If you are struck in the eye, particularly if the eye has been penetrated or your vision is in any way impaired, get to shore immediately. Don't touch your eye but cover it in a way that doesn't apply any pressure, put on sunglasses, and immediately go to an emergency room. The emergency room doctor will decide whether an eye specialist needs to be called in. If an operative procedure is required, remind the doctor that fiberglass fragments are often hidden in the wound and need to be carefully investigated. A strong argument can be made for using sunglasses as protection against eye trauma while surfing in remote tropical areas—it can be a long way to get decent emergency eye care.

## Case Study

Aussies Steve and Derek and Hawaiian transplant Peter each lost an eye from being struck by their boards, but all three remained hard-core surfers—presumably more careful surfers, though. Having one eye is not a reason to avoid surfing.

**EYE AND VISION PROBLEMS**

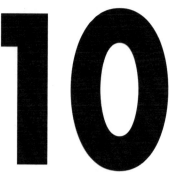

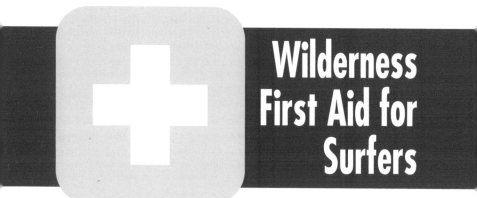

# Wilderness First Aid for Surfers

**E**ver since Bruce Brown's classic surf documentary *The Endless Summer* (1966), surfers have traveled to remote corners of the world in search of perfect empty waves. As surfing has become ever more popular, and local breaks ever more crowded, that search has

taken surfers farther and farther afield. From equatorial atolls in the

South Pacific to the icy waters of the poles, empty surf can still be found . . . if you search hard enough. Untapped surf breaks are often in remote, hard-to-reach places, accessible only by small plane, boat, truck, foot, or a combination of the above. While some of these uncrowded waves are located along desolate coastlines, others are near bustling population centers, but in developing countries with limited resources and little in the way of infrastructure. In either case, what could be termed definitive "modern" health care is often many hours or even days away, and local care, if available, may be substandard. As a result, surf travel often means that *you* will be ultimately responsible for your own medical care and may be called upon to treat fellow surf explorers. This book, and especially this chapter, was written to help you deal with medical emergencies should they arise during such travels, in places where calling 911 is not an option and health care is not readily available.

Emergency care in remote areas can pose challenges to physician-surfers, let alone those without medical training, because the resources and equipment available for diagnosis and treatment are generally quite limited. Whenever possible, we've tried to incorporate practical tricks of the trade that we've learned through personal experience and training to show you how to provide improvised care with items you are likely to have with you such as surfboards, plastic bags, and dental floss. Though we discuss how to manage common medical problems "in the field" (outside of a medical setting), we also try to make it clear when it is time to consider evacuation. The decision to evacuate from remote areas can be challenging because places that are hard to reach are often equally difficult to leave. Depending on weather, modes of transport, and other circumstances, the evacuation itself may pose a risk, not just to the victim but to others as well. We hope those kinds of decisions will be a little less difficult with this book in hand.

The treatment of other potential emergencies such as diarrhea and dehydration, marine stings, and selected infections can be found elsewhere in this book. Information about trip planning and first aid kits—both critical aspects in being prepared to effectively deal with a medical emergency—can be found in Chapters 14 and 16, respectively.

# Surf Rescue

### SURF-SURVIVAL STORY

On June 14, 1925, Duke Kahanamoku (the father of modern surfing and Olympic swimming champion) was on the beach in Corona Del Mar, California, when he saw that a yacht had capsized offshore in heavy surf. He immediately grabbed his surfboard and paddled out to the overturned yacht *Thelma*, where twenty-nine passengers were in the water clinging to the overturned hull amid pounding waves. Duke was able to save the lives of eight people, and other surfers rescued the remainder of the twelve survivors.

If you surf a lot, chances are pretty good that you'll be out on the water and encounter a surfer or swimmer in distress. Surfers can get knocked unconscious, lose their boards, or may simply be out in conditions that they can't handle. Swimmers frequently get caught in rip currents (80 percent of lifeguard rescues are due to rips) can be pulled out to sea and quickly tire out. The victim is often struggling and panicking, or worse yet, they may be facedown and not moving. Regardless of the scenario, if you are there, you will be called to action. Fortunately, as the Duke so aptly demonstrated, surfboards, particularly long boards, make excellent surf rescue tools. In the following sections, we describe tried-and-tested surf rescue techniques developed by lifeguards in Australia to show you how to bring surfer safely back to shore should the need arise.

## Rescue of the Conscious Victim

First and foremost, keep your own safety in mind.

Should you come across a swimmer (or surfer with lost board) in distress, approach cautiously, because in a panic they are prone to grab on and pull you underwater in a desperate attempt to keep themselves afloat. The safest tactic in this situation is to get off your board as you approach and extend it to them for use as a flotation device.

Allow the stricken swimmer to rest on your board and catch his or her breath. Offer calm reassurance—e.g., "You're going to be okay"—discuss a plan of action, and if conditions allow, help them to shore. If performing

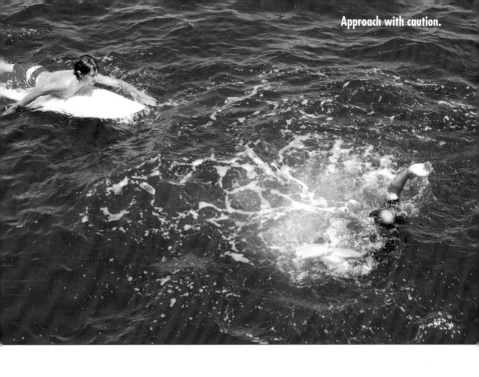

Approach with caution.

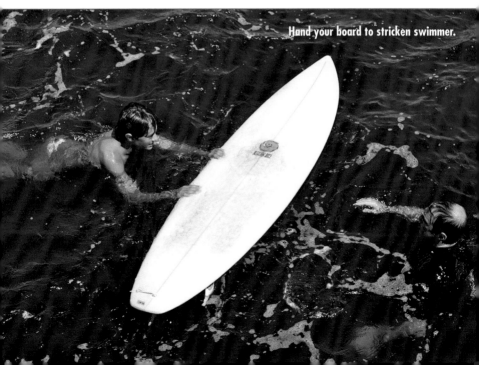

Hand your board to stricken swimmer.

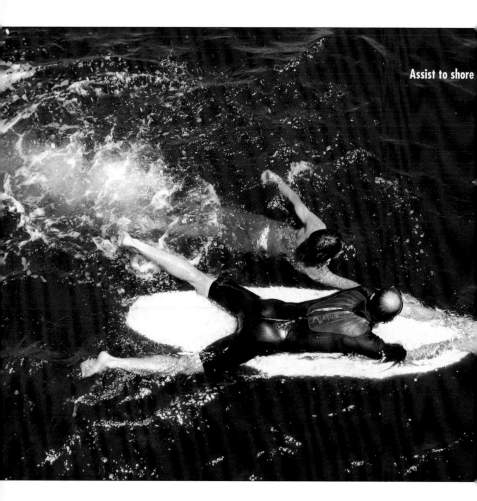

the rescue with a short board, you will need to swim them in as they lay atop your board, directing them to hold on tight in breaking waves. If you have a long board, have them splay their legs apart, get behind and on top of them with your chest between their legs (as if paddling for a tandem session), and paddle (see photo on page 170). If possible, put your leash onto their ankle so they do not get separated from your board and so you can locate them if they sink. Call for help and engage the help of other surfers whose assistance may be needed to get the victim through the shore break and on to land.

## Rescue of the Unconscious Victim

If you come upon an unconscious surfer or swimmer, there are a couple of techniques that can be used to get them onto a surfboard and back to land.

If it is clear that they are not breathing (no chest rise, no breath sounds), use their board as a rescue platform on which to give them five rescue breaths as soon as possible. Drowning victims are usually young and have healthy hearts which may still be beating despite respiratory failure. Therefore administering those first few mouth-to-mouth breaths in the water may be lifesaving. Chest compressions in the water are ineffective, and if there is no response to the first round of ventilations, and it looks like it may take more than two minutes before you can get the victim ashore, consider a second round of breaths. The best way to give rescue breaths is to position the board between yourself and the victim, perpendicular to the victim. Place the victim's head, face up on the board, and slide one arm under their armpit using your hand to gently lift their jaw. Use your other hand to pinch their nose.

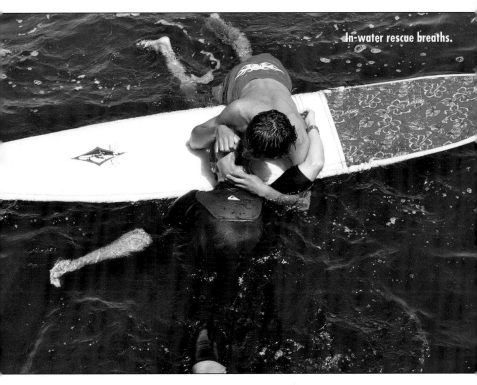

In-water rescue breaths.

Next, you need to get the victim onto a surfboard and back to land so you can initiate CPR. Flip their board fins up and place it perpendicular to their body, with the board between you and the victim. Reach across the upside-down board and grab both wrists, pulling the victim's head and arms onto the board.

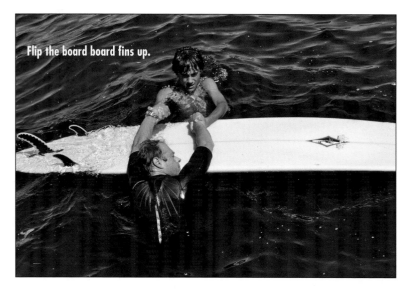

Flip the board board fins up.

Now here comes the tricky part. Lean across the inverted board and with your front hand, grab the far rail and, with your back hand, grab the victim's back wrist. Note the position of the rescuer's hands.

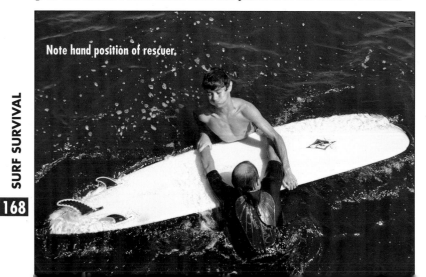

Note hand position of rescuer.

In one vigorous motion, pull the rail of the surfboard and the victim's wrist toward you as you lean backward. You will fall backward in the water as the board rolls over (fins down), and the victim's chest will lay across the board, with their arms and legs in the water.

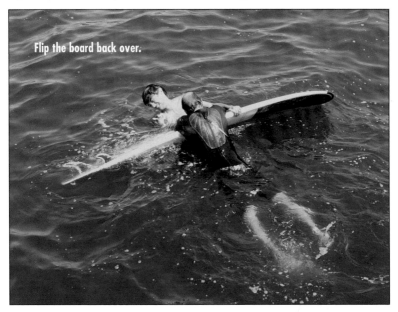

Flip the board back over.

The last step is to pivot them lengthwise on the board. If you and the victim are on short boards, you can place them on their board following the steps above, then put the front of your board on top of their board (and under their legs), and paddle in lying down on your own board.

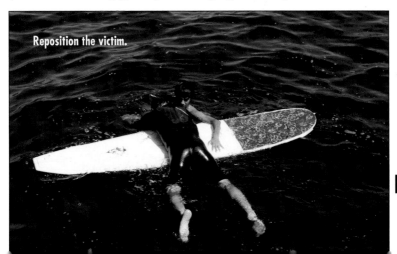

Reposition the victim.

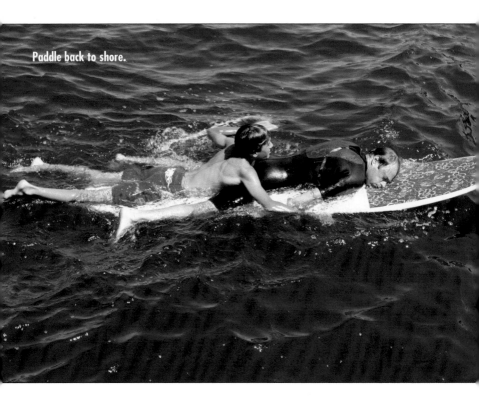

Paddle back to shore.

If rescuing the victim on a long board, get behind and on top of them with your chest between their legs. If you are alone, run the board and victim right onto the beach, then get behind them, put both of your arms under their armpits, and using one arm to support their chin, drag them up the beach. Immediately initiate CPR. If alone, proceed with CPR for two minutes, then call 911 if available. If you remember only two things about CPR for drowning, remember this: five rescue breaths in the water, followed by CPR on land: two breaths followed by thirty compressions in which you push hard and push fast.

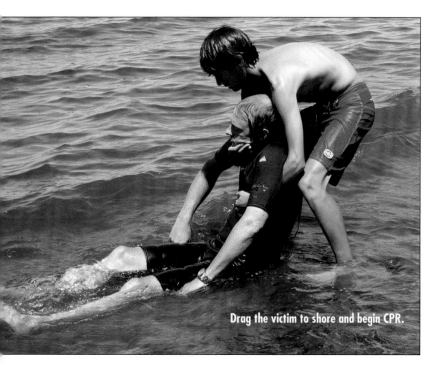
Drag the victim to shore and begin CPR.

Attempts at maintaining the victim's neck in a neutral position during rescue is nearly impossible and should not delay mouth-to-mouth resuscitation nor return to land. The focus needs to be on what is certain to kill the victim, namely drowning, versus the much less likely scenario that they also have a neck fracture. The overall incidence of spinal fractures in drowning victims is less than 1 in 1,000, though it is almost certainly higher among surfers. Use your judgment here; if the victim has an obvious cut to the top of the head, or was seen landing headfirst in shallow water, do your best to stabilize the neck.

When available, the best tool by far for surf rescue is a Jet Ski equipped with a rescue sled. When performing rescue of an unconscious swimmer/surfer on one of these, first hoist the victim as far onto the sled as possible by hooking your arm under his or her armpit and swinging them on board. Once you have driven out of the impact zone and away from danger, it may be possible to have a third person on the ski initiate chest compressions and recue breathing while you drive to shore. If you have a radio or cell phone, notify rescue personnel on land (if available) and arrange to meet them at a safe landing area that is accessible to ground transportation or helicopter.

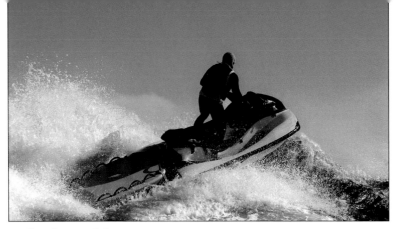

Jet Ski and rescue sled.

## Treatment for Near Drowning (Conscious Victim)

Once the person has been safely brought to shore, lay them down and roll them on their side if they vomit. Though you may be tempted to try to drain water out of the victim's lungs, such maneuvers are useless and potentially harmful. Surprisingly little water actually gets into the lungs of drowning victims, and most of it is quickly absorbed into the circulation. The stomach, on the other hand, is often full of swallowed water and attempts at draining water from the lungs often precipitates vomiting, which can lead to aspiration (inhalation) of vomited material.

Keep the person warm with dry clothing, a towel, or a board bag. Anyone who has blue lips and fingers, gurgling breath sounds, or vomits is likely to have inhaled seawater. People with any of the above symptoms should be evacuated to a medical facility where oxygen can be administered, oxygen levels can be monitored, and a chest X-ray can be obtained.

Despite initially appearing well, individuals who have inhaled even small amounts of water can deteriorate—up to twenty-four hours after the incident occurred. As a result, even those who look pretty well after a rescue should be closely monitored in a hospital setting for what has been termed "secondary drowning" and is due to injury of the delicate lining of the lungs and subsequent fluid buildup in the tiny air sacs called alveoli.

People whose only symptoms after a near-drowning episode are a cough that quickly resolves, should be okay, and generally should not require evacuation.

Phillipe Duhaime, a medical student at UCSD, was duck-diving his way out through solid eight-foot surf at Black's Beach in San Diego, California, when he encountered a man lying facedown in the water. Phillipe paddled over to the lifeless man, rolled him over, lifted his head out of the water onto his surfboard, called for help, and began administering rescue breaths. Off-duty lifeguard Dylan Jones was second to the scene and helped paddle the victim to shore. Once on land, Phil gave mouth-to-mouth resuscitation while physician-surfer Mark Bracker performed chest compressions. Within five minutes, one of the luckiest surfers alive, forty-nine-year-old goofy-footer Chris Ryan, came to life and started talking. He had been hit on the side of his head by his board after takeoff and knocked unconscious.

# Cardiopulmonary Resuscitation

Cardiopulmonary resuscitation (CPR) is a basic life-saving skill that should be acquired by all surfers. While we list the key elements involved in the adult CPR protocol below, this is no substitute for taking a hands-on basic life support course where you can practice the techniques of airway management, rescue breathing, and chest compressions under the supervision of a certified instructor. We highly recommend that you take such a course (offered by the American Red Cross, YMCA, and others) so, if the need arises, you will have already practiced these techniques on a mannequin and will be mentally and physically prepared to take immediate action.

*Adult CPR should proceed in the following sequence of assessments and actions:*

1.  **If the victim is in the water and needs to be rescued, above all else, ensure your own safety.** *Give five in-water rescue breaths if possible.* Use your surfboard as a rescue device. (See above.)

2.  Lay the victim faceup on the beach. *Clear the airway* of any seaweed or other obstructions. *Tilt the head back and gently lift up the chin* and look and listen for any breathing. (If there is a possible neck injury, such as a cut or scrape on the head or if the victim was last seen doing a header into shallow water, *do not* tilt the head back.)

3.  If the victim is not breathing effectively (not breathing at all, or only occasionally gasping), *pinch the nose and initiate mouth-to-mouth breathing. Give five rescue breaths.* If you find this too repulsive or are concerned about infections, you can do chest-compression-only CPR. White foam from the mouth is common.

WILDERNESS FIRST AID FOR SURFERS

173

4. If *vomiting occurs* (which it commonly does), *turn the victim's mouth to the side* and remove the vomit using a cloth or your finger. If there is concern for a neck fracture, turn the head, neck, and torso to one side as a unit (so there is no movement of the neck).

5. With two fingers, feel for the bottom on the chest plate (sternum). Place the heel of your other hand just above the two fingers. *Give chest compressions with the heel of your hand at a rate of* 100 *per minute* (to the beat of the old disco song "Stayin' Alive" — "Ha, ha, ha, ha, stayin' alive") *pushing down on the breastbone (sternum) about 2 inches. Give thirty chest compressions, then two breaths, and repeat.*

6. *After two minutes of CPR, call 911 for help* (if possible). The sooner a defibrillator and oxygen can be brought to the scene, the better.

Head tilt. Use this position to open the airway, listen for breath sounds, and perform rescue breathing.

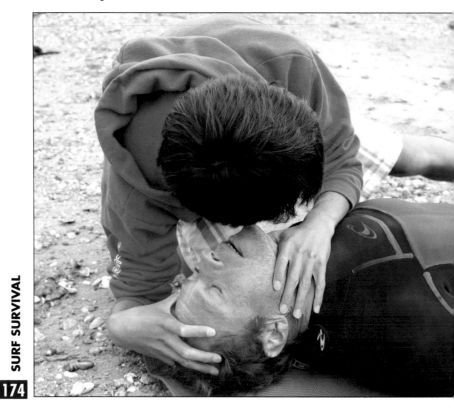

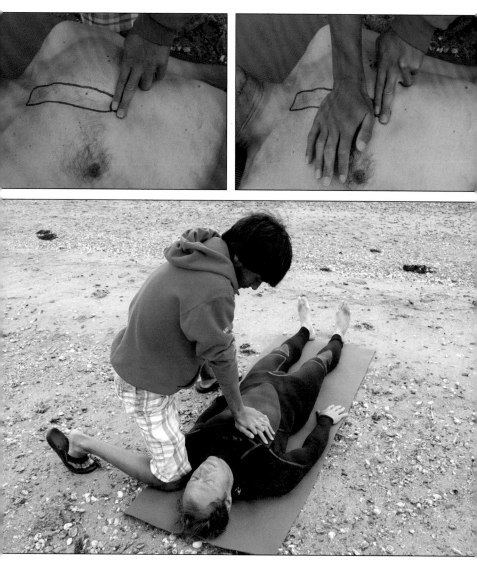

## Chest Compressions

Locate the bottom of the breastbone and place two fingers just above that point. Place the heel of your other hand above the two fingers. Lock your elbow and use your upper body to piston down the victim's chest wall 2 inches, at a rate of 100 compressions a minute.

# Hypothermia—the Cold, Hard Facts

It is easy to get hypothermic when you are surfing. Even warm ocean water is cooler than normal body temperature (98.6°F, 37°C), and heat is lost via conduction to water twenty-five times more quickly than it is to air. A significant amount of heat is also lost via evaporation from wet skin, rash guards, and wet suits, particularly on windy days. Usually heat loss is not a major issue because you simply head in to shore and warm up. Furthermore, as a warm-blooded mammal, there are a number of mechanisms by which your body maintains its normal temperature in cold environments. Shivering is one means by which extra heat is produced, and ramping up metabolism (up to fivefold) is another. Heat loss is also minimized in the cold by constriction of blood vessels in the skin (where most heat is lost) and diversion of blood flow to the body's central core organs, which are better insulated from the cold. However, at a certain point, one's ability to produce and conserve heat is overwhelmed by loss of heat to a cold environment, which, if allowed to continue unchecked, inevitably leads to hypothermia (body temperature below 95°F, 35°C). Hypothermia creates problems because all of your body's innumerable chemical reactions are set to perform optimally at around 98.6°F. With small drops in core temperature, down to about 94 degrees, your body attempts to compensate by increasing its rate of metabolism, shivering, increasing your heart rate, and increasing your respiratory rate. If your core temperature drops further, metabolism slows down, and the function of your vital organs—including heart, brain and muscle—gradually begins to decline. This results in a slow pulse, low blood pressure, impaired decision-making capacity, and weakness.

## Symptoms

Before actually becoming hypothermic, the first thing you notice is that you feel cold. This is a good thing. It is a warning sign, telling you to take action and seek warmth. Don't wait out there in the wind, rain, or snow for the perfect wave to come your way. Paddle in soon. Why? Because pretty soon you'll start shivering, and once the shivering really gets going, it will affect your fine motor skills. Your coordination will be off, making it difficult to catch waves and stand on your board. Once your core temperature begins to drop, your muscles lose much of their strength, and paddling becomes more exhausting. Your fingers will become numb and nearly useless, making it difficult to grip your board, take off your leash, or get into your car. Worse yet, with a further drop in temperature (around 93°F), you start getting confused and disoriented—not a good thing in cold surf. At these body temperatures, your heart rate, blood pressure, and breathing rate all slow down. With more pronounced hypothermia, your body loses its ability to shiver (and generate heat), and lethargy will set in. Eventually brain function declines to such an extent that you lapse into a coma.

Interestingly, most people in cold water don't die from hypothermia: they drown. In fact, an adult male who falls into ice-cold water (32°F, 0°C) could survive without a wet suit for at least forty-five minutes, but most people who fall into frigid water die in less than fifteen minutes because hypothermia robs their strength, coordination, and judgment, rendering them unable to stay afloat. Hypothermia has been implicated as a contributing factor in numerous drowning deaths among cold-water surfers.

## Prevention

While having the right wet suit (see below) is obviously a critical first step in avoiding hypothermia, listening to your body and paddling in at the first signs that you are cold is even more important. Winter sessions in cold climates should be time-limited because fatigue sets in more quickly than in balmy waters, and the risk of hypothermia leaves less of a margin for error. Extra effort is expended stretching out thicker neoprene with every paddling stroke, and considerable metabolic energy is expended simply generating heat.

Make your winter sessions (in cold climates) short but active by paddling for lots of waves as constant activity generates heat. Another key factor in keeping warm during winter surf is to eat plenty of food rich in carbohydrates a couple of hours before paddling out. Your body revs up its metabolism in an effort to keep you warm in colder climates and requires plenty of readily accessible fuel in the form of carbohydrates to keep the furnace stoked. Small thin surfers are significantly more prone to hypothermia than are large husky surfers whose ample layer of subcutaneous fat (think blubber) provides an excellent layer of natural insulation. If you are a hard-core year-round surfer in the Northeastern United States or the Pacific Northwest, consider putting on a few extra pounds in the winter months to help stave off the cold and allow for longer surfs. In bitter cold weather, make sure you have a good system for staying warm as you get into and out of your wet suit. You need to start out warm before you enter the water and don't want to freeze on the way out. A few surfers in remote northern areas have had close brushes with hypothermia when, upon returning to their cars, they could not find their keys and were literally left out in the cold.

# Assessment and Treatment of Hypothermia

Medical textbooks take great pains to distinguish between mild, moderate, and severe hypothermia as graded by body temperature. The idea being that mildly hypothermic individuals (90–95°F, 32–35°C) have the ability to generate heat by shivering and are able to rewarm themselves via shivering without additional heat sources, whereas the treatment of moderate to severe hypothermia hinges on warming up the victim's core, through modalities such as heated intravenous fluids, and other techniques. Because taking accurate (rectal) temperature readings in the field is impractical and requires a special hypothermic thermometer (normal ones only go down to 96°F), treating individuals on the basis of their symptoms outside of a hospital setting is often the only viable alternative.

The first step in caring for someone suffering from hypothermia is to prevent further heat loss. To minimize cooling from evaporation, dry the outside of the person's wet suit (but leave the wet suit on) and get them out of the wind. A car, tent, or even a board bag can provide a dry shelter and protection from the wind. Hypothermic individuals may have a clumsy gait (like a drunk), so they may require assistance when walking to ensure that they don't fall and injure themselves. Once in a sheltered environment, cover the person with as many insulating materials as are available and, if outdoors, place them on a sleeping pad or board bag to minimize conductive heat loss to the ground. If possible, provide external heat by turning on a car heater or building a fire. Chemical heat packs or hot-water bottles if available can be placed in the armpits or on the groin. Getting into a sleeping bag with the person can also provide warmth if other options are not available.

Warm drinks are comforting and provide hydration, but a half gallon of piping-hot liquid would be required to raise an average-sized adult's body temperature by only 1°F. Far more important for reversing hypothermia are food and/or beverages, which are rich in carbohydrates. These carbs are vital in supporting heat production via shivering and increased metabolism. Hypothermic individuals are often dehydrated, so liquids are beneficial, but never provide alcoholic beverages. Though alcohol may make you feel warm inside, it actually has the opposite effect on body temperature by dilating blood vessels in the skin, which promotes further cooling.

Anyone who is shivering and able to talk coherently should be able to generate enough metabolic heat to rewarm themselves so long as they are provided food, shelter, and insulation. Generally, those who are shivering and able to walk and talk do not require evacuation. Severely hypothermic individuals—those who are irrational, comatose, have slurred speech, or cannot walk—will not be able to rewarm themselves in the field and require evacuation to a medical facility where advanced rewarming techniques can be employed. Severely hypothermic individuals are critically ill and at risk for sudden cardiac death. Prior to evacuation, bundle the person up and lay them flat so blood can circulate to the brain and heart. The victim should be transported as gently as possible and not jostled about, as this has been known to precipitate fatal heart rhythms. At extremely low core temperatures (below 88°F), the person may appear to be dead due to an extremely faint, slow pulse, very shallow breathing, and lack of movement. Do not initiate CPR on a hypothermic patient until you have taken a full thirty seconds to be sure that he or she has no pulse and is not breathing. Do not terminate CPR on hypothermic victims until after thirty minutes (unless you are unable to, or at risk of injury) as there are rare cases of people having been successfully resuscitated after more than half an hour without a detectable pulse.

# Wet Suits

Wet suits should be viewed as important pieces of surfing gear. While their primary purpose is to keep a surfer warm, they also provide excellent sun protection, significant flotation, and some defense against abrasions from the seafloor. Not only have wet suits expanded the surfing season in temperate areas, turning it into a year-round sport, but they have expanded the surfable world. Vast tracts of coastline once considered off-limits to surfers due to inhospitably cold water and air temperatures are now fair game for those willing to don rubber. As wet suits continue to get warmer, more flexible, and more waterproof, it has become possible to surf in relative comfort even in the icy-cold waters of the far north and far south.

Key design features, which increase a wet suit's insulating properties, are the thickness of the neoprene (and any added liners like wool, etc.), the integrity of the seams, and the quality of the fit. Water temperatures below 50°F will require a wetsuit that is at least 5 to 6 mm thick. Smooth-skinned neoprene, though less durable than nylon-covered neoprene, is also desirable because it does not absorb water and thus decreases evaporative heat loss. The latest rage in surfing technology is the adoption of battery-heated wet suits, which may push the envelope of cold-water surfing yet farther, but it remains to be seen if they will catch on. Though many manufacturers state that their neoprene has better insulating properties than that of the competition (e.g., 30 percent warmer!), as of yet there is little objective evidence to back up these claims.

When buying a cold-water suit, invest in the most expensive one you can afford—as you'll get what you pay for. In terms of thickness, look at the manufacturer's recommendations; winter surfing in waters less than 50°F (10°C) will generally call for a suit that is 5 to 6 mm thick. Look for seams that are watertight, flexible, and durable. Of the wide variety of techniques currently used to join neoprene together, unglued flat-stitched seams are the most leaky, and stitched and liquid-taped are probably the best in terms of being watertight and retaining flexibility. When trying on a winter wet suit (which is about as much fun as trying on a tuxedo in the desert), make sure the fit is quite snug throughout, paying particular attention to the cuffs around the neck, wrist, and ankle. Keep in mind that it will expand slightly when wet. Because most zippers leak and don't stretch, zipperless or near-zipperless entry systems are best in terms of warmth and flexibility for winter suits. However, getting in and out of some of these suits requires the flexibility of a yogi and the patience of a Zen master. Impatient and not-so-flexible surfers have been stuck in these zipperless straitjackets unable get them off and, in a panic, have been known to literally cut their way out with scissors—so, buyer, beware.

# Head Injuries

Head injuries are common among surfers, accounting for up to 40 percent of all surf-related injuries. Fortunately most are minor bruises and lacerations. A few, however, are more serious—here's how to differentiate between the good, the bad, and the ugly.

The major risk in a head injury is the development of increased pressure around the brain caused by swelling or bleeding within the skull. Increased pressure can in turn force the brain downward, which can lead to brain damage, respiratory arrest, and death. This constitutes a major emergency, which cannot be handled in the field (unless you happen to be a brain surgeon with a drill close at hand), and requires immediate transport to a hospital.

So, how can you tell if someone who has received a blow to the head from their surfboard needs an ice pack or a medevac? Though you can't actually see bleeding or increased pressure within the skull from the outside, there are a number of ominous clues based on the history and symptoms that merit prompt evacuation.

# Worrisome Signs and Symptoms of a Head Injury

1. Prolonged loss of consciousness (greater than thirty seconds)
2. Altered mental status, including confusion, memory loss, incoordination, drowsiness, irritability, combativeness, or unconsciousness
3. Persistent vomiting
4. Severe headache
5. Seizures
6. Changes in vision
7. Bruising behind the ears or around the eyes
8. Clear fluid leaking from the nose or ears

If any of the above are present, the individual should be immediately evacuated and transported to a hospital equipped with a CT scanner. Those suspected of having suffered a significant brain injury should also be suspected of having a neck fracture and should be handled accordingly during transport (see page 183 for instructions on neck immobilization). Ideally the patient should be transported with his or her head elevated at 30 degrees to lower pressure in the brain (you can put a duffel bag or backpack under the head of the backboard) and log-rolled on to his or her side if they start vomiting.

Those who have suffered no more than a brief loss of consciousness (less than thirty seconds) and have none of the above worrisome signs or symptoms can be safely observed (with the exception of those on blood thinners like coumadin, Plavix, or eliquis). These individuals should be watched closely for a period of twenty-four hours for development of a headache, lethargy, vomiting, confusion, etc., and awoken when sleeping every two hours. If the person's condition deteriorates during this period of observation, they should be evacuated as above.

# Spine Injuries

Spine injuries are rare but potentially catastrophic injuries that can (and do) occur among bodysurfers, bodyboarders, and surfers, usually as a result of headfirst wipeouts into the seafloor. The human spine is made up of twenty-four mobile vertebrae, separated by fibroelastic discs, as well as the sacrum and coccyx, which are part of the pelvis. These vertebrae encase and protect the delicate spinal cord, which functions as the body's own information superhighway. All sensory input such as pain, temperature, position, and vibration flows up the spinal cord so it

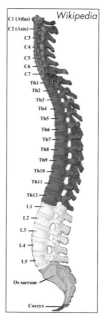

C1 (Atlas)
C2 (Axis)
C3
C4
C5
C6
C7
Th1
Th2
Th3
Th4
Th5
Th6
Th7
Th8
Th9
Th10
Th11
Th12
L1
L2
L3
L4
L5
Os sacrum
Coccyx

**Human spine.**

can be processed by the brain, and all motor output flows from the brain down the spinal cord, enabling you to move your arms and legs and perform other important bodily functions.

The seven vertebrae in the neck (cervical spine) are the smallest, most mobile, and least-protected bones in the spine and therefore are the most commonly fractured (broken). The cervical spine can be fractured from direct downward compression, excessive forward flexion, excessive hyperextension (backward), or rotation beyond the normal range of motion, any of which can occur from an ill-fated header into the bottom. Some spine fractures are stable, meaning that the integrity of spinal column is preserved and the spinal cord remains protected, while others are deemed unstable, meaning that broken parts of the vertebrae are free to move and damage the spinal cord. If the spinal cord has been damaged, the victim may have permanent loss of muscle function and skin sensation of legs and possibly arms as well, depending on the level of the injury.

---

### SURF-SURVIVAL TIP

**Any surfer with significant neck pain, numbness, or weakness of the arms or legs after a wipeout should be suspected of having an unstable neck fracture or spinal cord injury until proven otherwise.**

---

Though X-rays are needed to confirm a spine fracture, there are a number of worrisome signs and symptoms that suggest the presence of a fracture or spinal cord injury:

1. Severe midline back or neck pain
2. Tenderness along the midline of the back or neck
3. *Any* numbness or tingling in the arms, hands, legs, or feet
4. *Any* weakness or paralysis of the arms, hands, legs, or feet
5. Inability to control urine or bowels
6. Anyone with potential neck trauma who is unconscious or intoxicated

SURF SURVIVAL

A victim of a surfing accident with any of the above and any surfer seen floating motionless in the water should be presumed to have an unstable neck fracture until proven otherwise by X-rays and if possible an attempt should be made to immobilize the neck to ensure no further damage occurs.

The basic principle in caring for and transporting surfers who have potentially suffered a neck fracture is to immobilize the head, neck, and trunk so as to avoid movements of the neck, which could further injure the vulnerable spinal cord. Paramedics accomplish this by securing accident victims faceup on a rigid backboard and placing them in a rigid collar. As a surfer, you've already got a board at the ready, so all you'll need to do is fashion a collar. No problem. Fold a towel or wet suit so it is a few plies thick and wrap it around the front of the injured surfer's neck between his or her chin and the tops of his or her shoulders, keeping the neck in a neutral position (as if lying in a bed, staring at the ceiling). Use a tie-down strap or surfboard leash to secure this padding so the victim can't easily move his or her neck from front to back, or side to side. Place rolled-up towels on both sides of the head for added protection. Lastly, secure the victim's waist to the board so he or she won't roll off and so his or her body cannot move in relation to their head.

If the victim must be repositioned or rolled, make sure to move him or her as a single unit. For example, when a patient in the ER who is boarded and collared needs to vomit, a caregiver assigned to the head calls out to the rest of the team to roll on the count of three, and everyone simultaneously log-rolls the patient over to one side. In situations where the distance to the nearest vehicle is lengthy, assemble a team of four or more litter bearers to carry the injured surfer, using the surfboard as a makeshift stretcher. The front left litter bearer should be designated as the driver and is responsible for coordinating movements of the stretcher over, under, or around any obstacles.

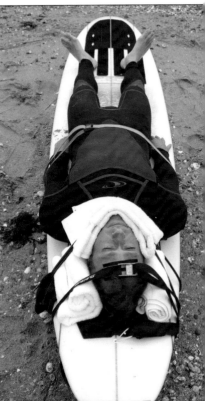

**Improvised backboard and collar to immobilize and transport a surfer with a potential neck fracture.**

# Wound Care for Surfers

Wounds, which include abrasions (scrapes), cuts (lacerations), or puncture wounds are the most common types of injuries you will encounter while surfing. With a little guidance, you should be able to manage many of these yourself in the field, so pay close attention to this section. While there are a variety of different ways to treat wounds, the goals are always the same: stop any bleeding (so you don't die), speed the healing process (so you can get back to surfing ASAP), decrease the risk of infection (so you don't fester), and have a satisfactory cosmetic result (so you can get a date).

## Bleeding

While bleeding is often alarming to the layperson, it can almost always be stopped simply by applying direct pressure to the wound. To do this, put pressure on the wound by wrapping a clean towel or T-shirt around two fingers or the palm of your hand and pushing firmly, directly on the area that is bleeding. Wear gloves or use a plastic bag to protect yourself if there is a concern about blood-borne infections such as hepatitis or HIV. Keep continuous firm pressure for a good fifteen minutes before taking a peek to see if the bleeding has stopped. Alternatively, you can place a stack of gauze pads over the bleeding area and make a pressure dressing by firmly taping the stack down or keeping it in place with a snugly applied Ace wrap. While still in the water you can use the ankle strap of a leash to fashion a pressure dressing around an injured extremity.

In the unlikely event that you encounter life-threatening hemorrhage that you can't control with direct pressure, such as from a shark attack or propeller strike, a tourniquet should be applied. *Do not hesitate* to use a tourniquet for life-threatening bleeding, amputations, or near-amputations.

Commercial tourniquets such as the C-A-T or SOFTT-W are the most effective and should be placed about 2 (5 cm) inches toward the armpit or groin from the wound. The tourniquet should be tightened until there is no more active bleeding, making it uncomfortably tight. Most make-shift tourniquets made from belts or surfboard leashes are simply not tight enough to fully occlude arteries (but do compress veins) and may actually increase blood loss. Creating an improvised tourniquet that can generate sufficient pressure to fully compress major arteries requires a windlass as described below.

Obtain a 3-inch (7 cm) strip of pliable non-stretch material such as a strip of towel, denim, or a bedsheet that is about 3 feet (90 cm) long. A surfboard leash, or rope, is too narrow— less likely to stop arterial blood flow and more likely to damage nerves and skin than a wider strip of cloth. Roof straps and belts are usually too stiff and difficult to tie. A screw driver, stout stick, or flashlight can serve as a windlass.

Begin by wrapping the material around the injured extremity about 2 (5 cm) inches above the wound, avoiding any joints. Tie a snug half-knot, like the first part of a shoelace, in the mate-

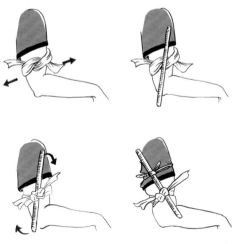

RENA RONG

**Improvised tourniquet using a windlass.**

rial. Next, place the windlass across the half-knot as illustrated and complete a square knot over the windlass. Twist the windlass tightly until there is no more active bleeding, then secure the windlass with another piece of cloth or string to keep it from unwinding. Note the time that the tourniquet was placed by writing it on the patient if possible.

Tourniquets can safely be left in place for about four hours before there is significant risk of damage to the limb. If medical help is not available after four hours, untwist the wand, leaving the tourniquet in place, to see if the bleeding has stopped or can be controlled with direct pressure. If bleeding cannot be controlled, re-tighten the tourniquet.

## Wound Cleansing

Wounds acquired while surfing are at high risk for infection for a wide variety of reasons. To begin with, seawater, even seemingly pristine crystal-clear seawater, is teeming with marine bacteria, many of which can cause nasty infections. Furthermore, many cuts and abrasions you get while surfing are caused by scraping against coral reef, barnacles, and other living creatures, which are often covered with bacterial organisms. Finally, the kind of warm, tropical, humid environments, which are favored hangouts for surfers (think Fiji and the Caribbean), are also favored hangouts for bacteria like *Staphylococcus* and *Streptococcus,* which are notorious for causing skin infections.

So what can you do to avoid an infection next time you get dragged over the reef in Recife? Basically, the answer lies in the old saying "The solution to pollution is dilution." You need to flush all those germs and bits of debris out of the wound by flooding it with a vigorous stream of irrigating fluid. Sterile saline solution is what we use in the hospital—but chances are slim (to none) that you'll have any of that lying around camp. Luckily, it turns out that clean drinking water or potable tap water is equally effective. The key here is to really hose the wound out with *at least* half a liter (four cups) of water using a fairly forceful spray. A shower or sink faucet works really well for this, but if those are unavailable, fill a clean plastic bag with water, poke a hole in it the size of a toothpick, and you can use that to generate a vigorous stream of water.

After irrigating the wound, be sure to remove any bits of material (fragments of reef, sand, etc.) still embedded in the wound, as these fragments are usually laden with bacteria and can form an abscess (pus pocket). The best way to get coral dust out is with a steady hand and a good set of tweezers or a needle. Prior to digging around a wound, be sure to sterilize your instruments with a flame or by placing them in boiling water.

*Do not* use seawater as an irrigating solution, because as mentioned above, it is home to many bacteria that may further contaminate the wound. *Do not* use alcohol, hydrogen peroxide, or undiluted providone-iodine (Betadine) to clean out a wound. While these chemicals kill bacteria, they are also toxic to the healthy tissues bordering the wound and paradoxically break down the body's natural barriers against infection.

Scrubbing wounds clean, once condoned by the medical establishment (no pain, no gain!), has recently fallen out of favor. In most studies, this practice has been shown to actually *increase* infection rates for many types of wounds, and current recommendations are that only *really* dirty wounds (like taking a digger off your scooter on a muddy road in Bali) be scrubbed to remove dirt or other embedded material.

Lastly, be sure your tetanus vaccine is up to date so as to avoid a dreaded case of lockjaw. Assuming you were properly immunized as a child (three shots), a booster shot is required for minor wounds unless you've had a tetanus shot within the last ten years. For major wounds, you need to get a booster shot unless you've had a tetanus shot within the last five years.

## Wound Evaluation

Halfway through a two-week sojourn in the Mentawis, your buddy hits the lip of yet another perfect glassy wave, and airs out. The trajectory is perfect, but during reentry something goes awry and he ends up with a significant fin cut on his forearm. The weathered boatman opens up a rusty first aid kit and pulls out some not-so-sterile gauze, which you successfully use to staunch the bleeding. Next you use your (flame-sterilized) multitool to bore a little hole through the top of an unopened plastic bottle of water, squeeze it, and direct the stream of water into his cut to clean it out. You are in full commando mode. Good.

But as the unofficial trip medic, how can you tell if this cut is something that you can just "hose and close" or a more complicated injury that requires him to cut his trip short (ouch!) and hightail it back to LA to see a real doctor? In paramedic parlance, do you stay and play, or do you scoop and run? To fully answer this question, you'd need to go to med school for four years, followed by three to six years of hard labor as a resident. We'll save you the trouble and summarize the key points in the next few paragraphs.

**Deep fin cut. Note the muscle visible beneath the layer of yellow/tan fat. This requires expert repair.**

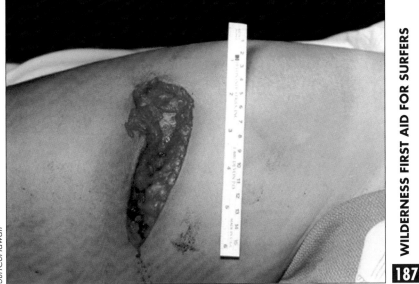

First, you need to peer inside the cut to look for damage to underlying structures such as tendons, muscle, nerves, blood vessels, and even bone. This is best done by putting on a headlamp and applying traction to the adjacent skin (or using sterile tweezers) to pull apart the wound edges. What do you see? Those glistening yellow-tan blobs are fat, which lies just beneath the skin. If you see dark red (think raw steak), that's muscle, sinewy white bands are tendons, and nerves look like yellow thread. Bone will look smooth and white. If you see anything more through the cut than a few blobs of fat, you are in over your head and need to seek the care of a doctor.

Visual inspection yields useful clues, but often does not tell the whole story because nerves are so tiny you usually can't see them, and tendons, once cut, often retract out of view. To get a more complete picture, you need to do a physical exam distal to (on the far side, away from the head) the laceration. In this particular case, you need to look for normal function of the wrist and hand.

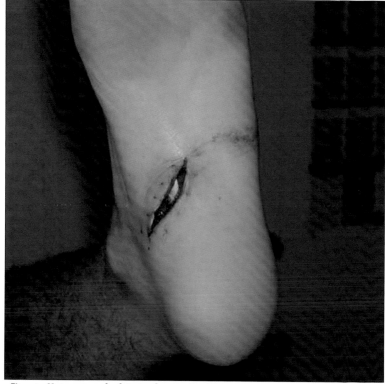

**SURF SURVIVAL**

Fin cut. Note exposed white tendon. Again, this requires expert repair.

Is there good strength and a normal range of motion in the joints distal to the wound? Does the wrist move properly? Do all the fingers open and close against force? If all the above are normal, then a complete tendon injury (but not a partial one) can be ruled out.

Is there normal sensation (feeling) past the wound and in all fingers? Normal sensation and good strength rule out any significant nerve injury.

Lastly, check the circulation. Feel the pulse in the wrist and compare it to the uninjured side. Feel the injured extremity to determine if it is cooler than the uninjured side (it should feel the same). Press on the fingertips until they blanch and then let go. The blanched area should pink up in less than three seconds if blood flow to the hand is normal.

In cuts to the leg, the same general principles apply, with particular attention paid to movement, sensation, and circulation of the foot.

If the motor and sensory function of the wrist and hand are normal, and the circulation appears to be intact, and all you see in the cut is a few blobs of fat, it is *probably* okay to stay and play. However, if you see tendons, muscles, nerves, or bone, or the bleeding is hard to control, you need to wrap up the cut and seek medical care. Ditto if there are any deficits of movement, sensation, or circulation in the hand or the wrist. Elevating the injured extremity above the level of the heart and putting it in a splint, if feasible, will minimize pain and bleeding and will certainly impress the folks back home. Note that while the repair of nerves and tendons is an urgent matter, surgery can be safely delayed for up to a week. Better to wait a few days and have a wound poperly repaired by a specialist (e.g., hand surgeon, plastic surgeon) than to have it botched up by a physician with little training.

Deep lacerations to the abdomen, chest, or groin mandate immediate evacuation. Anything worse than minor lacerations to the face, lips, and ear can be tricky to repair, may cause unsightly scars, and should be repaired by an experienced physician. Deep facial wounds can involve underlying structures such as nerves, tear ducts, muscles, etc.; and these, too, are best managed by experienced medical personnel. Minor lacerations (those that are less than a few inches long go no deeper than the fat layer) to the scalp, forehead, and extremities, however, can usually be safely managed in the field. If in doubt about the proper management of a laceration, it is always safest to seek a doctor's advice.

## Wound Closure

When most people get a sizeable cut, the first thought that comes to mind is, "I'm going to need stitches." After all, they reason, closing a wound keeps the germs out and decreases the risk of infection. Wrong. Closing a wound slightly *increases* the risk of infection because a wound can't adequately drain once it has been closed, and bacteria can get trapped inside and form an abscess (pus pocket). That is not to say that cuts should not be closed. In fact, in the ER, we repair wounds all the time because wound closure speeds the healing process, stops bleeding, and leaves less of a scar. However, the potential benefits of closing a wound (faster recovery, less bleeding, better cosmetic results) must be weighed against the increased risk of infection, especially outside of a hospital setting, where cleanliness may be an issue. Some injuries such as animal bites, puncture wounds (deep wound, small opening), and heavily contaminated wounds should *never* be tightly closed because the risk of infection is simply too great. Wounds less than half an inch (1 cm) long will generally heal equally well with or without stitches. Most clean wounds can be safely closed within the first eighteen hours, but waiting any longer than that significantly increases the risk of infection.

There are a variety of methods of wound closure, and we will go through the advantages and disadvantages of each one, particularly as they pertain to surfers.

## Wound Closure Strips

Adhesive tapes in the form of Band-Aids, Steri-Strips, cloth tape, and yes, even duct tape are easily applied, leave no suture marks, and can be successfully used to bring together the edges of a wound. These methods are best used on straight cuts whose wound edges are not gaping widely apart. You'll have the best success with this method of wound closure if you first apply tincture of benzoin to both sides of the wound and let it air-dry (for about thirty seconds). Benzoin is a very tacky material which will help the tape stay in place longer. Trim but do not shave any hair (shaving increases infection rates), which may interfere with adhesive strips. Never trim eyebrows, as they may never grow back.

Place Steri-Strips or tape perpendicular to the length of the wound, spaced at quarter-inch (6 mm) intervals. Begin by sticking down one end of the Steri-Strip and applying gentle traction to the other to bring the wound edges together. Once the wound edges are close together, the free end of the Steri-Strip can be tacked down to the other side of the wound.

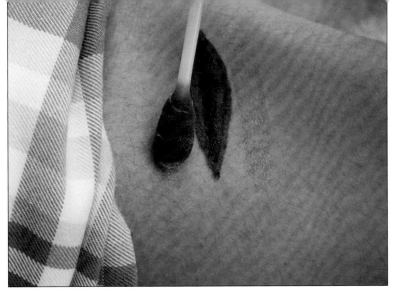

Apply benzoin with a swab stick (shown) or gauze. Benzoin will help keep
Steri-Strips and other adhesive tapes in place.

Once benzoin has dried, apply Steri-Strips as shown. Note: gloves should be worn when
repairing a wound.

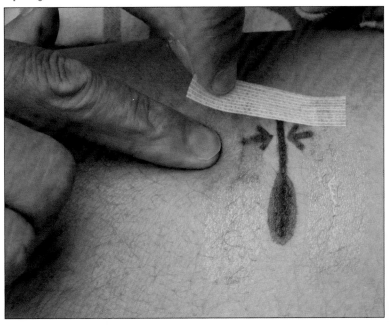

Unfortunately, even with benzoin, none of the above will reliably stay on through prolonged surfs. If you apply benzoin, then Steri-Strips, *and* put a good Band-Aid over the whole thing, you'll generally be able to get in a few good days of surfing before the whole thing needs to be redone. Tapes closures tend to fail across joints where there is excessive movement and on wounds that have a lot of tension pulling them apart.

## SURF-SURVIVAL TIP

Hair and dental floss can be used for the closure of scalp wounds. Bring together a bundle of hair from each side of the scalp wound, then use dental floss or thread to knot the bundles of hair together. Repeat the process a few times for long scalp wounds. If thread is unavailable, glue can be used to hold the bundles together.

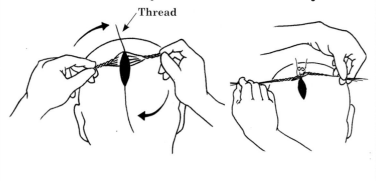
Thread

A variety of glues have been specially formulated for wound closure, and many are available without a prescription. Of these, 2-octyl cyanoacrylate (Dermabond, LiquiBand, etc.) seems best. Glues come in small cylindrical applicators that are easy to transport, are fairly easy to use, and cause no pain. Like tapes, they work best on small linear wounds that don't have a lot of tension gaping them open. Before use, the cut needs to be completely dry and nonbleeding. Have an assistant help squeeze the wound edges together and apply two layers of glue, waiting for one layer to harden, before applying another. Adhesive skin glues work by bridging both sides of a wound together, and care should be taken not to get any glue *into* the wound, which will impede healing, or into the person's eye. These glues inhibit bacterial growth, so there is no need to apply antibiotic ointment (which should not be used because it actually dissolves the glue). Glues do not work well on the hands, feet, elbows, or knees (too much motion, too moist), and their main limitation for surfers is that they do not hold up well when wet.

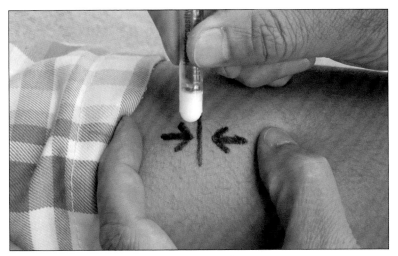

Squeeze wound edges together before applying adhesive.
Note: gloves should be worn (though they need not be sterile).

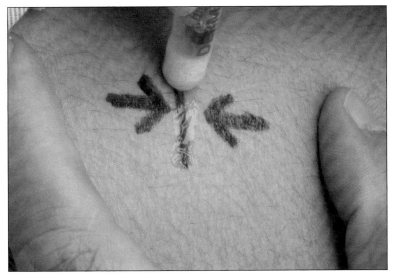

Crush vial to squeeze adhesive and saturate white applicator tip (which will turn blue). Apply thin layer of glue on top of wound to bridge wound edges together. Wait two minutes before applying another layer.

Surgical staples have been in use for many years and have cosmetic results that are indistinguishable from stitches. They come conveniently packaged in small staplers, require less skill to place than stitches, and are perfect for closing cuts on the scalp, arms, and legs. Putting them in only causes a little pinch (well . . . maybe not so little), so a few can be placed without the need for local anesthesia. To close a laceration with staples, hold the wound edges together and align a staple so it is centered across the wound. Press the stapler firmly onto the skin so

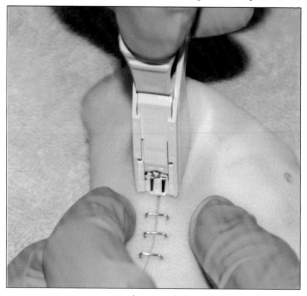

Staple gun technique.

the staple tips engage the skin surface and depress lever of the stapler. Place a staple approximately every quarter inch (6 mm) along the wound. The staples are stainless steel, hold up beautifully in the water, and will keep wound edges together even if they are under considerable tension. Don't forget to pack a staple remover along with the skin stapler for long trips.

The gold standard wound closure technique for surfers are sutures (stitches). They are good for irregularly shaped lacerations and can be used to pull the edges of a wound together despite significant tension. Furthermore, they are waterproof and are durable, even in the water. However, putting them in requires some training and experience, and a proper description is well beyond the scope of this book. If you are a physician or a physician's assistant, however, we highly recommend traveling with a suture kit, sutures of varying sizes, latex gloves, and local anesthetic. The three of us (authors) have had the opportunity to use our suture kits on multiple occasions.

Stitches, staples, and adhesive tapes should be removed after varying time periods according to where they have been placed: the face in five days, the scalp in seven days, the body in ten days, the hands and feet in twelve to fourteen days.

## Dressings and antibiotics

Once a wound has been cleaned (and closed if necessary), apply a topical antibiotic ointment such as Bacitracin to the injured skin. Not only will it help kill surface bacteria, but the petroleum jelly in these ointments also promotes faster wound healing. If antibiotic ointment is unavailable, honey has antibacterial properties and promotes wound healing, so it can be used as a substitute. Oral antibiotics, however, are only indicated as a preventive measure for heavily contaminated wounds, deep puncture wounds, and bite wounds—the same kinds of wounds we recommend you to leave open because they are at such high risk for infection.

Most medical authorities recommend that you keep a cut dry for a week or so postinjury, except to briefly clean it once a day with soap and water. After every cleaning, it is advised that you pat the wound dry, apply antibiotic ointment, and place a new dressing. The dressing serves to protect a wound from getting dirty, absorbs any wound drainage, and keeps the wound protected from the sun—which (surfer girls, take note) diminishes scarring. While the clean-and-dry approach works well for most people, to paraphrase Lieutenant Colonel Kilgore in *Apocalypse Now*, "most people don't surf!" Clean and dry is fine during a flat spell, but experience tells us that if you're in the middle of a two-week boat trip in the Mentawis and the conditions are epic, you won't exactly be following doctor's orders. You are going to go surfing no matter what they tell you, and what you really want is a bomber wash-and-wear dressing that will stay put through at least a couple of spin cycles.

### SURF-SURVIVAL TIP

For a surf-proof dressing, we recommend the following recipe: place a dab of antibiotic ointment on your wound, cover it with a clear flexible adhesive film like Opsite, or Tegaderm, and then cover the film with medical tape or duct tape. If the wound is in a place where it can be covered with a bootie or wet suit, better yet, as that will help keep the dressing in place and protect the wound from the sun and further trauma.

Having disobeyed doctor's orders by going surfing with a cut in the first place, you need to make up for it by compulsive wound care on land or you'll risk developing a sea ulcer (see "Sea Ulcers" in Chapter 7) or wound infection, either one of which could keep you dry-docked for weeks. As soon as you get out of the water, peel off your surf dressing, rinse off your wound with clean freshwater, and pat it dry with a towel. Now put on a fresh dab of ointment and apply a clean cotton gauze or appropriately sized bandage. Keep the dressing in place with medical tape or an Ace wrap. Make every effort to keep your wound as clean and dry as possible when out of the water. If there is drainage from the wound, change the dressings frequently. Take brief showers and don't go swimming. If the cut is on your foot, wear shoes and (horror of horrors) socks around camp. At night elevate the injured part and leave soupy wounds uncovered (except for a thin layer of antibiotic ointment) so they have a chance to dry out and form a protective scab.

For reef rash (reef-induced abrasions), a nonadherent dressing such as Telfa is preferable to cotton gauze because it can be removed more easily and with less discomfort. Aloe vera extract or even the juice squeezed directly from the plant can offer some relief for these extremely painful wounds and helps promote the healing process.

## Is There an Infection?

About 5 percent of wounds will ultimately become infected. Cardinal signs that a cut abrasion or puncture wound has become infected are redness around the area, swelling, worsening pain, warmth, and thick yellow drainage. While some clear, watery, yellow discharge is normal, a discharge which is thick, foul smelling, and yellow-white (pus) indicates infection. Pain from most wounds starts to improve by the second or third day after injury, and escalating pain may be an early warning sign of infection.

Most wound infections can be successfully treated with oral antibiotics, warm soaks, and elevation. Marking the perimeter of reddened skin with an indelible marker is a simple way to see if the antibiotics are working or if the infection is continuing to spread past the line you've made despite antibiotics. Warning signs that an infection requires evacuation to a hospital for intravenous antibiotics include the following:

1. **Red streaks running up an arm or leg toward the heart.**
2. **The infection is spreading despite oral antibiotics.**
3. **High fevers or chills.**
4. **Nausea, vomiting, and lethargy.**

If a wound that has been closed becomes infected, the first line of defense is to open it back up so it can drain. That's right, *remove* any stitches, staples, Steri-Strips, etc., that are keeping the wound closed and soak the wound twice daily in warm water, which will help loosen up and release any pus that is trapped inside. Put a moist gauze dressing *into* the wound to pack it open. This will help your body fight the infection by allowing bacteria to drain out of the wound. These moist dressings, which will draw out pus, should be changed at least twice a day. Elevate the wound above the level of your heart to diminish pain and swelling and promote faster healing.

While most surfing-related skin infections are caused by the same bacteria that cause land-based skin infections, namely *Staph* and *Strep*, some may be caused by bacteria that live in seawater. This is an important distinction, because antibiotics such as Keflex (cephalexin), which are routinely prescribed for skin infections, are going after *Staph* and *Strep* but are largely ineffective against marine bacteria (*Vibrio, Mycobacterium*). Similarly, the antibiotics that provide good coverage against marine organisms (doxycycline, Cipro, and Bactrim) are not very effective against *Strep*. Unfortunately, there is no immediate way of telling what kind of bacteria has caused your infection, so it is probably a good idea to use Keflex *plus* an antibiotic that works for marine bacteria. Alternatively, Levaquin (levofloxacin) provides pretty good coverage against both types of bacteria, but it is very expensive, somewhat restricted in its use, and should be reserved for major infections. When seeking medical care for an infection that you may have acquired while surfing, make it clear to your health-care provider that you spend a lot of time in the ocean so you can be put on the appropriate antibiotics.

# Fractures and Dislocations

## Fractures

Broken bones, also known as fractures, can often be difficult to diagnose in the field without X-rays. Fortunately, with proper prehospital care, most fractures can wait a few days for definitive diagnosis (X-rays) and treatment by an orthopedist. Fractures among surfers are relatively uncommon in comparison to other sports, and this section will concentrate on the types of orthopedic injuries most commonly sustained by surfers.

## Types of Fractures

The majority of fractures are closed, meaning that the skin above the broken bone is intact, as opposed to an open fracture, in which the sharp end of a broken bone pokes a hole through the skin. This is an important distinction, because with an opening to the outside world, the bone involved in an open fracture can become infected, and bone infections are notoriously difficult to treat. If there is a white piece of bone protruding from the skin, the diagnosis of an open fracture is obvious, but more often, the only clue to an open fracture is a small cut in the skin immediately above the injured area. This cut is the spot where a tip of the broken bone poked through the skin for an instant and then popped back under. Though a little cut on an injured (and usually deformed) arm or leg may seem like a minor issue, it is actually grounds for evacuation to a hospital for intravenous antibiotics to prevent the nasty bone infection known as osteomyelitis.

## Is It Broken?

In many cases, even the most astute surf docs cannot distinguish between a sprain and a fracture without an X-ray. There may be no difference in appearance, say, between a bad ankle sprain and a small ankle fracture. Fortunately, making an on-the-spot diagnosis of a fracture is not critical, because the initial treatment for most fractures and bad sprains is the same, and even those fractures requiring surgery can usually wait a few days without adverse consequence.

Though ruling out a fracture may be difficult without X-rays, there are a number of clues that are suggestive of a fracture. Most fractures will have surrounding swelling, are tender to the touch, and develop bruising in a day or so. Unfortunately, all these findings are also common with sprains and strains. However, a number of additional clues can help confirm the presence of a fracture:

1. **If the limb appears deformed or is bent at an impossible angle, it is likely broken. Look at the uninjured side for comparison.**

2. **Crepitus: a rice-crispy-like grinding between broken ends of a bone felt by the patient or examiner can only be caused by a fracture.**

3. **Did the person feel or hear a crack? This suggests a fracture or tendon rupture.**

4. **Can the person use the injured extremity? Most (but not all) cannot walk on a broken leg and will not use a broken wrist.**

# Treatment of Fractures

The mainstay of the initial treatment of a fracture is a splint or sling to immobilize the injured part, which diminishes pain and protects against further injury from movement at the fracture site. Before applying a splint, make sure to remove any rings (or other jewelry) from the injured extremity because they can cut off circulation to fingers or toes and may be very difficult to remove once swelling becomes more pronounced. Rest, ice, compression (Ace wrap), and elevation (RICE) are mainstays of treatment for fractures (as they are for sprain and strains) and help diminish swelling and relieve pain. Make sure to provide the injured surfer with pain medicine such as Motrin (ibuprofen) 800 every six hours with food, or Vicodin 5 mg/325 mg (oxycodone/acetaminophen) one to two tablets every four hours.

Setting a displaced or angulated fracture in the field is unnecessary in most cases. However, if the fracture is bent at an angle (angulated) *and* is compromising blood flow downstream of the injury (e.g., hand or the foot), then straightening of the fracture is important, particularly if medical help is more than a couple of hours away. If the hand or foot on the injured extremity is pale, cold, and you cannot feel a pulse, then

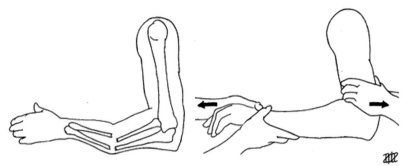

**For visibly deformed extremity fractures, apply longitudinal traction as shown, before splinting. This will improve circulation and relieve pain.**

have the victim chew on surf wax as you pull gently straight along the axis of the injured arm or leg. The risk of making the injury worse is negligible. After the limb has been aligned in a more anatomically correct (i.e., normal) position, then place it in a splint. Check the temperature, color, and pulses of the affected body part after realignment to see if the circulation has improved.

If you see a cut that is suspicious for an open fracture or see white bone protruding from a wound, irrigate the area with sterile water (boiled and cooled) or sterile saline solution and then cover the wound and any exposed bone with a moist sterile dressing. Place the extremity in a splint and seek emergent transport to a medical facility.

## Making Splints and Slings

Splints are used to immobilize fractures and sprains. They should be rigid and well padded and for extremity fractures they should cross the joint above and below the fracture site. For fractures involving a joint, the splint should include the long bones on either side of the joint. As a general rule, joints should be splinted in a position of function. This means that the elbow is splinted at 90 degrees, the ankle at 90 degrees, the knee ever-so-slightly bent, and the wrist and hand should be placed in what is referred to as the beer-can positions—that is, the position in which one would hold a can of beer (and no, we surf docs didn't make that up for the book . . . honest).

Splints can be improvised from a variety of rigid materials such as tent poles, fishing poles, pieces of wood, and sleeping rolls in combination with an Ace wrap, which holds the rigid members in place and also provides compression. Be sure to use plenty of padding between the skin and rigid members of the splint. If you don't have an Ace wrap, take your least-favorite rash guard and, starting at the bottom hem, cut around in a spiral fashion to fabricate a long three-inch-wide elastic bandage. Often it is helpful to fabricate a splint on the arm or leg of an uninjured person, before placing it on the injured surfer. Ultimately, the injured person is the best judge of weather a splint is properly stabilizing a fracture, is adequately padded, or is too tight.

You'll save some major headaches with improvised splint-making by carrying a lightweight, compact, rolled-up SAM Splint in your first aid kit. We recommend the 4.25-inch-by-36-inch version as a convenient and versatile splint, which is relatively easy to apply and can be molded for use on wrists, ankles, knees, and elbows. It is essentially a long flat thin strip of malleable aluminum backed on both sides with foam. When a length of the material is bent into a gutter shape, it becomes stiff and suitable for use as a splint.

Below are instructions on how to make an ankle splint and a wrist splint, which are among the most common types of splints you'll need to make as a surfer.

# How to Make Wrist and Ankle Splints

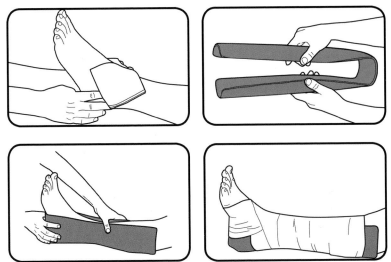

First, place padding on bony prominences. Then mold splint as shown. Apply elastic bandage to keep splint in place and to generate compression.

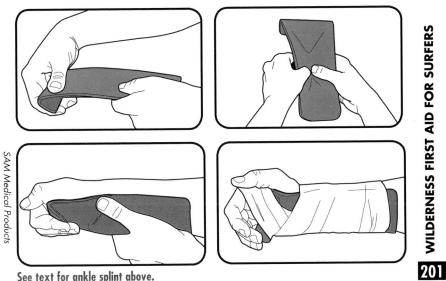

See text for ankle splint above.

**WILDERNESS FIRST AID FOR SURFERS**

## Dislocations

A dislocation occurs when a bone forming a joint gets pulled out of its socket. Usually the ligaments and tendons that hold the joint in place are stretched or torn in the process. The surfer will generally know that something is out of place, and movement about the joint is severely restricted and painful. On inspection, the joint often appears distorted or squared off in comparison to the opposite normal joint. Sometimes dislocations are difficult to differentiate from a fracture, and occasionally joints are dislocated *and* fractured.

## Treating Dislocated Joints

If treatment will be significantly delayed, it is best to attempt to fix (reduce) a dislocation in the field. Reducing (fixing) a dislocation quickly has a number of advantages. To begin with, reducing a joint provides significant pain relief to the patient. Furthermore, joints left out of socket for a long time can result in injury to nerves and blood vessels and are harder to pull back in place if they've been out for a while. Lastly, some return of function in a splinted position will facilitate travel. While there is a theoretical risk that you are pulling on a fracture and not a dislocation, the risk of making the situation worse is minimal. Luckily, the most common dislocations, namely, the shoulder, finger, and kneecap, are relatively easy to put back in place with a little guidance.

Once a joint has come out of socket, the surrounding muscles tend to tighten up, which keeps the affected body part (finger, arm) shortened compared to its normal length. In order for the bone to get back into place, the limb needs to be pulled out to length (overcoming the force of the muscles), which will allow the bone to freely pop back into its socket. The tricks to reducing a joint are first to get the patient to relax their muscles and, second, to pull very, very gradually. Sudden yanking causes involuntary muscle contraction, which is exactly the opposite of what you are trying to achieve.

## How to Reduce a Shoulder Dislocation

Let's start with shoulder dislocations, because they are fairly common among surfers. Shoulders are usually dislocated when the arm is overhead and gets rotated outward and forced backward. This can easily happen when getting axed by the lip of a big wave while trying to dive forward to get away from your board in a wipeout and even while paddling, particularly if you had a prior history of shoulder dislocations. The individual with a dislocated shoulder will usually support the injured arm with the uninjured hand, keeping the elbow of the injured

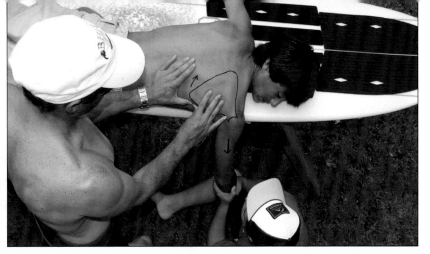

To reduce a dislocated shoulder, gradually pull the arm downward with steadily increasing force as an assistant pushes the tip of the scapula as shown.

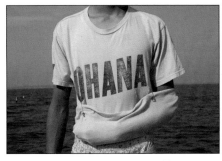

Use safety pins to make an effective shoulder sling.

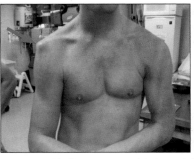

Note squared-off appearance of dislocated shoulder.

side slightly in front of and away from the body. The contour of the shoulder will have lost some of its rounded appearance and look different than the other side. They will not be able to touch their good shoulder with the hand of the injured side. Usually the surfer will know that the shoulder is out.

The sooner you try to get the shoulder back in, the easier it will be. Have the person lie facedown on an elevated surface such as a table, with the injured arm hanging over the edge. Try to create a relaxed atmosphere so the person (who will be in significant pain) can relax. If available, have the person take pain medications (Vicodin 325/5 mg, Motrin 800 mg) or muscle relaxants (Valium, diazepam 5 mg) or both. One assistant should pull very, very gently downward, while the other assistant pushes the tip of the scapula (shoulder blade) toward the spine as illustrated. The downward force should be increased very gradually (over a few minutes), but steadily. This will cause some discomfort, but the person needs to keep those muscles relaxed. Firmly massaging the shoulder muscles helps keeps them relaxed and greatly facilitates successful reduction. We often will tell the patient something like, "Relax, close your eyes, breathe slowly . . . give me your arm." The downward traction may eventually need to be quite forceful, particularly if the surfer is big and strong. If this is a first-time dislocation, the traction may need to continue for a good five minutes or longer until you hear (and the patients feels) a gratifying clunk. Generally there is no mistaking that the shoulder is back in. As a test, see if the person can touch the uninjured shoulder with the hand of the injured side. If they can do so, the shoulder is in. If they can't, give the meds a half hour or so to sink in and give it another go.

Once the shoulder is back in place, the surfer should be put in a shoulder sling, which can easily be improvised with a couple of safety pins and a shirt. The sling should be worn for two weeks, but should be occasionally removed to gently straighten and flex the elbow and wrist joints to prevent them from stiffening up. This type of sling can also be used for collarbone fractures and elbow injuries.

## How to Reduce a Finger Dislocation

Each finger (except the thumb) has three joints, but it is usually the middle joint that gets dislocated. This happens to surfers who get the leash twisted around a finger during a wipeout or if the fingers of an outstretched hand get jammed into the seafloor. The finger joint will appear deformed, and there will be little to no movement about the joint. Because there are few muscles to overcome, reducing a dislocated finger joint is usually pretty easy.

Use one hand to pull the finger out to length, while pinching the base of the dislocated bone with your other hand as illustrated in the diagram below. Use your thumb to apply downward pressure to the base of the bone, as your other hand pulls lengthwise until the joint clicks back

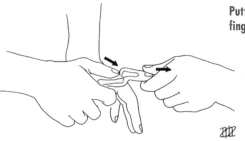

Putting a dislocated finger joint back in place.

into place. Once reduced, buddy-tape the injured finger to a neighboring finger for support using a few strips of tape. Occasionally, a dislocated finger, once reduced, will refuse to stay put and pops right back out of socket again. This is because a piece of connective tissue is in the joint, blocking the bone from fitting back into its proper place. This type of dislocation generally will require surgical repair by a hand surgeon.

## How to Reduce a Dislocated Kneecap (Patella)

The kneecap (patella) is dislocated more frequently in women than men. These injuries occur when the leg is straight, and the knee gets twisted as might happen when landing an aerial. The kneecap pops to the outside of the knee, the person will not be able to walk, and the knee will be held in a slightly bent position. The patella can be felt on the outer part of the knee, as opposed to in front of the knee where it belongs.

To reduce these, try to straighten the person's leg. Sometimes that's all it takes, but usually you need to apply pressure with both of your thumbs on the outside edge of the kneecap and push it toward the center. Once reduced, the individual should be able to straighten and bend their leg, although there will continue to be some residual discomfort. A knee brace and crutches (if available) will provide added comfort and speed the healing of torn ligaments.

## Allergic Reactions

Allergic reactions can be caused by exposure to a huge variety of substances either from ingestion (food or medicine), a sting, or skin contact. Fortunately, regardless of the cause of an allergic reaction, the treatment protocol is the same.

Individuals suffering from an allergic reaction generally develop itchy, red, slightly raised patches on the skin called hives. Hives can vary in size and location and may disappear from one place and reappear in another. Hives from a sting (e.g., jellyfish, bee) often begin right at the site of the sting and then may spread outward.

The majority of allergic reactions are limited to hives, which though extremely itchy and bothersome, are not dangerous, and can be treated with Benadryl (diphenhydramine) 25–50 mg every six hours. Benadryl is a safe drug whose main side effects are sleepiness and dry mouth. If you find Benadryl too sedating, you can use Claritin (loratadine) 10 mg once a day. If Benadryl (or Claritin) does not seem to be doing the trick, a more potent drug is the steroid prednisone, which can be taken at

60 mg daily for four days, though some physicians will prescribe a tapering dose (e.g., 60 mg on day 1, then 40 mg, 20 mg, 10 mg).

In some cases, particularly if the person has had allergic reactions to the same allergen before, the symptoms can quickly progress over the course of a few minutes and cause swelling of the lips, tongue, and throat. Some people with severe allergies will also develop wheezing, shortness of breath, and become light-headed or even faint due to low blood pressure. Any symptoms beyond simple hives constitute a true medical emergency because significant swelling of the airways can result in airway obstruction and death. As soon as it becomes clear that an allergic reaction is causing swelling of the lips, tongue, throat, or wheezing, epinephrine 0.3 mg should be administered intramuscularly into the victim's thigh. After epinephrine, Benadryl 50 mg and prednisone 60 mg should be administered by mouth. Epinephrine spring-loaded autoinjector kits (EpiPen) are available via prescription and should be a component of any advanced first aid kit and carried by anyone known to suffer from severe allergic reactions. People suffering from a severe allergy may develop a return of symptoms when the epinephrine wears off (thirty minutes) and may require a second injection. Transport the person to a medical facility once treatment has been initiated.

## Treatment of Allergic Reactions

| Symptoms | Treatment |
|---|---|
| Mild hives | Oral Benadryl 25–50 mg every six hours |
| Severe hives | Oral Benadryl 50 mg every six hours, plus oral prednisone 60 mg daily for four days |
| Hives and swelling of airway | Intramuscular epinephrine injection 0.3 mg, plus oral Benadryl 50 mg every six hours, plus oral prednisone 60 mg daily for four days |

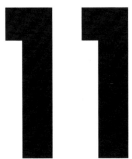

# 11

## Dangerous Marine Animals

The oceans are by far the largest wilderness areas on earth, covering 71 percent of the planet's surface. While the fringes of these oceans are our surfing playgrounds, they are also home to thousands upon thousands of species of marine animals. In fact, four-fifths of all life-forms live in the sea, and each has adapted unique ways to protect themselves from predators, reproduce, and gather food. While the vast majority of marine creatures are harmless, a few are not.

The true waterman is familiar with the marine ecosystem in which he/she surfs and takes a particularly keen interest in the behavior and habits of any native species that can bite, poke, or sting. For the traveling surfer, this often means obtaining local knowledge from surfers or fishermen in the area so as to avoid unnecessary run-ins with sea urchins, stingrays, jellyfish, and toothy creatures, which may be lurking beneath the surface. This chapter discusses how to best avoid injury from dangerous marine animals and reviews the specific treatment of animal-related injuries should they occur.

 A few general principles apply. Because many sharp and spiny creatures reside on the seafloor, make every effort to avoid touching bottom in order to prevent painful cuts, scrapes, and stings. If you wipeout in shallow water, avoid the temptation to stand up when retrieving your board—swim over to it instead. Paddle your board over the shallows, instead of walking—particularly when surfing tropical reef breaks, where the bottom is frequently jagged and may be littered with sea urchins and other hazardous critters. When walking through the water is unavoidable, tread as lightly as possible by using your floating board (fins up) to support some of your weight and to balance yourself. Hard-soled booties can provide significant protection from reef cuts and other injuries (though they are no guarantee against stonefish and stingrays), and wearing them is a good idea if you are surfing over a shallow live reef at an unfamiliar break.

Bites, stings, and cuts acquired in the marine environment are particularly prone to infection, especially if they result in puncture wounds, or if foreign matter (sand, coral bits, or spines) becomes embedded in the wound. Even seemingly pristine, crystal-clear ocean water is home to thousands of species of marine bacteria, and a few of these bacteria (e.g., *V. vulnificus, V. parahaemolyticus, E. rhusiopathiae*) can cause some pretty nasty infections. The best way to steer clear of such infections is to vigorously wash out any surfing-related wounds by forcefully irrigating them with at least half a liter of either normal saline solution or tap/drinking water (which is equally effective). Removing any particles remaining in the wound after irrigation is key to avoiding infections, but don't butcher yourself trying to get out sea urchin spines (more on that later). For more details on wound care and wound infections, see "Wound Care" in Chapter 10.

Marine stings, just like insect stings, have the potential to cause allergic reactions. Most of these reactions are minor, causing only local redness and itching, but occasionally allergic reactions can be severe, causing widespread raised itchy red welts (hives), wheezing, swelling of the lips and tongue, and even low blood pressure. It is important to keep a close eye on anyone suffering from an allergic reaction, because you'll need to be prepared to initiate treatment immediately if there are signs that the reaction is spreading beyond the site of the sting. The most serious reactions involve wheezing and swelling of the lips, tongue, and throat, because they can progress to airway obstruction and death if untreated. (See Chapter 10.)

Lastly, surfers from all corners of the globe seem to share the widely held belief that urine is the universal antidote for all manner of marine stings. The thought seems to go . . . if it is a jellyfish sting, piss on it. Fire coral sting: piss on it. Sea urchin, stonefish, whatever: piss on it. Unfortunately, this time-honored remedy is not supported by a single shred of scientific evidence, and while this treatment may provide considerable relief for the guy "providing" medical care, it does nothing (except perhaps add insult to injury) for the victim of the sting.

# Sharks: The Good, the Bad, and the Ugly

## SURF-SURVIVAL STORY

Kenny Doudt was on dawn patrol one chilly November, near Oregon's Haystack Rock, surfing a rare, clean northwest swell. It was a weekday, so the spot was uncrowded with surfers (though the sea lions were plentiful).

Without warning, Kenny was pulled underwater by a fifteen-foot great white shark that had both he and his board sandwiched in its mouth. The shark then surfaced and vigorously shook Kenny from side to side for about twenty seconds as his buddies watched in horror. Then the massive fish released its grip and slipped away. Miraculously, Kenny paddled back to shore alive despite the fact that he had four broken ribs, a collapsed lung, shredded muscles, and had lost many pints of blood. After over five hundred stitches, hours of surgery, and multiple blood transfusions, he made a full recovery, and has returned to surfing.

(Adapted from *Surfing with the Great White Shark* by Kenny Doudt, 1992)

**DANGEROUS MARINE ANIMALS**

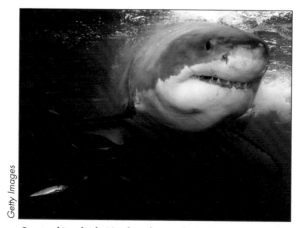

*Getty Images*

**Great white shark (*Carcharodon carcharias*).**

While encounters such as these are extremely rare, they are well publicized and send shudders through the collective psyche of the surfing community. While well-informed surfers need to have a healthy respect for sharks, shark phobia—a fairly common malady among surfers—is, for the most part, unfounded.

Sharks are prehistoric predators whose design is so perfect they have changed little in the last 400 million years. They are fast, agile swimmers equipped with flexible cartilaginous skeletons, a tough outer skin, and a keen sense of smell, vibration, and motion. The business end of these apex predators is well suited to the task at hand. Many species have powerful jaws lined with rows of replaceable razor-sharp teeth, which enable them to tear out large chunks of flesh out of their prey with each bite.

Fortunately for us, sharks do not regard humans as attractive food items and attacks on surfers are extremely rare. In fact, in US waters, with an estimated population of three million surfers, there are an average of only thirty shark attacks on surfers annually with only one shark-related fatality per year. Worldwide, there are an average of eighty documented shark attacks per year and roughly five fatalities, but only 60 percent of those involved surfers. Supporting the theory that sharks don't regard us as sources of food is the fact that over 90 percent of surfers survive shark attacks, and the majority of those attacks involve only a single bite. It has been estimated that your chance of being attacked by a shark when entering North American waters is one in five million. You are ten times more likely to be killed by lightning.

Of the 375 species of sharks, only 20 or so pose a threat to man, with the great white, tiger, and bull sharks being responsible for the vast majority of bites. Because species identification is difficult, any shark over six feet in length should be regarded as potentially dangerous. Theories abound as to why humans are occasionally attacked. Some scientists postulate that from below a surfer looks like a seal, and we are victims of mistaken identity. Sharks may mistake a splashing foot or hand for a fish, especially in water with low visibility (their underwater vision is about the same as ours). Others feel that sharks use their mouths as a means of exploring their environment (they have no hands) and take bites of unfamiliar objects to get more information. Whatever the reason, it is this bite-first-ask-questions-later behavior that has given sharks such a bad reputation over the years.

It comes as no surprise that the majority of shark attacks on surfers take place in areas where surfers come in close proximity to large populations of sharks. Sharks are known to frequent surf breaks near seal-breeding colonies, river mouths, and steep drop-offs, where food is abundant. Regions that are notorious for shark attacks include the coastlines of South Africa, much of Australia, Florida's Atlantic Coast, the Hawaiian Islands, and Northern California.

Attacks are most likely to occur to isolated surfers near dawn or dusk in murky water. If a large shark is spotted, it is best to leave

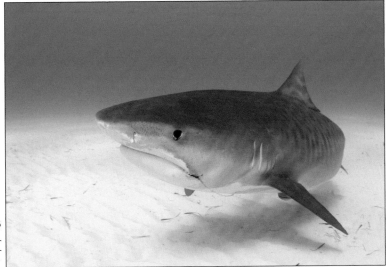

iStockphoto

Tiger shark (*Galeocerdo cuvier*).

the water calmly and slowly, as sharks are attracted to splashing and commotion. Just prior to attack, sharks often posture with an arched back, elevated snout, and depressed pectoral fins, and may begin swimming erratically. Unfortunately, because of their camouflage and stealthy style of approach, most surfers never see a shark before it hits. Despite a ferocious demeanor, sharks are opportunistic predators that try to avoid injury when feeding (most close their eyes just prior to attack to avoid eye injury) and appear to respect an opponent's size and power. If attacked, do not react passively; aggressively fend off the shark by striking it as hard as possible on their sensitive snout, eyes, or gills. Although many shark-repellent systems for surfers have been developed, none have proven to be practical and reliable.

The victim of a shark attack should be assisted to shore immediately. Rescuers are almost never attacked, and rendering assistance earns you major (and well-deserved) bragging rights in the lineup. When rendering assistance, lay the victim flat with the injured body part elevated, and apply direct pressure to any area that is bleeding. This is best done using the heel of one's palm covered with a towel or wet suit. Ten to fifteen minutes of continuous direct pressure will almost always stop bleeding, even if it is squirting out of an artery. For an extremely large bite, bigger than your hand can compress, cover the area with a folded-up towel and wrap a leash around it to make a pressure dressing. After bleeding has been controlled, immobilize the injured part with a splint (see section on splints in Chapter 10) and elevate it above the level of the heart. If direct pressure fails to stop the bleeding, you may need to apply a tourniquet to the injured extremity as described in Chapter 10.

Any exposed organs should be covered with a clean moist towel. The victim should be transported to the nearest hospital as soon as possible. Shark bites are at high risk of infection and require professional medical attention—which includes generous irrigation of wounds; repair of tendons, nerves, and blood vessels; loose closure; and appropriate antibiotics.

SMA archives

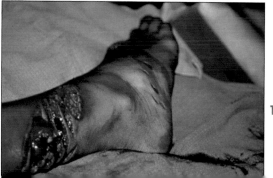

Typical shark bite.

Here are a few pointers when surfing in waters where sharks are known to reside to help ensure you are the only one in the water who is shredding:

1. Be wary of surfing at dawn or at dusk; sharks feed during these times so you may not be the only one on dawn patrol.

2. Avoid murky waters; they may mistake your hand or foot for a fish.

3. Avoid surfing in river mouths or near sewer drains or in groups of seals or other marine mammals, particularly rookeries; sharks often feed in these areas.

4. Avoid bleeding into the water; most of a shark's brain is devoted to smell (though it has never been shown that menstruating women are at increased risk of shark attack).

5. Be wary if you see schools of baitfish jumping out of the water and gulls squawking for leftovers. The big fish eat the little fish. And be wary of surfing near a floating seal or whale carcass.

6. Surf near other surfers, as sharks are more likely to attack isolated individuals.

7. If a large shark appears, leave the water with calm, slow movements—do not splash.

8. Do not wear shiny watches or jewelry or bright colors in the water—sharks are attracted to bright, shiny objects.

9. If attacked, try to repel the shark with sharp blows to its eyes, gills, or snout.

## In Defense of the Sharks

Many species of sharks are in danger from overfishing. Each year over 100 million sharks are killed for use as fertilizer, food, and for sport. Simply put, we kill ten million sharks for every human they kill. In Asia, sharks are slaughtered for their fins, which are made into soup, and in Polynesia for their teeth, which are used to make jewelry. In the United States, more than 90 percent of captured sharks are discarded. Though unlikely to replace panda bears as World Wildlife Fund poster children, sharks are an integral part of the marine ecosystem, culling out weak and diseased prey and preventing overpopulation. As surfers we need to be advocates for the marine environment and should lead by example. Any efforts at slaughtering sharks are grossly misguided. Sharks are among the most graceful and majestic creatures of the deep. For the most part, they leave us alone, so let's do the same for them and respect the real locals in the lineup.

**DANGEROUS MARINE ANIMALS**

# Stingrays: Avoidance and Treatment of Stings

Stingrays are shy, nonaggressive bottom dwellers that burrow into the sandy bottoms of tropical and semitropical waters worldwide, feeding on worms and mollusks. Their excellent camouflage can make them difficult to see, particularly when they lie on the bottom, partly covered with sand.

As a purely defensive weapon, stingrays possess one or two three- to six-inch-long serrated barbs located on the back of their thick, muscular tail. When stepped on or disturbed, a stingray will reflexively whip its tails back, often inflicting a puncture wound or jagged laceration to the hapless victim's foot or ankle. Adding insult to injury, the barb is encased in a thin venom-filled sheath, effectively making it a poison-tipped spear. The pain from a sting is sudden and severe, often described as an electrical or burning pain; it reaches its peak of intensity in thirty to sixty minutes and often radiates up the leg. Other symptoms such as vomiting, diarrhea, weakness, muscle twitching, and dizziness may occur, but are uncommon. Stings to the abdomen, chest, and arteries are extremely

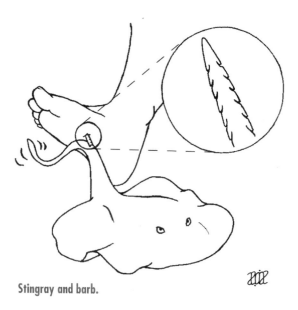

Stingray and barb.

rare but can have fatal consequences, as was the case with "crocodile hunter" Steve Irwin.

When surfing in waters known to contain stingrays, the best way to avoid being stung is to do the "stingray shuffle" when walking in shallow water, which will frighten these timid creatures away. Because their bony stinger is sharp and serrated like the edge of a knife, neoprene booties and wet suits offer little protection.

Stingray wounds should be vigorously irrigated with clean freshwater or saline solution to wash away bacteria, reducing the risk of infection. Next, soak the foot in nonscalding hot water (114°F, 45°C) for twenty to thirty minutes, which deactivates the venom and provides significant pain relief. If the pain returns, soaking the injured extremity again is usually helpful. Analgesic medications such as (Vicodin 325/5 mg, Motrin 800 mg) may be needed for adequate pain relief. Sometimes the stinger, fragments of the stinger, or its sheath are left in the wound and will need to be removed to prevent infection. If available, an X-ray or an ultrasound should be obtained to exclude the possibility of a retained barb. Because stingray wounds are so highly prone to infection, they should routinely be treated with antibiotics such as the combination of Bactrim (trimethoprim/sulfamethoxazole) and Keflex (cephalexin) for five days as a preventive measure. These wounds should *not* be closed tightly, because it turns out that stitching or taping a contaminated wound closed traps bacteria in the wound, *increasing* the risk of infection. After the wound has been irrigated and soaked, apply an antibiotic ointment such as Bacitracin and cover it with a clean gauze dressing. The injured foot should be elevated above the level of the heart to prevent swelling and reduce pain. Individuals suffering from symptoms other than just local pain (e.g., vomiting, diarrhea, dizziness) should seek prompt medical attention.

## Sea Urchin Injuries and Stings

Sea urchins are nonaggressive, slow-moving animals whose squat round bodies are covered with sharp, brittle spines. Because they inhabit crevices in shallow, rocky, and reefy waters over a wide range of latitudes, injuries to surfers from these spiny creatures are very common. The spines may be solid, hollow, or clawlike (pedicellariae), with the hollow and clawlike types capable of injecting venom. Of the 750 known species of sea urchins worldwide, approximately 80, found predominantly in tropical waters, are known to be poisonous.

Most injuries resulting from encounters with sea urchins are simple nonvenomous puncture wounds of the foot, often containing retained spine fragments. These wounds cause burning pain that generally subsides in the first few hours, but may persist for up to a week. A purple pigment left behind in a puncture wound frequently causes tattooing of the skin, but does not always mean that an embedded spine is present. X-rays or ultrasound are the most reliable way of determining the number and location of retained spines.

The majority of sea urchin injuries heal spontaneously, with gradual absorption or expulsion of retained spine fragments. Because the spines are so brittle, removing the deeply embedded ones is almost impossible, and attempting to dig them out often causes more harm than good. Our advice is to try to pull out any spines protruding from the skin and leave the rest alone, with the exception of those that have entered joints. Spines embedded in joints (usually fingers or toes) can lead to permanent pain and stiffness of the affected joint, and these should be removed by a surgeon. Occasionally, sea urchin injuries can become infected (warm, red, swollen, increasingly tender), and these, too, will require surgical excision and antibiotics such as Bactrim (trimethoprim/sulfamethoxazole) and Keflex (cephalexin).

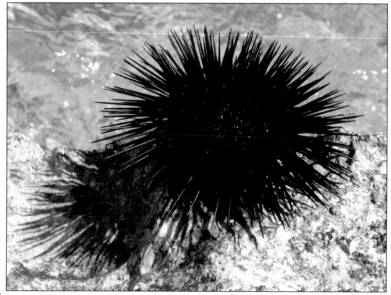

Venomous sea urchin.

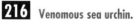

SURF SURVIVAL

Shutterstock

If an intense itchy rash develops a week after contact with a sea urchin spine, this is probably a delayed allergic reaction. Treat this with a steroid cream such as 1 percent hydrocortisone; for severe cases, oral steroids may be needed. Rarely, sea urchin spines will cause small, firm purple bumps (doctors call them granulomas), which appear months after the original injury. If these are in the sole or the palm, they can be painful and annoying, and also call for surgical removal.

Poisonous sea urchin stings cause an immediate and severe burning or aching pain, not only near the site of the wound, but also radiating up the afflicted arm or leg. Stings can also cause redness and swelling within hours of injury. Severe reactions may include dizziness, light-headedness, tingling of the skin, weakness, and temporary paralysis. For injuries caused by venomous sea urchins, first scrape off any

**Sea urchin tattoo.**

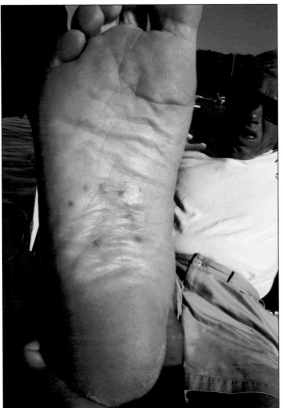

Nathanson

adherent pedicellariae (stubby three-clawed venomous spines) using a knife edge or credit card. Then soak the injured body part in non-scalding hot water (114°F, 45°C) to deactivate the venom. Elevate the injured part to alleviate pain, and reduce any swelling. Severe pain can be treated with ibuprofen (Advil, Motrin) or Vicodin. Victims suffering from light-headedness, tingling, weakness, or paralysis should be cared for in a hospital setting.

Sea urchin injuries are best prevented by not standing or walking on the seafloor. Whenever possible, lay on your board and paddle, and if you wipeout in shallow water, avoid the temptation to stand up; instead of walking, swim to retrieve your board. Hard-soled booties provide sufficient protection against sea urchin spines, but some spines are able to penetrate through neoprene booties.

## Coral Reef—"Reef Rash"

Athough coral reef may not generally be considered a dangerous marine animal, we surfers know otherwise. Abrasions from encounters with coral reef are so common among surfers as to merit their own medical diagnosis in surfer parlance—namely, reef rash. Considered by some hard-core tube chargers as a badge of honor, abrasions from coral reef are painful and have a tendency to get infected if not properly cared for. Wounds do not heal well when embedded with organic (once living) material such as fragments of coral reef, and any self-respecting reef rash will leave at least a few fragments of reef in your sorry hide. Furthermore, the reef itself is often covered with slime, bacteria, and viruses many of which can cause skin infections. No great surprise, but research has shown that the higher the local human population in the area, the higher the concentration of reef-dwelling bacteria, which likely translates into higher rates of infection from reef rash.

The key to avoiding infections from reef rash is to

**Tavaruan Reef Rash**

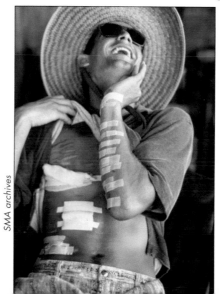

"I don't hurt .... "

thoroughly irrigate these abrasions with large volumes (at least one-half quart/500 cc) of clean freshwater (or saline solution), following the adage "The solution to pollution is dilution." A vigorous stream from a shower or sink faucet works well. Thoroughly scrubbing the wound as you irrigate it will serve to remove any retained particles of "coral dust" that are not visible to the naked eye. After the scrape has been meticulously cleaned, apply a layer of antibiotic ointment such as Bacitracin and cover it with a nonadherent dressing such as Telfa.

## Jellyfish, Sea Anemones, and Other Stingers

In contrast to many menacing-looking animals such as sharks, stingrays, and sea urchins, jellyfish and sea anemones are graceful, attractive, and often flowerlike, but they too are dangerous carnivorous predators. Instead of teeth, they rely on potent venoms delivered by microscopic stinging harpoons called nematocysts to stun and kill their prey. Nematocysts discharge on contact with skin, but only a small percentage of the millions of stingers on a jellyfish tentacle will actually deploy. The rest remain toxic, even when the tentacle has been torn from the body of the jellyfish, so treatment (described below) involves deactivating the venom of nematocysts that have fired, as well as the removal of undischarged nematocysts, so as to prevent further injury. Even dead jellyfish that have been lying on the beach for days should be avoided, because they, too, are capable of delivering a nasty sting.

Jellyfish, Portuguese man-of-war, sea anemones, and fire corals are all members of the phylum Cnidaria, which contains over ten thousand species. Among these primitive life-forms are over one hundred species whose nematocysts are powerful enough to penetrate human skin. Stings range in severity from the skin irritation that occurs when brushing against fire coral, to the potentially fatal sting of the Australian box jellyfish. Always be on the lookout for any signs of an allergic reaction due to a jellyfish sting, particularly if the victim has a prior history of allergies to the same species, as these reactions have been known to be fatal. (See "Allergic Reactions" in Chapter 10.)

Jellyfish often drift around in large swarms, mostly at the mercy of winds and currents, and inhabit all oceans, though the most poisonous species live in the tropics. While near-shore jellyfish swarms are usually unpredictable, some species come ashore at predictable intervals, like the Hawaiian box jellyfish, which congregates in protected bays on the island of Oahu seven to ten days after a full moon.

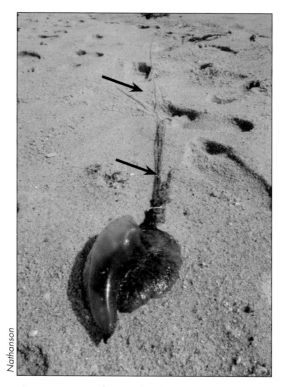

**Portuguese man-of-war *(Physalia physalis).*
Note the length of the tentacles.**

Most jellyfish stings are relatively benign and self-limited. The majority of species cause an immediate prickling or burning pain that typically lasts less than an hour, followed by itching and a tingling sensation. A reddish brown rash may quickly develop in the area of contact, often leaving temporary whiplike tentacle prints on the victim's skin. This type of sting is typical of the Atlantic Portuguese man-of-war (*Physalia physalis*), which is technically not a true jellyfish but a colony of hydrozoans; its smaller Pacific cousin, the blue bottle; and the enormous cold-water lion's mane jellyfish (*Cyanea capillata*). Large surface-area stings and those from the more poisonous varieties cause more intense pain lasting a few hours and often cause a raised rash that will eventually blister and leave a scar.

The box-type jellyfish (cubozoans), named for their four-cornered bell, are armed with some of the most potent venoms known to man and are capable of inflicting much more severe stings. The most deadly jellyfish, the Australian box (*Chironex fleckeri*), can be encountered

**Nematocyst in Action**

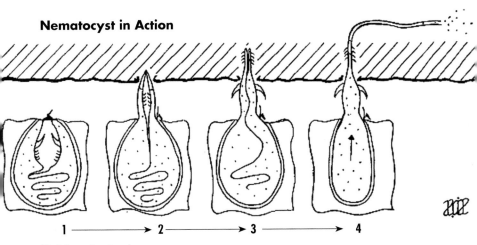

1 ──────→ 2 ──────→ 3 ──────→ 4

1) Trigger is tripped
2) Barb explodes outward through skin
3) Thread deploys by turning inside out
4) Venom is injected

along the northern coast of Australia, as well as in Indonesia and the Philippines. Stings from these species cause immediate excruciating burning pain and may cause breathing difficulty, low blood pressure, and rapid collapse of the victim. Tentacle prints from the Australian box jellyfish often blister, cause ulcerations through the skin, and can leave permanent scars. Death, which has been known to occur in as little as five minutes after the sting of a box jellyfish, is uncommon, but more deaths worldwide have been attributed to jellyfish stings than to shark attacks. Most of the fatalities are small women and children who have a large surface-area sting from a big jellyfish. The highest risk period for Australian box jellyfish stings is between October and May, during which time many beaches are netted off in an effort to protect bathers.

The less-dangerous but still fearsome Hawaiian box jellyfish (*Carybdea alata*) has a sting so painful that even macho surfers along Oahu's south shore will resort to wearing pantyhose to avoid being stung when these jellyfish swarm the lineup. The symptoms of the Hawaiian box are generally self-limited to a painful rash, but severe allergic reactions have been reported, and particularly severe stings may require intravenous medications for adequate pain relief.

The tiny and nearly invisible Indo-Pacific Irukandji jellyfish (*Carukia barnesi*), another cubozoan, has a nearly painless sting but can cause severe muscle cramps, breathing difficulty, nausea, and vomiting. These symptoms generally resolve within twenty-four hours, although deaths have been reported from this species as well.

Sea anemones are attractive, brightly colored flowerlike animals that are anchored by their stalks to the seafloor. Short fingerlike tentacles surrounding the mouth of the anemone are covered with nematocysts and are capable of stinging passing fish or unwary surfers. The sting from sea anemones is similar to that of a jellyfish, causing an immediate burning pain, which may be followed by tingling or itching. The less toxic species cause raised red hives, while more toxic species may cause blistering, ulceration, and may become infected. Treatment using vinegar is identical to that of a jellyfish sting.

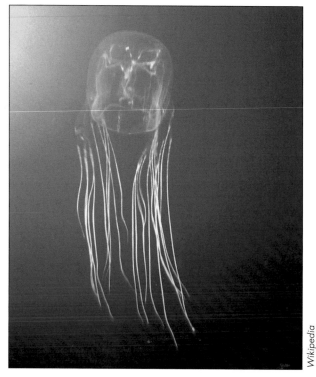

*Wikipedia*

Australian box jellyfish *(Chironex fleckeri).*

# Treatment

The treatment of all jellyfish stings involves removing loose tentacles from the skin, deactivating undischarged nematocysts, and finally, scraping off any residual tentacle fragments. The best way to remove adherent tentacles is to rinse them off with seawater and then carefully pick off any that remain using your fingertips (the skin there is too thick for most nematocysts to penetrate). Nematocysts of many species (including the Australian box) can be deactivated using household vinegar (acetic acid), but this is ineffective for the Portuguese man-of-war, blue bottle, and Hawaiian box, and will actually trigger nematocysts to fire. For those latter species, use nonscalding hot water (114°F, 45°C) for five to ten minutes from a shower or tub. Irrigate stings to the eye by blinking underwater or with a stream of saline solution or contact lens solution. Never use vinegar in the eye. Rubbing the skin or rinsing with freshwater, alcohol, ammonia, papain, or urine should be avoided, as this will cause more nematocysts to discharge, exacerbating the sting. Once the nematocysts have been deactivated, any adherent material

## Range of the Deadly Australian Box Jellyfish

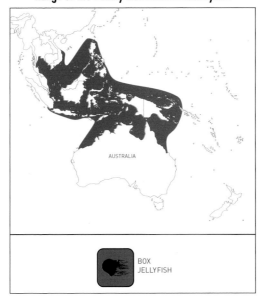

AUSTRALIA

BOX
JELLYFISH

should be shaved off with a knife, razor, or even a credit card. Any victim suffering from more than just a painful local reaction should seek medical attention.

For skin irritation that persists for more than twelve hours, a topical steroid cream and oral Benadryl (diphenhyramine) are often useful. An injectable Australian box jellyfish antivenom is available in some lifeguard towers and hospitals in Northern Australia and should be administered as a shot or given intravenously for any severe box jellyfish stings.

## Prevention

When surfing in jellyfish-infested waters, a wet suit or rash guard provides excellent protection for covered areas. Whole-body rash guards and stinger suits provide full-body protection in warm water (from jellyfish stings and the sun) and make sense if surfing in northern Australia or parts of Indonesia during the summer months. For protection of areas not easily covered by a rash guard (hands, feet, and face), a creme called Safe Sea has been shown to be very effective. Safe Sea is an innovative new product based upon the protective slime of the clown fish, which enables them live among anemones without being stung. This sting repellent is also available in combination with a sunscreen!

### SURF-SURVIVAL TIP

#### For Jellyfish Stings

1. Exit the water to assess the sting.

2. Flush affected area with saltwater (not freshwater, alcohol, or urine).

3. Remove adherent tentacles carefully with fingertips.

4. For most species, bathe the sting in vinegar.

   • For stings from Portuguese man-of-war, blue bottle, and Hawaiian box jellyfish, bathe the sting in nonscalding (114°F, 45°C) hot water for five to ten minutes.

5. Scrape off any remaining nematocysts with a knife edge or credit card.

6. If there are any systemic effects such as difficulty breathing, vomiting, lethargy, or confusion, call 911 and seek immediate medical care.

7. If a rash persists longer than twelve hours, apply 1 percent hydrocortisone cream to the affected area and take diphenhydramine 25 mg (Benadryl).

# Seabather's Eruption a.k.a. Sea Lice or Pica Pica

As the common name "sea lice" implies, seabather's eruption is an extremely itchy bumpy rash, caused by a tiny critter. The critters in this case aren't insects, but jellyfish or sea anemone larvae, too small to be seen by the naked eye, that get trapped in or under bathing suits or wet suits. Unlike jellyfish stings, which almost universally affect unclothed areas, these tiny larvae, which are armed with nematocysts like their adult counterparts, tend to sting parts of the body that *are* covered by a rash guard or bathing suit. While the free-floating larvae don't cause stings on exposed skin, when trapped in a bathing suit, wet suit, or surfer's hair, their nematocysts can be triggered by mechanical friction or changes in salinity as occurs with evaporation or when rinsing off in freshwater.

Along the Eastern Seaboard of the United States, seabather's eruption is either caused by the larval form of the thimble jellyfish (Florida) or the larvae of a sea anemone (Long Island) and causes an itchy, red, bumpy rash that doesn't appear until hours after exiting the water. While in the water, there is no itching, pain, or visual cue to give you any warning that you are, in fact, in the midst of a giant swarm of larvae.

Irritation develops along areas of friction with surf wear, such as the collar of a wet suit, a bathing suit waistline, or bathing suit top. The rash is mainly caused by an allergic reaction to the sting, as opposed to the sting itself, so itching, rather than pain, is the predominant symptom and, like the rash of poison ivy, it can last for a week or more if untreated. Once you've had seabather's eruption (and are sensitized to the allergen), subsequent exposures tend to cause more intense reactions.

In tropical waters, such as Fiji, there lurks a more painful form of this invisible menace. This variety causes an obvious sting while you are still in the water, often inflicting pain on everyone in the lineup. It is likely that some of these more painful forms of seabather's eruption are due to tiny bits of adult jellyfish tentacles that have been torn to shreds by heavy surf.

Because the stinging cells are trapped in your clothing, you can avoid the Atlantic variety of seabather's eruption by removing your bathing suit while still in the water! Or by rinsing yourself off with saltwater as opposed to freshwater (which activates the nematocysts). Treat the rash and itch of seabather's eruption with a topical steroid (1% hydrocortisone creme) and, if needed, an antihistamine such as Benadryl.

DANGEROUS MARINE ANIMALS

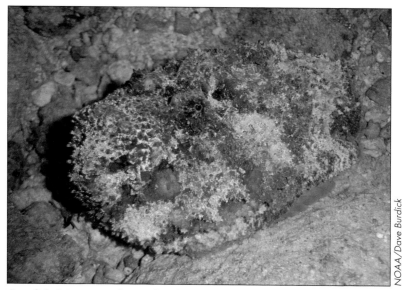

NOAA/Dave Burdick

Stonefish: Poisonous, well camouflaged, and looking like a stone.

## Stonefish and Other Stinging Fish

The family Scorpaenidae are a group of squat six- to fourteen-inch-long tropical reef fish that lay nearly motionless in the shallows awaiting passing prey. These bottom dwellers can be so sedentary that seaweed will grow on their backs, making them virtually indistinguishable from the seafloor. A common feature of this rather ugly group of fish—which include the likes of the toadfish, lionfish, and the wharty ghoul—are numerous venomous dorsal spines, which are erected when the fish is threatened. Injuries commonly occur when an unsuspecting surfer steps on a scorpion fish, and the stout, sharp, dorsal spines penetrate through the sole of the victim's foot, injecting venom. The sting causes an immediate intense burning pain, which lasts for a few hours and radiates up the leg. Swelling of the foot and blister formation at the site of the sting are common. Wounds from stinging fish may become infected, particularly if spine fragments remain embedded in the wound. The pain from the sting of the dreaded Indo-Pacific stonefish (*Synanceia horrida*), the most dangerous of the lot, can last for days if untreated and may cause vomiting, diarrhea, delirium, and heart problems. Occasional deaths have been reported.

## Range of the Stonefish

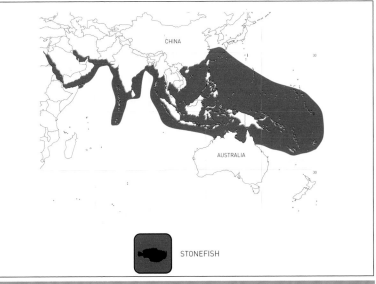

STONEFISH

Weaver fish, found on the sandy bottoms of many surf breaks in France, Spain, and England, are also armed with venomous dorsal spines, but are slightly less toxic than the scorpion fish. As opposed to merely sitting on the seafloor, these fish bury themselves in the sand, leaving only their poisonous spines exposed. Step carefully in Europe!

## Treatment

Like the venom from stingrays, the venom from all stinging fish can be partially deactivated with heat, by immersing the affected foot in nonscalding hot water (114°F, 45°C) for five to ten minutes. After a hot-water soak, the small puncture wound should be cleaned with soap and water and irrigated with a vigorous stream of freshwater. The affected foot should be elevated above the level of the heart, and the puncture covered with clean gauze. Pain can be treated with Motrin (ibuprofen) 800 mg, every six hours, but a stronger prescription medication like Vicodin may be required, particularly in the case of stonefish stings. Any symptoms beyond localized foot pain and swelling warrant a visit to the hospital. If there is suspicion that fragments of a spine remain in the wound (i.e., if the victim complains of a foreign-body sensation), then an X-ray should be obtained. Stonefish antivenom (CSL Australia), which is produced from purified sheep serum (bahhh!), is indicated for severe stonefish stings but is manufactured in limited quantities and is generally only available at a few hospitals in Australia.

## Sea Snakes

There are over fifty-five species of sea snakes that inhabit the tropical and semitropical near-shore waters of the Indian and Pacific Oceans, including Fiji, northern Australia, and southern Mexico. The good news is that they are generally nonaggressive and have small mouths with poorly developed fangs so that most bites (approximately 80 percent) do not deliver venom. The bad news is that they are among the most poisonous animals known to mankind, and bites can be fatal. Sea snakebites, like terrestrial snakebites, are usually not surprise attacks. Most bite victims see the snake and are messing with it (or clearing their fishing nets) before they are bitten. As taught to us back in medical school, those at risk for snakebites can best be described by the "the five Ts"—toothless, T-shirt, tattoo, tequila, and testosterone. While not exactly politically correct, you get the idea that Darwin's survival of the fittest is at

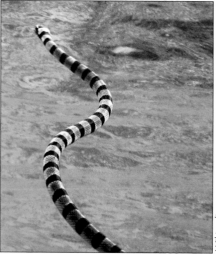

*Wikipedia*

**Yellow-lipped sea krait (Laticauda colubrina). Don't tread on me.**

work here. Generally, if you don't mess with a sea snake, it won't mess with you.

Unlike the bite of terrestrial snakes, which really hurt, sea snakebites cause so little pain that the victim may not even be aware that they *were* bitten. The onset of symptoms is anywhere from thirty minutes to four hours and include muscle aches, weakness, slurred speech, trouble swallowing, and blurry vision. Symptoms can progress to coma, respiratory paralysis, and death.

## Treatment

Initial first aid includes having the victim lie down and remain as still as possible, because any muscle activity will act to pump venom toward the heart and into the circulation. Next, wrap an Ace bandage snugly around the length of the bitten extremity and use a SAM Splint to immobilize it. If these materials are unavailable, cut a long three-inch-wide strip from a wet suit or rash guard to make an elastic wrap and use a tent pole or stick for support (as illustrated below). Keep the limb at the level of the heart. This "pressure immobilization" technique puts light pressure on the veins, sequestering venom in the bitten limb so it can't spread to the rest of the body.

Sea snakebites are life-threatening emergencies, and after a constricting splint has been placed, the victim should be immediately transported to the nearest medical facility lying faceup, preferably a hospital with the ability to provide intensive care. Sea snake antivenom can be lifesaving and should be administered to anyone with a suspected sea snakebite that is experiencing any symptoms.

The pressure immobilization technique used to treat sea snakebites.

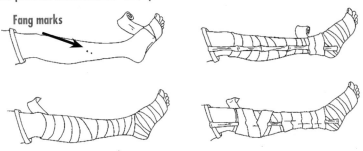

Fang marks

# Saltwater Crocodiles

"Everyone who spends a lot of time in Costa Rica has some horrific croc stories. The ones I heard about and the one I saw with my own eyes include the kid who got killed at Tivives (the story I heard is four gringos paddled out, three paddled in), the guy who got bit at Tivives (he showed me the scar . . . over and over), the croc I saw swim up the face of a wave at the Tulin rivermouth . . . eight-foot face . . . six-foot croc, and the Israeli dude in Tulin whose dog got eaten by a croc about thirty yards from where we were sleeping . . . on the ground . . . under mosquito nets. He walked past us with his dog's leg in his hand . . . we got a hotel room." (Tim's blog)

As a kid, did you ever daydream about what it would be like to live in the age of the dinosaurs, trying to survive amidst huge carnivorous reptiles? Well, saltwater crocodiles are modern-day dinosaurs, and judging by their appetite for human flesh, we would not have fared well. There are only a handful of animals that can truly be considered man-eaters (even sharks usually swim off after the first bite), but crocodiles are certainly among them.

The largest of all living reptiles, the saltwater crocodile (*Crocodylus porosus*) routinely reaches eighteen feet in length and weighs 2,200 pounds or more. They have a broad geographic range, from northern

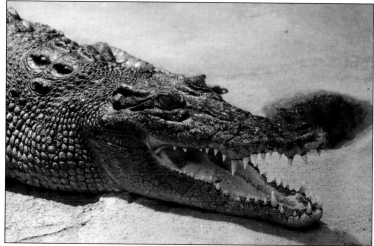

*Wikipedia*

**SURF SURVIVAL**

Saltwater crocodile *(Crocodylus porosus)*—A true man-eater.

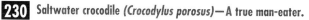

Australia to Southern India (including parts of Indonesia, Malaysia, and Borneo), and inhabit brackish rivers and estuaries, often swimming out to sea. Though sluggish in appearance, crocodiles are fast, powerful swimmers and surprising quick and agile on land. These apex predators are capable of taking down water buffalo and can generate enough jaw pressure to crack the skull of a cow. The slightly smaller American crocodile (*Crocodylus acutus*) inhabits both coasts of the Americas from northern Mexico to Venezuela and Peru, including many islands in the Caribbean, and has also been known to attack man (see above).

Crocs are well-camouflaged stealthy swimmers that often appear to be floating logs (if you fail to notice the beady eyes), and most attacks occur on unsuspecting swimmers and those camping near the edges of rivers and marshes. Crocodiles have been known to attack, kill, and eat surfers. Attacks most frequently occur at twilight or at night, and their usual MO is to grab the victim by the leg and twirl them underwater until they drown. Then they'll leave their kill in the sun for a few days to ripen up prior to consumption. If you're not scared of crocodiles, you should be. Those who do survive an attack often suffer extremity fractures and puncture wounds, which have a high incidence of infection. Treatment is similar to that for shark bites.

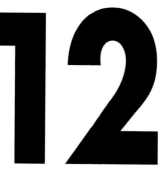

# 12

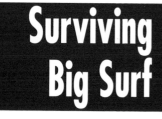

# Surviving Big Surf

The focus of this chapter is on safely riding truly big surf. Fraught with danger, yes, but you can safely coexist with big surf, just as you can readily drive down a highway with semis thundering toward you just the other side of a double yellow line. You can survive big surf if you take care to learn where that double yellow line is, and not cross it.

It is estimated by action sports advertisers that there are about twenty million surfers worldwide, but that includes anyone who has ever surfed, even just once, and all forms of surfing, including bodyboarding. The number of active, stand-up surfers is a lot lower—perhaps only four million people worldwide surf at least once per month. While 90 percent of those have probably ridden waves that were at least head high, maybe only 10 percent of active surfers, or about four hundred thousand, have ever ridden waves double overhead or bigger. Bigger than that and the proportion drops radically—figure less than three thousand surfers have ever ridden waves four times overhead or bigger. Eight to ten times overhead, and you're looking at less than a hundred, though more have done it on Jet Skis. 2009–2010 was a watershed season, with a dramatic shift away from towing-in back to paddling in, even in waves over forty feet in height.

The reason there are so few big-wave surfers is not that surfers worldwide are chicken: it's more about access and the chance to gain enough experience—big surf is a rare event, occurring in only a few places in the world and on only a limited number of days per year.

## Size Matters

If you are lucky enough to be present where truly big surf is arriving, the question naturally arises: *Am I up for surfing it, or will I be watching this swell from the shore?* The starting point for that internal conversation is to ask, *How big is it really, and how dangerous?* Answer that and then you can make your determination of whether you're up to it.

> "You're telling me it's only six foot out there? Well, if that's six foot, then your dick must only be an inch long." —Bob Wise (owner of Wise Surfboards, Ocean Beach, San Francisco)

There is no commonly agreed-upon way to judge wave height by sight alone. Nonsurfers are continuously perplexed when they happen to be looking out at big waves that, to their eyes, look at least twenty feet high, but the surfer standing next to them is calling it ten feet.

It wouldn't be so bad if all surfers similarly saw it as ten feet, but they are just as likely to call it twelve to fifteen feet or six to eight feet or even three to four feet. The important thing to remember is that many surfers undercall wave height, often absurdly so.

It is not worth trying to understand why, other than to realize that, since surfing originated in Hawaii, the dominant method of judging wave heights comes from there. It is referred to as the North Shore method. Adherents to this venerated system claim to measure wave height from the back, not the front of the wave. In other words, not the face of the wave, where one actually rides, but the back of the wave—never mind that the back of a wave is all but invisible from where they are standing onshore sizing up the waves. Furthermore, for big waves breaking over shallow bottoms, such as Teahupoo, in Tahiti, the back of the wave may only be two feet high, but the front of the wave could be over twenty feet! Truth be told, most surfers using the North Shore method aren't even considering the height of the backs of waves; they're just trying to be macho and love getting a rise out of you.

### SURF-SURVIVAL TIP

**Do everything you can to not fall prey to the North Shore wave height system—it will only get you or someone else in trouble.**

Big waves tend to break far from shore and can be hard to see, much less to judge their size. So, how to know? Don't rely solely on newspaper, TV/radio, the Internet weather report predictions, or buoy readings, which are mainly based on open-ocean sea-wave heights. Although buoy readings somewhat correlate to inshore breaking wave heights, they can be dangerously misleading for long-period swells (thirteen seconds or longer): an eight-foot buoy reading for a sixteen-second interval swell may result in breaking waves that are twice as big as an eight-foot buoy reading for an eight-second interval swell!

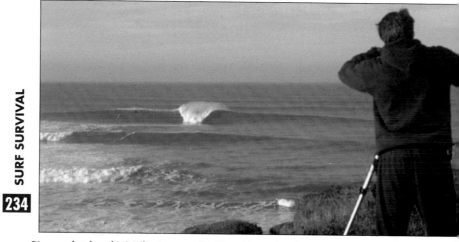

**Big, yes, but how big? What's your call?** *Hint: this is a big day at Maverick's.*

We call surf big, but not tall, which means we are also talking about the volume and mass of a wave—how thick and mean it is. Every surfer should be able to calculate wave interval (also called wave period), which is how long it takes for two consecutive waves to pass the same spot: start counting seconds (one, one thousand; two, one thousand; etc.) right after you first see a wave break until the next wave breaks in approximately the same spot. It is most relevant to do this during a set that is a group of two to five (or more) bigger waves, which may only arrive every few minutes. Know, too, that it can be useful to measure the time between sets: if getting shorter, the swell is building; if sets are less frequent, the swell is dropping.

Most online surf forecasters and wave reporters skirt the wave height issue by going to a simpler system based on how tall the wave looks when someone is riding it. It assumes the rider is standing up straight and is gliding along the bottom of the wave. By that system, the wave can be reasonably said to be chest-high or head-high or double overhead and so forth. (Just for the record, you can convert to height in feet: a double-overhead wave is about twice your height or about ten to twelve feet of wave face height.) The overhead system is probably the safest way to judge and speak of wave height. Note: using this system requires that someone is out there riding the waves!

## Top Big Wave Spots in the World

| Name | Where | When | Hazards |
| --- | --- | --- | --- |
| Maverick's | Half Moon Bay, California | October–April | Kodak courage, cold water, crowds, rocks, sharks |
| Todos Santos | Island off Ensenada, Mexico | November–March | Isolated, Jet Skiers |
| Waimea Bay | North Shore, Oahu | November–March | Crowds, currents, shore break |
| Outer Reefs | North Shore (multiple spots) | November–March | Distance in, currents |
| Jaws | Maui | November–March | Jet Skiers, off-shore winds |
| Dungeons | Cape Town, S. Africa | May–November | Sharks, kelp, beach crime |
| Nazare | Portugal | October–April | Shore break, rocks, Jet Skiers |

# Fear and Allure

One of the most exciting moments for any surfer is to be the first person to paddle out, particularly on big days, when all other surfers are staying ashore, jittery, and unsure and making excuses. That is when one comes up against a more universal method of judging wave height, by looking into yourself and deciding if you feel comfortable with not only how big it looks, but also the entire situation: the vibe on the beach, how wicked the ocean seems, how your recent big-wave surfs worked out, what kind of day you've been having, suddenly remembering you forgot to run an errand. It's nothing objective or rational—are you freaked out or feeling confident?

> **"Big waves are measured not in feet but by increments of fear." —Buzzy Trent (North Shore, 1963).**

Perhaps the only thing those silly beach blanket movies got right about surfing is that for most surfers, it really is about sitting out there and waiting for a "big one." Even if it is only a head-high day, if a set is coming in that includes a clearly bigger wave, you better believe that every surfer out there has their eyes on it and will soon be scrambling to position themselves to claim it as their own. A bigger wave has unbelievable allure, and for the chance to catch such a wave, surfers will sometimes sit for hours, no matter how cold they are or how late it will make them for a land-based obligation.

At some point, though, in big surf, the big waves they are seeing will have the opposite effect, such that an internal invisible fear line is crossed. At that point, a surfer begins to physically (and mentally) position themselves a bit to the sidelines, where they aren't likely to have to try to catch the biggest one but still might catch something—they still crave being out there, sharing in the excitement of being around big waves. At some point, if it gets bigger still, the allure will be overridden by fear, and they will likely finally beat a retreat to shore, however gradually (hoping to catch a smallish big one on the way in).

Big surf doesn't occur rapidly, usually taking six to eight hours to fully build—it would be unusual for overhead surf to double in size in less than two hours, but in open-ocean and exposed places like Hawaii, it can happen. In general, though, you don't have to worry much about suddenly being ambushed by giant surf. Oceanographers speak of extreme or rogue waves (greater than two and a half times average wave height during a big swell), but they are rare as hen's teeth. And tidal waves, also extremely rare, are irrelevant when discussing big wave surfing, which is mainly done in greater water depths than the more dangerous inshore, shallow depths where tidal waves wreak havoc.

It is a different story if you are onshore, hanging out or perhaps camping. Learn from the February 2010 experiences of surfers in Chile: if there is a large earthquake and you are on the shore, head immediately for high ground—leave all your belongings behind, you may only have seconds before the tsunami hits.

> "On any given day in front of my house on the beach up from Pipeline, I see surfers limping along like zombies, with swollen arms, legs, and scratches from head to toe."
> —Fred van Dyke

## How Risky Is Big-Wave Surfing?

Throughout the evolution of big-wave surfing, from Greg Noll and the Boys at Waimea in the late '50s to the Outer Reefs in the '80s and finally to the '90s and beyond at Jaws and Maverick's, there has been a jaw-dropping stepping up in the size of waves being ridden. What hasn't changed is that, with each step forward, there is a chorus of experts certain there will be an epidemic of deaths among that new breed of big-wave riders. But that just hasn't been the case. Yes, nonsurfers regularly are swept off a high-berm beach and drowned by big surf, and beginners and inebriates may drown, but very few experienced big-wave surfers have died in big surf. In the past fifty years, there have been so few, probably less than fifteen, that each death has become a legend. Amazingly, there has yet to be a death involving tow-in surfing (though many injuries, some severe).

Overview of Big Waimea Bay at the Eddie.

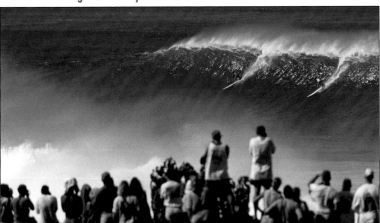

iStockphoto

## The Legend of Dickie Cross

In 1943, seventeen-year-old Dickie Cross, eager to learn how to ride bigger waves, went out with big-wave veteran thirty-plus-year-old Woody Brown at Sunset Beach. It was a rapidly building swell, and when Sunset started closing out, they reasoned the safest way back in was to paddle three miles to the deeper Waimea Bay, but when they reached Waimea, it too was showing signs of closing out. It was getting dark, and Dickie hastily tried to paddle in, lost his board, and disappeared—never to be seen again. Brown waited longer, better timed his paddle, and made it in, but just barely—washing ashore unconscious. (From Matt Warshaw's *The Encyclopedia of Surfing*, 2003)

Pay attention to the Dickie Cross/Woody Brown story: (1) they knew an escape route, (2) they thought nothing of paddling three miles down to Waimea, (3) they were involved in self-rescue and weren't expecting anyone else to rescue them, and (4) the younger, less-experienced surfer apparently lost his head and his life.

The two main ingredients to successfully and safely ride big surf are conditioning and experience. No surfer should be out in well over-head surf unless they, too, could at any time (even at the very end of their session) paddle three miles, if prompted by any such Cross/Brown emergency situation. Keep in mind that before the early '70s, surfers were in far better shape, if only from carrying and paddling such big, heavy boards, and since surf leashes weren't in use yet, they regularly had to swim after lost boards. Also, the ideal in those days was to be a well-rounded waterman, able to swim fast and for long distances, paddleboard and dive, as well as surf. Few surfers today measure up to that waterman ideal, but it isn't hard to at least achieve and maintain sufficient paddling and aerobic fitness. A Dickie Cross/Woody Brown three-mile paddle benchmark would seem a reasonable goal for any surfer wanting to ride big waves. If you regularly surf for several years at least twice a week, no matter the surf height, you're probably fit enough.

One of the last vestiges of that golden era of surfing is that, at least when it comes to big-wave surfing, younger surfers still look to learn how from older surfers. Again, because there are so few days of big surf, it can take many years to gain enough experience to ride (and enjoy) big surf. It would be extremely rare for someone who has only surfed for two years or less to comfortably be out in and ride double overhead or bigger surf—by three years, maybe. The majority of big-wave surfers are older, with an average age of above thirty.

Doctors speak of mortality (death) and morbidity (injury), and while big waves rarely kill surfers, they certainly injure them. Higher velocities—especially on the drop and being on bigger boards—is a recipe for traumatic injuries, particularly to the neck, lower back, and shoulders.

> **"There are old bar pilots and bold bar pilots, but there are no old bold bar pilots."**
> **—Sailors' maxim.**

The key predictor to how many big-wave surfing injuries you will get is how bold you let yourself be. Bold big-wave surfers tend to get the most spectacular rides, but also tend to be caught inside more, wipeout more often, and tend to make fewer waves; bold surfers also have the most injuries. A perfect day of big-wave riding is to make every wave and come in with your hair still dry. Safe big-wave surfing is about more than not having any wipeouts, but also about avoiding dangerous situations, such as getting caught inside. There are double yellow lines out there you just shouldn't cross.

If you are not making at least 90 percent of your drops, then either your wave-selection ability is not what it should be, the spot is beyond your skill level, or you are on too small of a board (the most likely explanation—though sometimes a board can be too long and not fit the wave face). Otherwise, if you are not making at least 90 percent of your waves to the end, you are either not using proper lineup markers (taking off too deep), are trying too many maneuvers (show off!), or don't particularly care if you get hurt or washed in.

There is an interesting phenomenon known as Kodak courage, which also explains why there is photographic documentation of so many truly horrifying wipeouts on the biggest days. Kodak courage more often affects younger surfers (e.g., sixteen-year-old Jay Moriarty's Iron Cross Mavs wipeout in 1994) and those who don't regularly surf a given big-wave spot but have come for the first time, often with a photographer in tow. Locals cringe—it is surfing's greatest horror show.

## Work Up to Big Surf

For any surfer who has learned how to surf reasonably well in small surf, there needs to then be a stepwise approach to work up to big surf. Rather than just wait for bigger surf to come to your favorite small-wave spot, seek out spots elsewhere on the coast that are known as big-wave spots, but start at first with the softer, easier spots, the places where the waves are considerably bigger than you are used to but that are actually fairly gently breaking.

# Learning How to Survive Big Surf

When contemplating going out in big surf, wise surfers try to spend at least a few minutes watching it and judging its size, frequency of sets, wind direction and signs of a possible coming storm (common on the heels of a big swell), far offshore and inshore currents, tidal changes, hazards such as rocks and exposed reefs, difficulty of takeoffs, places the wave is sectioning, and most importantly, escape routes in. For those who are extremely familiar with a given big-wave spot and it is a more usual-sized swell, they often forsake such study and have few problems. But prior knowledge can be an impediment: if the day is remarkably bigger or the conditions are different than usual, those who are relying on past knowledge can make colossal mistakes, due to expecting it to be as it always has been, unaware that it now isn't (i.e., choosing the wrong place to paddle out). In general, though, younger and less-experienced surfers will be rewarded by at least following the routes in and out of the surf that the older, more experienced surfers are using. It is also perfectly acceptable to ask questions: "That channel over there looks like a good place to paddle out, but is that the best place to come in too?" Or, "The lefts look makeable, but why isn't anyone taking off on them?" While you'll drive someone crazy if you ask too many questions, if you can't think of any to ask, it means you're probably not being observant enough.

## Case Study

On a particularly big and vicious day at Waimea Bay, Ken Bradshaw lost his board and began swimming in. Before he could reach shore, a current swept him far down the beach toward a treacherous set of rocks. Instead of panicking and trying to swim harder or faster to get into the beach, he instead swam back out to sea and all the way back to the lineup to try again. On his second try, he also couldn't get in and so swam back out again. He wasn't freaked out; in fact he said it was kind of interesting: "Hmmm, how will I get in?" On his third try, he let himself be pounded by a big set, which pushed him closer to the point, and from there he was able to swim in to the beach.

With big-wave surfing, you always need to hold a lot in reserve—Ken wouldn't have been able to do what he did if his gas gauge was on empty. When you are out there, and especially after a particularly bad drilling or wipeout, ask yourself and honestly answer, "How much gas do I have left?" If you're near empty or even a quarter full, it is time to go in. Keep in mind that big-wave sessions usually last longer than small-wave sessions, sometimes up to four or more hours—it just takes so much longer to paddle out and manage to catch even one wave.

And while you're out there, you'll be so pumped up with adrenaline that you may not recognize signs of fatigue or dehydration (which is a given if you're out longer than two hours). Jet Ski big-wave riders can more easily rehydrate (on the ski, and can even make a meal!), and SUP riders can use camel-back fluid dispensers. Big-wave surfers stay out longer sometimes by sticking an energy bar and soft-pack container of water or juice into their wet suit (just beneath either collarbone is a good stash place).

Wipeout technique is crucial in terms of conserving your energy and not getting hurt. The great advantage of big-wave over small-wave surfing is that once you realize you are going to fall or not make a wave, you have an extra second or two to decide how you want to wipeout. Seek to (1) not be hit by your board (best to jump backward from your board, i.e., not be on the land side of it), (2) try not to end up where you will be close to or hit another surfer or their board, (3) get forward of the lip and let it explode behind you and then sit back into the white water, (4) consider proning out and belly-riding toward the channel, (5) if you are falling hard, try to penetrate the water as cleanly as possible and not bounce or skip across the water.

A similar dilemma and of sometimes greater worry than wiping out is when you get caught inside. Put out of your mind the idea that you will try to duck-dive your board to get through it; a truly big wave can only rarely be duck-dived, and that is only if you are trying to get through it just before it breaks. You could be severely hurt by your board trying to duck-dive serious white water. Don't even think to try it. (Those who have may account for a goodly number of those who won't go into big surf.) While there are still a few big-wave die-hards who refuse to use or rely upon a leash, it is okay to use and rely upon a leash. (The leashless ones at Makaha sometimes clip a swim fin to their waist for emergencies.)

A wet suit, even a vest or spring suit, is actually a flotation device, and it will help you come to the surface. As it lifts you upward, it will help you orient to where the surface is without having to open your eyes (not an option for those wearing contact lens). The thicker the wet suit, the more the flotation; a 5mm or 6mm full wet suit will get you to the surface pretty quickly.

In recent years, flotation vests have become commercially available. The simpler, more trouble-free vests contain foam panels measuring up to 22 mm. thick, and cost about $100. The more sophisticated vests are $CO_2$ cartridge inflatable, are variously called personal surf inflation vests, cost $500 to $1250, are worn inside or outside a wet suit (depending on the design), are not trouble-free, and require signing a

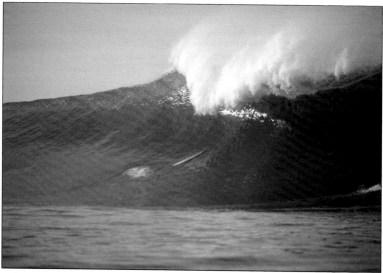

Doug Acton

Oblivion or proper abandon-board and dive-though technique, your choice. Serious Maverick's.

disclaimer. Inflatable vests are increasingly being worn in surf over fifteen to eighteen feet by the majority of surfers.

If you can manage to swim through a giant wave's face before it breaks, it is better to swim through the lower half than to aim for the top half, which sometimes is on its way to becoming a lip, and you could be pulled backward over the falls with it. Also, trying to punch or swim through the lip will put the greatest strain on a leash and the board as it is ripped backward and carried over the falls. That is when most leashes (and boards) break. If you dive through the base of the wave and don't have too long a leash, you often get through unscathed.

If you have to throw your board away and dive, it is essential to be relaxed and controlled. Once you realize you are caught, it does little for your situation to use up breath or energy by frantically paddling. It is better at that moment to stop and look around you: see that no one is behind or close to you, then safely slide your board behind you, and dive forward, headfirst, well before the wave gets to you. The bigger and meaner (and long period) the wave, the deeper you'll need to dive. Try to get at least ten feet down before the wave rolls over you. To get deeper, you need to dive earlier. Those who wait until the last second to dive are the ones most physically and mentally thrashed. Some don't swim down headfirst, but instead do a jumping-jack maneuver with their arms, trying to send themselves down feetfirst, which sure seems like a way to not get very deep, and it puts your head in a vulnerable position. Others will try to use their board as a kind of diving platform to stand on and dive down—good luck!

Whether you've wiped out or been caught inside, now we are at the acid test of big-wave surfers: breath-holding. Surfers who avoid big-wave surfing often say it is because they can't hold their breath long enough, but there has never been a physiological study of surfers that has borne this out. Most surfers can hold their breath plenty long enough. Even in the event of a two-wave hold-down (which is uncommon, happening to only a minority of big-wave riders throughout their surfing career), it is extremely rare to be held down longer than thirty seconds—and most everyone can hold their breath that long. So why is breath-holding such an issue?

If your pulse is even 25 percent higher than what is normal for you, your breath-holding ability will be diminished. Sometime, while you are walking down the beach carrying your board, try holding your breath—you'll find it difficult to last even thirty seconds (shorter if you have a heavier board), are in dry sand, or were walking fast. Big-wave surfers, as do most surfers in general, learn to never let themselves get even remotely out of breath. They want always to be ready in case they have a long hold-down. That means doing everything possible to not let your heart rate get too high or to be out of breath.

Try not to be in a hurry in big surf. Try to think of it as a more qualitative experience rather than a quantitative one: it's not about how many waves you catch or how big they are. If you only end up catching one wave every two hours or no waves at all, so be it—you were out there and part of it.

While there is good medical literature on training yourself to hold your breath longer, the more important first step is in training yourself to not become afraid or anxious, which will push your pulse higher and

**SURVIVING BIG SURF**

use up more oxygen. Yoga and relaxation training can go a long way toward learning to control your pulse and breathing.

As for deliberate breath-holding training, there are what are called "breath-holding" or "apnea courses" occasionally offered in heavily surfed big-wave regions. The essence of these courses is that it is possible to train yourself to override the body's usual cues to breathe. For instance, after twenty seconds of your lungs not exhaling, your brain will frantically tell you to breathe by flooding you with adrenaline (which jacks up your pulse and makes you want to breathe even more). Some can learn to mentally override this, but also you can fool your brain into thinking you took a breath if you just contract your chest wall and abdomen. There is another brain alarm that goes off at about a minute, but again, you can learn to mentally override it too. The point of passing out is longer than that, up to eight minutes or longer in professional free divers.

Except in safe circumstances (not while underwater), it is not recommended that any surfer practice carbon dioxide–depletion methods, such as by deep, rapid breathing (hyperventilation) before holding their breath. It is true that hyperventilation allows you to hold your breath longer, because you blow off carbon dioxide, and it is a building carbon dioxide level that stimulates the urge to breathe. The danger is that with low carbon dioxide levels, you won't notice you've run out of oxygen, so you may pass out. This is what is called a shallow water blackout, which is what Jay Moriarty is thought to have died from while practicing deep water breath-holding during a trip to the Maldives.

One thing for all surfers to consider practicing, though, is surviving a two-wave hold-down. This can be easily simulated on even the smallest day. Let yourself be caught inside, dive down, and stay under until a *second* wave passes over you while underwater. In a typical thirteen-second swell, that means you'll have had to stay down for only about twenty-six seconds. Then you'll know you can survive a two-wave hold-down (and you will have highly amused your friends).

As for becoming more comfortable in bigger surf, particularly at the start of each season, when one of those big days appears that you might think a bit too big or wild for you, grab a pair of swim fins and swim out in it and try to bodysurf, or at else let it bounce you around a bit, to where you begin to feel comfortable out there. Plus, it is superb conditioning.

# The Right Equipment

The biggest mistake most surfers make when it comes to big-wave surfing is that they try to do it on far too short or thin a board, which means they are likely to only be able to catch and stand up on a big wave after it has become extremely steep and critical. Looking down that sheer wall, they freak out and usually pull back—or else they go and have a brutal wipeout. Either way, it's a formula for scaring oneself into not wanting to ride big surf. A good rule of thumb is to take out a board that is six inches longer than you think you need. Until you own a board that is a true big-wave gun, in the 9'6" to 10' range, you'll have trouble progressing beyond double-overhead waves.

You need your board with you in big surf, if only as a self-rescue tool. That means it is crucial to have the best possible leash. Yes, thicker is better, with special attention to the connection points and how thick and fresh the tie cords are and how heavyduty the swivels and ankle strap are. Beyond personal safety, a good leash will save your board from being swept into rocks and being destroyed. Spend money on good leashes and check them for wear and nicks often. In an emergency (e.g., leash caught on the ocean bottom), it can be nearly impossible to pull the strap off your ankle, and so some big-wave leashes have an easy-to-grab pull-ring—or you can beef up the ankle strap tab with a ball of duct tape or attach your own pull-ring.

Given that big-wave sessions tend to be long ones, use a thicker, more full wet suit than you might think necessary. Consider stashing some sunscreen up your sleeve or ankle and try to remember to use it.

Helmets are a good idea in big surf, especially if you are surfing alone, in extracrowded conditions, or if it is offshore (your board may spin out of sight high in the air, then come crashing down onto your head). An optimal helmet for big-wave surfing has not yet been designed. The problem is that most helmets' wider profile prevents your head from entering the water smoothly. This can result in a whiplash-type injury to your neck, but worse, it may amplify wipeout-associated acceleration-deceleration brain microtrauma. Such repeated head trauma over many years, probably more common in big-wave riders, may lead to a slowing of brain function and has been called shaken surfer syndrome. It is similar to what is seen in boxers and football players from repeated head trauma. To lessen your number of wipeouts is to lessen your chance of getting shaken surfer syndrome.

Every surfer should at least mentally think through or actually practice (if they get the opportunity) big-wave rescue with a Jet Ski, boat, or helicopter.

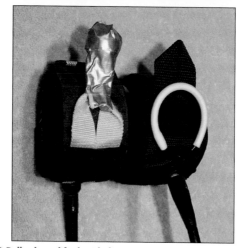

**(L) Pull tab modified with duct tape. (R) Quick release leash.**

And every surfer should know how to precisely position themselves so they don't get caught inside and run down by big sets. Most big-wave spots overlie an uplifted ocean bottom that causes car-sized boils to roil to the surface after (and sometimes in advance of) large sets. Each boil for each swell is a signature for a precise location in the water and can be relied upon to locate yourself as to where best to sit for takeoffs and where not to sit lest you be run over.

You should also consider using a method known as triangulation. Here's how: when you are sitting precisely where you want to be in the lineup, look either way down or up the coast and try to find two landmarks (a rock, a lighthouse, a distant dip or a rise in a hill), one closer and one farther away, chosen so that they line up with each other. Then look about 90 degrees in from there (i.e., straight in to shore) and try to find another set of lineup markers (one closer, one farther) that also line up with each other. Whenever you are able to have both sets of lineup markers lined up, it means you are again sitting where you want to be, and more importantly, you can know you aren't sitting past the double yellow line, where you could be in harm's way.

Lastly, on a smaller day and on an extremely low tide, go out on the reef or into the rocks and create permanent mental maps of where all the hazards are and the escape routes you could use if you were pushed into there on a big day on a higher tide.

Because of recent drowning and near-drowning episodes, key individuals in the big-wave and surf rescue communities, such as Brian Keaulana, Danilo Couto, and Greg Long have begun offering one- to two-day courses in big wave survival training. The courses include CPR training, uses of Jet Skis in big surf, big wave risk-assessment measures, and the effective use of life guards on Jet Skis assigned to specific surfers during particularly harrowing days.

Remember, it is all about prevention, of learning where the double yellow line is out there, and doing all that you can not to cross it.

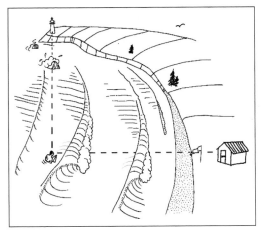

**Use landmarks to triangulate your position in the water.**

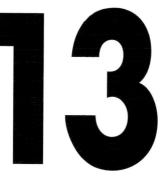

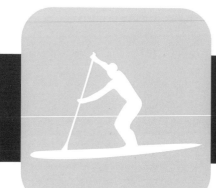

# Stand-Up Paddle Surfing

Stand-up paddling (SUP) is one of the fastest-growing sports in the world and has broadened surfing's field of play by opening up access to hard-to-reach breaks, marginally breaking waves, and flat water locales like bays, lakes, and rivers. It has been embraced both by longtime surfers seeking new challenges in the surf, and newcomers eager to get out and play on the water. Whether practiced in the surf or in calm waters, the ergonomic, upright paddling stance involves almost every muscle in the body and is among the best symmetry-intensive workouts around. As more and more people get involved in the revival of this ancient Polynesian sport, previously quiescent muscular imbalances will begin to act up among those with poor technique, and injuries will occur among those riding waves, sending both novice and die-hard enthusiast to the sports medicine clinic.

 Compared to a riding a regular surfboard, a stand-up paddle board's length and width give it the ability to get into waves early, the upright stance enhances wave selection by improving the vantage point over the horizon, and the paddle provides an added means of maneuverability. However, the large board and paddle pose a unique set of safety issues. In the hands of a beginner, these boards steer more like a '70s Cadillac than a modern sports car, and they can be hard to rein in and control after a wipeout, so the rider carries a significant responsibility for the safety of nearby surfers. The size of the board combined with the fact that one hand must be devoted to hanging on to a paddle make recovery from wipeouts awkward, putting stand-up surfers at risk of injury from their own equipment.

We will begin this chapter by discussing strategies that can be used to prevent acute SUP surfing injuries, and then shed some light on how to avoid and rehabilitate overuse injuries commonly seen among SUP'ers.

## Acute SUP Injuries and Their Prevention

### Getting into the Water

Let's start with the challenges involved in getting the big stick safely off the roof rack and into the water. For boards without a handhold, balancing the board on top of your head with paddle in hand and walking down to the water's edge can be a tricky proposition. Add a strong wind and slippery rocks to the mix and the prospects of a nasty fall increase dramatically. Strongly consider taking your gear to the water's edge in

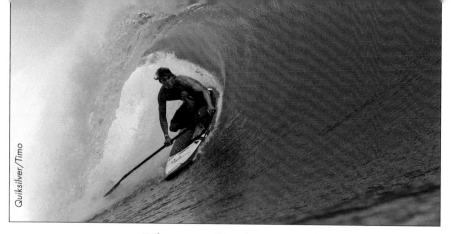

**"Who are you calling a broom sweeper?"**

two trips if (1) you are small, (2) it's windy, or (3) the footing is sketchy. Make sure to walk with the nose of your board pointing into the wind so you don't get thrown off balance by a gust, and never let your leash drag behind as it is apt to snag on something and trip you up.

Okay, you (and your board) made it to the water's edge in one piece. Before jumping in, take a while to observe the wave heights, wind speed, wind direction, tide, and crowd. If there is a thumping shore break, leave your leash off when entering the water so if you lose control of your board in the shore pound, you'll have a better chance of dodging a mow-down from your own board. Wait at the water's edge for a lull in the waves, then scoot in with your board, and paddle. If the water is shallow, plop your board into the water fins up and use it for support until you reach water deep enough to accommodate the fins. Once in deeper water, flip the board, get into a stable knee-paddling position, and paddle through any breaking waves until you are clear of the shore break. Once in a safe zone, you can put on your leash and hop up to a standing position. Because you can easily cover distance on a SUP board, opt for the safest launching area, as opposed to the one closest to the break where surfers (who can duck-dive) may be getting in.

## SUP-SURVIVAL TIP

Legendary shaper Dave Parmenter, who was among the leaders of the modern SUP revolution, relates how to survive a beach landing in big shorebreak:

"Hit the shore like an infantryman on Omaha Beach, as fast and in control as possible. Ride up onto the sand on the back — not the face — of a smallish wave, and get up onto the sand as far as you can. Then jump off, still holding the paddle in one hand, and firmly grab the leash railsaver and let the board pivot nose-first on the wet sand back toward the surf; then, run up the sand, towing the board out of harm's way."

# Up-standing Citizenship

Unless you are an accomplished surfer, rarely wipeout, and have full control over your board when riding waves, stay clear of crowds. With a board big enough to take out the whole lineup, those new to wave riding should stick exclusively to surfbreaks devoid of other surfers, their out-of-control boards present a safety hazard to anyone within a twenty-foot radius (ten feet of board plus ten feet of leash). The significant advantages imparted by long hull and paddle mean that it only takes a few weeks of learning before you're able to get out there and catch waves, waves that would literally require years of experience to catch on a shorter board. But even though you can catch those waves, learning how to ride them properly is a whole different story. The ability to "read" waves, stay in the pocket, and surf with style and control takes years to master—no way around it.

Prone surfers will be envious of your ability to see waves from afar and easily paddle into the best set waves. As a result, they will be more than eager to call you off of what had traditionally been "their" surf break. Don't ruin the vibe for other SUP'ers by being a kook, wiping out in the impact zone after your takeoffs and running into other surfers. Surf on less-crowded and at hard-to-get-to breaks until you've spent time paying your dues, worked your way up the skill ladder, and can ride in full control. Likewise, if you are already a good surfer, be respectful of others in the water when stand-up paddling and avoid the temptation of hogging all the best set waves.

# Paddling Offshore

Before going for a long offshore paddle, check the marine weather forecast, particularly as it pertains to wind, rain, and fog, any of which could affect your ability to make it safely back to shore. As a stand-up paddle surfer, you are much more at the mercy of the winds than is a prone surfer because your upright body, and to some extent even your paddle and board, present a large surface area to the wind and act like a sail. Paddling straight into a stiff breeze can be exhausting, and if the wind blows hard enough, you won't be able to make any progress at all. Beware that offshore winds (winds blowing straight out to sea) will get progressively stronger as you make your way away from the lee of the land, and that the wind strength in the protective lee (downwind side) of a tall bluff or cliff will be deceptively light as compared to what the conditions are really like out at sea. In offshore wind conditions, plan on the fact that the paddle out will be literally be a breeze, but that the upwind slog back in will be much more difficult. In seriously hard offshore winds, such as Southern California's Santa Ana's, the risks of getting blown out to sea are great enough that you should avoid going out altogether. If you ever do find yourself struggling to make forward progress against a strong headwind, try paddling from a kneeling position to decrease windage and increase stability. If you still find yourself losing ground in a headwind, try lying prone on your board and paddling like a surfer. To do this, secure the paddle by tucking the blade under your chest with the shaft pointed forward and upward. Even if you are being blown out to sea, *never* abandon your board, as it provides flotation and makes you much easier to spot in the event of an aerial search.

When cruising or racing offshore, strongly consider bringing along a communication device and a water bottle. A cell phone in a waterproof cover can work if you'll always be in close proximity to a cell tower, but is less reliable than handheld marine VHF radio. The VHF is more rugged, has a five-mile range (around you, not a land-based tower), and emergency channel 16 is continuously monitored by Coast Guard, fishing vessels, and recreational boaters who can come to your aid if needed. During a search, the coast guard can also use your radio signal to home in on you by using a radio directional finder (RDF), which can't easily be done with a cell phone. When touring along a coastline, or from island to island, make sure you have a GPS/compass and navigational charts.

## Wave-Riding Injuries

Though the true incidence of SUP injuries is unknown, undoubtedly many are caused by mechanisms similar to those seen in prone surfing, i.e., getting hit by your own board, hitting the bottom in small surf, and getting axed by the lip of waves in larger surf. However, in SUP, injuries are compounded by the effects of a heavier board, a longer leash (if a leash is used), and a sharp-bladed paddle. After a wipeout, the inability to duck-dive and the added recovery time in getting righted and back up on the board increase the chances of taking a whole set on the head, all the while holding a paddle and getting dragged by the board. In order to avoid injury to yourself and others, good wave selection and positioning is critical, particularly in hefty surf where a badly timed wipeout may entail getting worked all the way into the beach. That being said, stand-up paddlers do have the distinct advantage over their prone counterparts of being able to see sets approaching from afar, catch waves early, and paddle with speed to stay out of harm's way. Thus, the experienced SUP'er, like a good chess player, plans a few moves ahead and has few excuses for getting caught inside where there is risk of injury to self or other surfers.

Like prone surfers, SUP'ers' biggest source of injury stem from collisions with their own boards, and given the added weight and volume of a stand-up board, those blunt force injuries can be severe. Pair the difficulty of wrestling such a big board in the white water, with the fact that one hand is occupied holding on to a paddle, and the probability for broken noses, concussions, and facial trauma from being hit by one's own equipment becomes significant.

The paddle is another potential source of injury. The long lever-arm of the shaft can exert a tremendous amount of torque on the wrist of the paddler as he/she attempts to cling on after a wipeout, which can lead to sprained wrists and dislocated fingers. During wipeouts, the paddle's blade can live up to its name and cut the rider (or someone else), and the rigid T-bar and shaft can break ribs and rupture spleens.

---

## SUP Survival Tip

When getting pummeled underwater in big surf, learn to use your paddle as a steering device. Do this by holding firmly on to the paddle with both hands, keeping your bottom hand close by your side and the blade trailing behind. As you get pulled feet-forward by your board, utilize your paddle like the tail flaps (elevator) of an airplane to stabilize yourself in the turbulence and control your ascent to the surface.

---

While being connected to one's board by a leash is usually a good thing (swimming after your board while holding on to a paddle is difficult at best), there are occasions where leashes can be problematic. The long leash of a SUP board can wrap around a leg, arm, finger, or even neck, creating boa constrictor–type injuries. Even more concerning is a long leash's ability to get snagged on an underwater overhang, kelp, or a crab trap, possibly tethering its user underwater, in which case the rider has but a few moments to disengage from his/her leash. Another scenario where quickly unfastening your leash can be critical is if you're being pushed by breaking waves into a dangerous shoreline (e.g., a wave-pounded cliff). In this case, getting free of your board and swimming to a safe landing zone might be your best option. For these reasons, we highly recommend that you invest in a leash equipped with a quick-release pin, which allows the leash-cord to disconnect from the leg/ankle strap with a simple upward yank on a pull tab (see leash photo in Chapter 12). Broken leashes are common among SUP'ers in big surf due to the tension imposed on them, so invest in a heavy-duty SUP-specific leash.

STAND-UP PADDLE SURFING

# SUP Overuse Injuries

The bio-mechanics and paddling stance for SUP surfing and prone surfing are completely different, and as a result, the overuse injury patterns seen in the two sports are dissimilar. Upper extremity injuries in SUP, seen primarily among those with poor paddling form, are surprisingly similar to injuries seen in racquet sports. Lower-extremity overuse injuries can arise from the constant micro-adjustments required to maintain balance on an unstable surface. Many of these balance muscles are little used during routine daily activity, and after a long day on the water leg, soreness will serve to remind you of their presence.

A more complete description of sprains, strains, and the general principles of rehabilitation can be found in Chapter 5, but we will recap some of the highlights here. Healing from an overuse injury involves three phases: an inflammatory phase, a phase where scar tissue forms, and a maturation phase where scar tissue shrinks while functional capacity recovers. The goal of any rehabilitation program is to accelerate a return to functional capacity so you can get back up on your board and in the water as soon as possible.

Several approaches can be used to accelerate return to functional status, including icing and ice massaging the area up to four times daily. Additional treatments can be obtained from a doctor's visit. These include the following: judicious fourteen-day use of anti-inflammatory medicine, risk versus benefit analysis of injection treatments, or physical therapy. As with rehabilitation for surfing overuse injuries, treatments such electrical stimulation with corticosteroid cream (iontophoresis), or electrical stimulation alone (TENS unit) can be of additional benefit. The following section describes common SUP overuse injuries and rehab.

# Iliotibial Band (ITB) and Patellar Tendon Syndromes

These are overuse problems often seen in hikers, bicyclists, runners, backcountry skiers, and now SUP'ers. They manifest themselves as nagging pain on the outside of the knee just above and below the knee joint and can be problematic. The discomfort may be so intense as to discourage you from participating in long and rewarding sessions of SUP and other endeavors. So what can be done about to treat these issues?

Ice and friction massage are the best initial therapies for ITB syndrome or any overuse injury. Hold a cube of ice in a napkin and massage the inflamed area crosswise until the cube has melted. It could take up to twenty minutes. Do this once or two times daily. A Cho-Pat strap or similar compression tape may help moderate inflammation at the bone-tendon junction, but ultimately it comes down to adjusting biomechanics and muscle balance. Try to limit locking the knees, flexing the knees over the toes, and excessively twisting the knees during paddling. Additionally, the following exercises should help:

## Iliotibial Band Stretch

### Standing
Cross one leg in front of the other leg and bend down and touch your toes. You can move your hands across the floor toward the front leg, and you will feel more stretch on the outside of your thigh on the other side. Hold fifteen to thirty seconds, contracting the muscle briefly for about two seconds midstretch to facilitate muscular biofeedback in the stretch. Return to the starting position. Reverse the positions of your legs and repeat.

### Side-Bending
Cross one leg in front of the other leg and lean in the opposite direction from the front leg. Reach the arm on the side of the back leg over your head while you do this. Hold this position for fifteen to thirty seconds. Return to the starting position. Repeat three times and then switch legs and repeat the exercise. This exercise can be made even more challenging by standing on an Indo board with the IndoFLO cushion.

## Clam Exercise

Lie on your uninjured side with your hips and knees bent and feet together. Slowly raise your top leg toward the ceiling while keeping your heels touching each other. Hold for two seconds and lower slowly. Do these as many times as possible until proper form cannot be maintained working from fifteen repetitions per thirty seconds toward a goal of sixty repetitions per minute. This works the hip abductors that stabilize the iliotibial band.

Strong yet limber quadriceps, hamstring, and gluteus muscles buttress the knee and hip joints. Try the following prevention and rehabilitation program:

## Hamstring Tree Stretch

Lying on your back, place the heel of each leg on a tree or lifeguard tower until you feel a gentle stretch. Stretch twenty to thirty seconds for each leg.

## Side-Lying Leg Lift

Lying on your uninjured side, tighten the front thigh muscles on your top leg and lift that leg about a foot away from the other leg. Keep the leg relatively straight and the tempo slow. Do as many as possible, focusing on the gluteal muscles.

## Piriformis and Gluteal Syndromes

Piriformis syndrome refers to possible irritation of the sciatic nerve as it passes through or next to the piriformis muscle located deep in the pelvis and buttock area. Inflammation of the sciatic nerve, called sciatica, causes pain in the back of the hip that can often travel down the back of the leg. How does this occur? The piriformis muscle is located deep in the buttock and pelvis and allows you to rotate your thigh outward. The sciatic nerve travels from your back into your leg by passing through or next to the piriformis muscle. If the piriformis muscle is unusually tight, or if it goes into spasm, the sciatic nerve can become inflamed or irritated. This is a controversial sports medicine topic. Sciatica should be evaluated by a physician, and the butt muscles need to be stretched and strengthened for peak SUP conditioning. There should be no controversy about that.

You may do all of these exercises right away in addition to ice and friction massage as well as foam rolling.

## Gluteal Stretch

Lying on your back with both knees bent, rest the ankle of one leg over the knee of your other leg. Grasp the thigh of the bottom leg and pull that knee toward your chest. You will feel a stretch along the buttocks and possibly along the outside of your hip on the top leg. Hold this for fifteen to thirty seconds. Repeat three times.

## Partial Curl

Lie on your back with your knees bent and your feet flat on the ground. Tighten your stomach muscles. Tuck your chin to your chest. With your hands stretched out in front of you, curl your upper body forward until your shoulders clear the ground. Hold this position for three seconds. Don't hold your breath. It helps to breathe out as you lift your shoulders up. Relax. Do these as many times as possible until proper form cannot be maintained working from fifteen repetitions per thirty seconds toward a goal of sixty repetitions per minute.

## Prone Hip Extension (Bent Leg)

Lie on your stomach with a pillow underneath your hips. Bend one knee, tighten up your buttocks muscles, and lift your leg off the ground about six inches. Keep the leg on the floor straight. Hold for five seconds. Then lower your leg and relax. Do these as many times as possible until proper form cannot be maintained working from fifteen repetitions per thirty seconds toward a goal of sixty repetitions per minute.

Repeat this exercise for the other leg.

## Quadruped Arm/Leg Raise

Get down on your hands and knees. Tighten your abdominal muscles to stiffen your spine. While keeping your abdominals tight, raise one arm and the opposite leg away from you. Hold this position for five seconds. Lower your arm and leg slowly and alternate sides. Do this ten times on each side.

## Rotator Cuff Strains, Impingement, and Tears

A rotator cuff injury is a strain or tear in the group of tendons and muscles that hold your shoulder joint together and help move your shoulder. Overuse of your shoulder in sports with repetitive overhead movements, such as swimming, surfing, tennis, and SUP, tend to gradually stretch the tendons of the rotator cuff, which can progress to tendinitis and eventually tears of the rotator cuff. A paddle that is too long, improper paddling technique, and poor shoulder posture compound this problem. A fall while desperately holding on to the paddle with an outstretched arm has also been known to cause an acute traumatic rotator cuff tear. To preserve your shoulders, avoid flexing them far overhead when initiating the SUP stroke and choose the right length of paddle; if you stand up and place the paddle handle on the ground, the intersection of the shaft and blade should be at eye level or slightly above. And if it comes between holding the paddle and your rotator cuff, let the paddle go!

The ergonomic Tahitian paddling stroke generates most of its power from the rotation of the torso, the quadriceps in the front of the leg, and a slow forward punching action of the upper arm, using a relatively straight lower arm as a fulcrum. The hand of the upper arm need not rise much above shoulder level, and shoulder of the top arm moves thorough a relatively short range of motion. The proper stance is fairly upright and relaxed, and almost all of the muscles in the body are engaged, which is what makes SUP such an excellent workout. Done properly, there should be little strain on the shoulders. For a detailed description of proper stoke mechanics, see some of paddling guru Tom Bradley's excellent YouTube instructional videos.

Just as in surfing, overdeveloped paddling muscles contribute to impingement and strain, where the muscle literally becomes pinched under bone and frays away until it tears. Think of muscle-bound individuals with their shoulders hunched forward. This leads to a chronic posture of the shoulders being rolled forward accompanied by tight chest muscles leading to shoulder impingement. Impingement can be thought of as muscular imbalance of the shoulder that causes pain either by compression of the rotator cuff tendon or subacromial bursa (lubricating sac in shoulder) leading to strain or bursitis, respectively. There are posture shirts, such as IntelliSkin from Dr. Tim Brown, that can assist in correcting this dysfunction. Most of all, good preventative medicine for SUP shoulders involve preserving shoulder balance and avoiding paddling with repetitive overhead impingement arcs of motion. Because up to 50 percent of middle-aged people will experience a rotator cuff tear from repetitive overhead activity, be sure to concentrate on the proper ergonomic technique outlined above as you sweep your way across the water.

## Rehabilitation Exercises for the Shoulder

### Scapular Squeeze

Just like the surfing neck rehabilitation sequence (Chapter 5). While sitting or standing, squeeze your shoulder blades together as many times as possible.

### Thoracic Extension

Just like the surfing neck rehabilitation sequence, contract shoulder blades back and look up toward the sky several times per day.

### Mid-trap Exercise

Lie on your stomach with your elbows straight, fingers pointing toward feet, and thumbs toward the sky. Slowly raise your arms toward the sky while squeezing your shoulder blades together. Lower slowly. Do as many as possible.

## Biceps Stretch

Stand holding your SUP board or paddle with both hands behind your back like the vintage Hawaiian photos for twenty to thirty seconds several times after your surf session. You should feel a stretch in your biceps and pectoral muscles.

## Scaption

Stand with your arms at your sides and with your elbows straight. Slowly raise your arms to eye level. As you raise your arms, they should be spread apart so that they are only slightly in front of your body (at about a 30-degree angle to the front of your body). Point your thumbs toward the sky. Hold for two seconds and lower your arms slowly. Do these as many times as possible until proper form cannot be maintained working from fifteen repetitions per thirty seconds toward a goal of sixty repetitions per minute.

## Lateral Epicondylitis (SUP or Tennis Elbow)

This is the name for a condition in which the bony bump at the outer side of the elbow is painful and tender. The elbow joint is made up of the bone in the upper arm (humerus) and one of the bones in the lower arm (ulna). The two bony bumps at the bottom of the humerus are called epicondyles. The bump on the outer side of the elbow, to which certain forearm muscles are attached by tendons, is called the lateral epicondyle. Inflammation of the attachment point of those tendons is called lateral epicondylitis or, more commonly, tennis elbow, but we prefer to call it SUP elbow. How does this occur?

SUP elbow results from overusing the muscles in your forearm that straighten and raise your hand and wrist. It is a result of an improper paddling technique wherein recovery of the paddle from the stroke overwhelms the wrist extensors. When these muscles are overused, the tendons are repeatedly tugged at

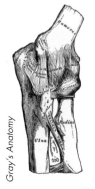
Gray's Anatomy

**Elbow front view.**

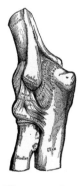

**Elbow rear view.**

the point of attachment (the lateral epicondyle), causing tiny tears in the tendons, inflammation, and pain. Other activities that can cause this condition are tennis and other racquet sports by the same mechanism of overloading the muscles with poor technique. Fix the technique and thus fix your elbow! Finesse the paddle out of the water rather than wrenching it from your previous stroke's momentum.

If you have had this elbow condition for a long time, scar tissue can develop and compound the situation. Address it sooner rather than later. Counterforce (tennis elbow braces) can help by taking the pressure of the bone-tendon junction while the injury heals. Ice and friction massage after a SUP session can immediately decrease the inflammation and break up potential scar tissue. Better yet, do both at the same time. Hold an ice cube in a towel and friction massage crosswise at the point of maximal tenderness until the cube has melted.

Strengthening and rehabilitation exercises include wrist flexion and extension as well as forearm internal and external rotation. With palm down, bend your wrist upward, then downward, and twist left and right as if opening the door. Do these as many times as possible throughout the day toward a goal of sixty repetitions multiple times a day (see Chapter 5 for more on elbow rehab exercises.

## Balance and Stability Training (Simulated SUP)

### 1. Dome trainer, dome side down with paddle, medicine ball, or body bar

Go barefoot so you can really get the feel of the movements of the dome like a board on the water. Step on safely, feet parallel to the plug, posture nice and tall, relaxed looking ahead. Take your paddle, medicine ball, or body bar and start to paddle two strokes each side. Switch off to mix it up. As you move your arms out and to the side, notice how sensitive the dome becomes.

### 2. Balance board on top of dome

Place the board itself on top of the dome. Have a little less board off the back to pretend heading down the line. Or if you're more comfortable to start, place the board so it's nicely balanced in the center. Change it up. You can place your feet side by side as if you're cruising and do it that way, or if you're charging some waves, assume the surf stance (see Chapter 5 for more on elbow rehab exercises).

# Foiling

Foiling is taking off, both literally and figuratively. Airplane shaped, hydrofoiling fins generate enough to lift to raise board and rider out of the water, significantly decreasing water resistance. Diminished forward resistance, in turn, allows the foiler to glide over the water's surface with minimal wave-energy. As a result, even marginal, mushy, on-shore conditions allow for long high-speed rides. Lame conditions become epic. Even large, open ocean swells can be ridden. The flying sensation has been described by Pro-SUP'er Chuck Patterson as akin to gliding across the water like a pelican wing-tipping along a wave's updraft. Even in choppy water the ride is buttery smooth. (See photo on page 318.)

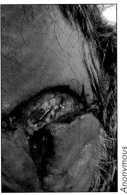

Curses, foiled again! (Without a helmet.)

But all is not perfect in foil-ville. Not only is the equipment expensive and the learning curve steep, but the potential for severe injury to the rider and others is significant. If fin-related injuries are the most common types of injuries among traditional surfers, imagine the potential consequences of having a much longer, four-pronged appendage hanging from the bottom of one's board. In fact, despite the sport's near-infancy, a slew of nasty lacerations has already been reported. To reduce the risk of foil-related injury, see the list of safety recommendations below.

## FOILING SURVIVAL TIPS

1. Avoid crowds. Start out at a small, crumbly break, far away from other surfers.

2. Wear a helmet and an impact vest. Consider booties to protect feet and ankles.

3. Dull the sharp, trailing edges of mast and wings with fine-grit sandpaper.

4. Use a long leash (some favor the coiled variety).

5. Get comfortable carrying your board on land before your first surf.

6. When paddling in the shallows foil-up, brace mast on shoulder so it can't slide back and hit you (like the guy in the photo above).

7. Start off with a short mast before progressing to a longer one.

8. Avoid steep waves and beach breaks.

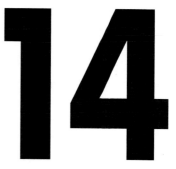

# 14

## Surf Travel Medicine: The Surfari

**S**urfers have a long history of rugged exploration and self-sufficiency. This tradition has its roots among the very first surfers, Polynesian voyagers, who traveled for thousands of miles across the open Pacific in double-hulled sailing canoes in search of new settlements, subsisting only on what they brought with them and the fish they caught. It continued with the boom of modern surfing in the '60s when crowded local surf breaks forced those seeking empty waves and new challenges to venture farther down the coast, down dusty rutted tracks, deep into the Baja peninsula and mainland Mexico, eventually on to the rest of Latin America, Africa, Indonesia, and elsewhere in their quest for the endless summer. Aided by advanced forecasting tools and satellite imaging, today's hard-core surfers continue to pioneer new breaks along remote shorelines, in heavily populated developing nations, and even offshore of their own home breaks. As evidenced by the proliferation of surf camps in such far-flung surfing outposts as Papua New Guinea, Micronesia, and Nicaragua, the spirit of the surf travel has never been greater than it is today.

 Successful surf travel, however, like surfing itself, requires planning and preparation and is not entirely without risk. The hazards involved vary widely depending on the destination, modes of transportation, lodging arrangements, geopolitical climate, and even time of year. The experienced traveler assesses the risks he is most likely to encounter and prepares for them so as to maximize the time doing things he enjoys, like pulling into a clean barrels, and minimize the time doing things he doesn't enjoy, like crouching over dirty squatters with a vicious case of Montezuma's (cursing for having forgotten to pack the toilet paper). The goal of these next two chapters is to help you spend more time surfing and less time squatting.

## Pretrip Planning

A couple of months prior to departure, browse the web and talk to other surfers to educate yourself about travel risks associated with the region(s) you'll be visiting. Probably the single best online resource for this is the Centers for Disease Control and Prevention (CDC) website CDC.gov/travel, which has excellent and up-to-date regional information regarding travel-associated health risks; take a read through the CDC Yellow Book on that site, which is updated yearly. Get an early start on this, because travel to some warm-water destinations will require vaccinations for entry into the country (e.g., yellow fever vaccine), some of which take weeks to become effective or are given in a series of shots over a period of time. When traveling to a less-developed country in the tropics, visiting a travel clinic (find one near you at istm .org or astmh.org) will be your best bet, as they generally have the most current travel recommendations and stock vaccines that won't be readily available at your doctor's office.

And don't forget to make sure your at-home vaccinations are up to date.

## Here is what you need for routine vaccinations:

- Tetanus booster every ten years.
- Measles booster may be needed if born after 1956.
- Rubella (German measles) booster for women if low antibodies or if never vaccinated.
- Polio booster if low antibodies (need blood test to know).
- Hepatitis A vaccination if traveling in high-risk areas (requires two doses).
- Hepatitis B vaccination if high-risk work or activities (requires three doses).
- Periodic tuberculosis skin test (PPD) if exposed to persons who may have tuberculosis.

If you are on any medications, store them in containers labeled with your name, bring an extra supply in case your return is delayed, and be sure to pack them in your carry-on luggage. Bring copies of your prescriptions or a list of meds, including their generic names, on official-looking letterhead from your doctor to avoid any hassles with border officials. This is particularly important if you are carrying any injectable medications, narcotic painkillers, or sedatives.

Many of the world's best waves, particularly those that remain uncrowded, are far off the beaten path, where medical care is rudimentary at best. Travel to the nearest hospital may be hours to days away, so medical self-sufficiency is the rule. Bring your own first aid kit (see The Surfer's Medical Kit, Chapter 16), a copy of this book, and plan on the fact that you'll need to take care of yourself (and perhaps others). Take a wilderness first aid course, an EMT course, or a CPR certification course so you can practice any procedural skills under supervision and will feel more confident and prepared when called to action.

# Travel-Related Injury, Illness, and Death

Encountering health problems on trips abroad is not all that uncommon; in a recent study of travelers to developing countries, roughly 65 percent reported having had a health-related problem, 8 percent were sick enough to seek medical care, and 5 percent sustained injuries. The most common issues were relatively minor self-limited illnesses such as diarrhea, respiratory infections, motion sickness, and rashes, which, while not life threatening, can certainly put a damper on a good trip. However, more serious problems can and do occur.

## Road Kill

Though catastrophes such as tsunamis and terrorist attacks make headlines and most travelers focus their efforts on the prevention of tropical diseases such as malaria, yellow fever, and the like, the leading cause of death among healthy travelers is accidents. A study of US tourists in Mexico found that half of all deaths were due to accidents such as car crashes, homicide, and drowning, while less than 1 percent were due to infectious diseases. The likelihood of an accidental death in Southeast Asia and Africa has been found to be two to three times higher than it is back home.

Despite the fact that many surfers will hesitate to take a late drop at Uluwatu (particularly at low tide), most think nothing of hopping in the front seat of their buddy's rickety VW bug at night (after a few Bintangs) and racing off to the clubs in Kuta. But the risk of death while surfing is miniscule compared to that from a car crash, particularly in developing countries where it has been estimated to twenty to forty times higher than in the United States. An analysis of fatal car crashes among Americans abroad revealed that most were not from crashes between vehicles, but rather single car accidents due to operator error. Contributory factors included small vehicles lacking seat belts or air bags, driving at night along poorly lit roads shared with livestock and pedestrians, and that old standby, alcohol. Also to blame were lack of familiarity with local roads and signage, sketchy roads lacking shoulders and protection from cliffs and curves, and confusion when driving in countries with right-hand drive. To avoid becoming road kill, have a local drive you around when possible, rent as decent car as you can afford, and don't drive at night along unfamiliar roads or under the influence of drugs or alcohol.

Similarly, motorcycles and scooters are common sources of carnage for surfers, many of whom have little riding experience and all

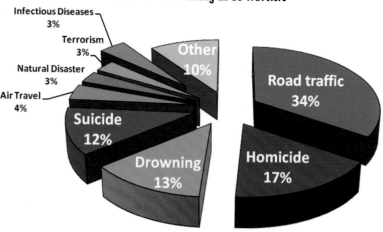

**Accidental Death among all US Travelers**

Infectious Diseases 3%
Terrorism 3%
Natural Disaster 3%
Air Travel 4%
Suicide 12%
Other 10%
Road traffic 34%
Drowning 13%
Homicide 17%

*U.S. Department of State, 2002–04*

too frequently cruise around with a board (begging for liftoff) tucked under one arm. Injuries and death related to aviation accidents also occur at a higher proportion abroad than in the United States, with surfers flying in small planes on unscheduled flights at particularly high risk. If possible, stick to twin-engine planes with more than fourteen seats, as their safety regulations are considerably more stringent than for smaller aircraft.

Tourists are frequent targets of crime. After traffic accidents, homicide is the second leading cause of accidental death among travelers and is the leading cause in some countries like Guatemala and Colombia. Regardless of your own self-perception, in many countries just the presence of a board on your roof pegs you as a naive, wealthy Western tourist who is likely to have cash and valuables on hand. In some countries, like Mexico, you are just as likely to be shaken down by corrupt police looking for a bribe (*la mordida*) as you are to be robbed by criminals. To avoid being victimized, try to attract as little attention as possible by wearing local clothing, not flaunting your wealth, and respecting local traditions (e.g., no surfing on Sundays in the Maldives). Steer clear of high-poverty areas, areas of civil unrest, and don't cruise around at night unnecessarily. Buying and using drugs abroad increases your odds of getting killed (or arrested and imprisoned) exponentially.

## Medical Care and Evacuation Abroad

Like it or not, if you get really sick or badly injured on surfari, you'll probably need to seek medical care from whatever local resources are available. To get help weighing your options, contact the nearest US consulate (get the phone number and save it on your cell phone) or visit the US Embassy website (usembassy.org), which provides recommendations for doctors and hospitals under the citizen services tab for each country. A more current and updated list that includes recommended English-speaking, Western-trained doctors is available from the International Association for Medical Assistance to Travelers (iamat .org) but access to this data requires membership registration (free of charge). Another option is to subscribe to a US-based telemedicine service, which can provide you with online or telephone-based consultation during your travels. If you end up by being admitted to a hospital, these services (some of which are bundled with travel medical insurance) will help coordinate your care by collaborating with local doctors; reviewing your CT scans, X-rays, and blood tests; and providing the advice of specialists in the United States. Of course, this type of remote medical consultation requires Internet or cell phone service, which may not be universally available. If you are planning on being way, way out there, for an extended surf adventure (e.g., a boat trip in the Tuamotus), you may want to consider renting a satellite phone for truly global communication.

Even when traveling well prepared, if the shit really hits the fan—for example, you take a header off your motor scooter in the Dominican Republic or start vomiting blood—you'll probably want a medical evacuation to whisk you off to a major medical center, preferably in a developed country. Should you ever find yourself in this unfortunate predicament, you'll soon learn that an air ambulance staffed with a physician and nurse will cost upward of $40,000, is not covered by your regular insurance, and if you don't have the money, they won't come get you. To make matters worse, even local medical care in a foreign country may not be covered by US health insurers. To prepare for this contingency, we recommend purchasing travel medical-evacuation insurance (not to be confused with travel insurance), which can be obtained from a variety of sources (e.g., International SOS, Medex) for just a few dollars a day. Make sure to read the fine print of these policies. Some include telemedicine services, most will only come get you if you are hospitalized (i.e., you have to get yourself to a hospital), and some have clauses excluding those participating in extreme sports. Some will repatriate you, meaning that they will take you back to a hospital in the United States, whereas others will save money by transporting you to the closest major medical facility until you are well enough to fly home via a commercial airline. As of this writing, Global Rescue (globalrescue.com) is one of the only companies that will provide field rescues and evacuations from remote locations.

## Seasickness—Chumming and Bumming

A boat-based surf trip is perhaps the epitome of surf travel and is most surfers' ultimate fantasy. From exploring new breaks and surfing all day long, to eating fresh-caught fish, and talking story, all the ingredients for an epic adventure are there. But as the *Pura Vida*, the sixty-foot steel trawler you'll call home for the next ten days heaves rhythmically through a much-anticipated ground swell, you note the smell of diesel fumes and fish heavy in the still air of the galley. Pretty soon you have a mild headache and an uneasy, queasy feeling in the pit of your stomach. A cool sweat breaks out on your brow, and the next thing you know, as your friends are popping open the first beers of the voyage, toasting to the good life, you are doubled over the rail blowing big chunks of chow. After three hours of unrelenting dry heaves, you assume a pitiful fetal position on deck, wishing you were back home in New Jersey. Your ten-day dream trip has just begun.

If this sounds familiar, you are not alone. In moderately rough conditions, seasickness affects 15–30 percent of experienced sailors and as many as 60–90 percent of landlubbers. For unknown reasons, a wide range of susceptibility exists between individuals; while some seem to feel sick as soon as they set foot on a dock, others can go below deck in a gale and eat cold pizza. However, given rough enough conditions, even the crustiest sea-salt will eventually succumb.

Seasickness is a type of motion sickness (like car, air, and even space sickness), and its exact cause is not entirely understood. The sensory conflict theory maintains that conflicting information between what you see with your eyes, sense with your inner ears (organs of balance), and feel with body-position sensors in your trunk and neck, activates the vomiting center in your brain. For example, when below decks in a heavy swell, your eyes see no movement of the immediate surroundings, but the fluid in your inner ear (that is getting sloshed all around) and your body-position sensors tell a different story, as the boat moves up and down and rolls side to side. One way to minimize this sensory conflict is to stay on deck and to stand or sit upright and focus on a stable point of reference such as land, or the horizon, so your eyes see what your body feels. Just as the driver of a car rarely gets carsick, taking the helm is often helpful because by anticipating a vessel's movements, your brain can more readily adapt to the unfamiliar motion environment. Closely focused tasks such as reading a navigational chart down below or looking through binoculars add to the sensory conflict and should be avoided in those prone to seasickness. If you must go below, go into your bunk (so long as it is not above my bunk), lie on your back, and close your eyes. Hopefully you are one of those people in whom seasickness induces sleepiness.

Other things to avoid include enclosed, poorly ventilated spaces, foul odors, and alcohol, all of which worsen the symptoms of motion sickness. It is the relatively slow frequency up and down motion of a boat (appropriately known as heave) that most provokes symptoms of seasickness, so it is best to stay in the middle of the boat and avoid the bow or stern of a vessel where heave is most pronounced. Though it has been said of seasickness that "first you think you're going to die, and then you wish you would," after about three days, the symptoms of motion sickness gradually abate as the individual gets adapted to the vessel's movement (assuming sea conditions don't deteriorate during the period). Though you feel absolutely miserable, other than mild dehydration and the inability to function as a useful crewmember, there are no major complications associated with this unpleasant condition.

## Medications and Alternative Therapies for the Prevention of Seasickness

If you are particularly prone to motion sickness, it is wise to take medications for the first few days of travel to give your body a chance to adapt to a life at sea. It is important that medications used to prevent motion sickness be taken at least a few hours before travel if not the day *before* travel, because once the symptoms begin, the condition is very hard to treat. Furthermore, seasickness itself delays the absorption of medications, and vomiting may preclude the use of pills entirely. The night prior to departure, avoid alcohol, have a meal high in carbohydrates, and if you are highly susceptible to seasickness or the forecast calls for rough weather, begin treatment with one of the medications listed below. Prior to embarkation, make sure you are well hydrated and have had a small snack, because your enthusiasm for food and drink is likely to be diminished once under way.

For nonmedical intervention try the Sea-Band, a wristband with a large bead that applies pressure on the P6/Neiguan acupuncture point and is purported to prevent nausea induced by seasickness. The Reliefband, a wristwatch-like device uses a battery to deliver electrical stimulation to the P6 point, causing a tingling sensation (or even twitching) of the palm and fingers. Many people swear by these devices, and the medical literature supporting their use has shown some positive results, so they are certainly worth a try, and unlike medications cause no drowsiness. Ginger is a nutritional remedy that is touted by some (try cutting a dime-sized piece of raw ginger and placing on the tip of your tongue), and studies have found mixed results—some studies showed a benefit, and others showed no difference from placebo. Regardless, ginger is not harmful and has no significant side effects. The bottom line is to try the different options and see what works best for you.

Bon voyage!

## Medications for Seasickness

| Medication | Dosing | Comments |
|---|---|---|
| Dramamine (dimenhydrinate) | 50 mg capsule Every 4–6 hours | Drowsiness, dry mouth Over the counter |
| Bonine (meclizine) | 12.5/25 mg tablet Every 6–8 hours | Drowsiness (less than Dramamine), dry mouth Over the counter |
| Stugeron (cinnarizine) | 15 mg tablet Every 6–12 hours | Drowsiness, dizziness Not available in the United States |
| Phenergan (promethazine) | 12.5/25/50 mg tablet/suppository/ IM Every 6–12 hours | Drowsiness, dizziness Muscle stiffness, neck spasms, tongue spasm, anxiety (if these rare side effects occur, give Benadryl 50 mg) Can be given as an injection for severe vomiting. Needs a prescription |
| Transderm-Scop (scopolamine) | Skin patch Apply behind ear every 3 days then stop. One day break before applying a second patch | Drowsiness, dry mouth, some blurred vision. Wash hands after applying patch (if it gets in your eye, vision will be extremely blurry). Urinary retention in senior surfers. Contraindicated for those with glaucoma Probably the most effective medication Needs a prescription |

# 15

*A repo man spends his life getting into intense situations.*
—***Repo Man**, 1984*

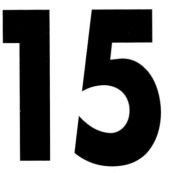

# Surf Travel-Related Infections: Prevention, Diagnosis, and Treatment

Traveling the world these days—especially into the less-developed parts of the world—feels dangerous to many people, if only for fear of terrorists, much less the potential to contract malaria, cholera, or

AIDS. Surfers, however, by time-honored tradition, are ever willing to go widely forth looking for waves. The following section walks you through each of the major diseases that traveling surfers need to understand to better their chances of preventing. Mostly, though, it comes down to avoiding mosquito bites, and funky food and water.

## PREVENTING MOSQUITO BITES

 Malaria, dengue fever, Rift Valley fever, chikungunya fever, Japanese encephalitis—even though you may not have heard of all of these diseases, they are not all that rare. What these diseases have in common is that each is transmitted by mosquitoes. Though not all types of mosquitoes carry diseases, it is safer to assume they do and to not let yourself be bitten by even one mosquito. Let's start there.

Dusk to dawn is when most mosquitoes feed, so during those hours you want to go out of your way to be covered up by clothes: a long-sleeved shirt, long pants, and socks, all of which, if sprayed with the chemical called permethrin, will be evermore repellent to mosquitoes. And just to be extra safe, put some mosquito repellent on the face, ears, neck, and any exposed skin areas. When it comes time to sleep, have a mosquito net around your bed, ideally impregnated or sprayed with permethrin.

Unfortunately, that time around sunset when mosquitoes become so active is also a treasured time to surf, with many surfers staying out until last light. So if that describes you and you're then going to run the mosquito gauntlet at near dark back to your tent, car, or hotel, frantically (and ineffectively) waving your hands around your head to ward them off, give consideration to carrying a stash of mosquito repellent in your trunks or wet suit to slap on even while in the water or for sure at the moment you hit the beach running. What's the best repellent, you might ask?

The United States Centers for Disease Control (CDC) recommends you use one of the following four types of mosquito repellents:

DEET, picaridin (a.k.a. KBR 3023), oil of lemon eucalyptus (a.k.a. PMD), or IR3535. The best and least expensive way to apply mosquito repellents is to smear some on your palms, rub them together, and apply a thin layer to your face, ears, and neck. There are also mist sprays and hand wipes, but hand application is most effective. Here is some information to help you decide which to use.

*DEET* (diethyltoluamide) is a synthetic chemical that was developed in 1940 and has been in general use since about 1950, so its safety and toxicities are pretty well understood. The more concentrated DEET is, the longer it lasts, with concentrations of 20–35 percent providing about twelve hours of at least 95 percent protection from mosquito bites. You can buy DEET in up to 100 percent concentrations, even as a sustained-release type, but higher concentration DEET products are not necessarily more effective—they just work longer and cost more. A product with at least 5–35 percent DEET will work just fine in most circumstances, but if bushwhacking or exercising, use higher DEET concentrations, since sweating and rain can reduce DEET-protection time by as much as one-half. Avoid DEET use in newborns, and for children over two months of age, do not use concentrations greater than 30 percent. DEET can irritate sensitive skin. Don't apply DEET over a wound or rash. Simultaneous use of DEET and sunscreen will decrease sunscreen's effectiveness by as much as one-half. It is the chemical smell of DEET that puts most people off—that and the fact that it melts plastic, so don't spray it on your tent or sleeping bag.

*Picaridin* is an interesting more recent alternative to DEET; it was only introduced into use in Europe in 2000 and the United States in

Female *Anopheles* mosquito, the malaria vector.

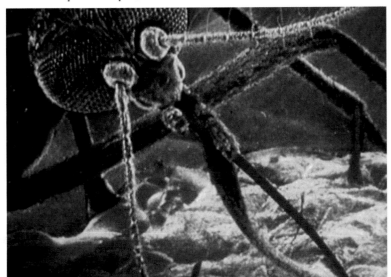

2005, so most people have never heard of it. It is a natural chemical in the piperidine class, meaning it is derived from the pepper plant. It has only minimal odor, and what you can smell is pleasant. It causes very few skin reactions and is favored over DEET for people with sensitive skin and for children. As with DEET, higher concentrations work for longer, but cost more. A picaridin concentration of 5–20 percent can be expected to work just fine. An advantage to picaridin over DEET is that while both will repel mosquitoes well, picaridin repels ticks better, particularly at lower concentrations. As with DEET, there are many brands, including nifty individually wrapped tissues (Natrapel Picaridin Wipes).

*Oil of lemon eucalyptus* is also a natural product (from leaves of lemon eucalyptus trees). It is also known as PMD (p-menthane-3,8-diol). Again, most people aren't aware of it—it wasn't commonly sold as a mosquito repellent in the United States until 2002. It, too, is easier on the skin than DEET and would be favored in children. There are varying concentrations, and again, the higher the concentration, the longer it works. It may not work as long as DEET. It is safe to swallow—there are many brands of lemon eucalyptus cough drops. Though lemon eucalyptus oil smells like citronella oil, which is also sold as an insect repellent, it is a more effective mosquito repellent than citronella, which is not recommended by the CDC. Again, there are many brands; it can be found in health food stores.

*IR3535 (3 [N-butyl-N-acetyl] aminopropionic acid)* is, by name alone, the dark horse of the CDC recommendations. Introduced to the United States in 1999, who's ever heard of it? Well, maybe by some of the brand names that contain IR3535: Bullfrog's Mosquito Coast and Skin So Soft Bug Guard Plus IR3535 (which also comes combined with a sunscreen). It may not work as well or as long as DEET; again, the higher the concentration, the better it works. It is chemically similar to the amino acid alanine, so it is agreeable to the body—easy on the skin, kids, and you can even swallow it! IR3535 also works well against tics and gnats and no-see-ums.

## Mosquito-Transmitted Illnesses

### Malaria

Malaria is one of the world's worst diseases, with close to 500 million cases and 1 million deaths each year. The malarial belt extends worldwide across the equator, reaching to 40 degrees north latitude,

45 degrees south latitude, and up to 2,500 meters elevation. Though location is a big variable, poverty plays a big role too: most developed countries have eradicated malaria by mosquito control, but most undeveloped countries are still struggling to control it, if only by providing permethrin-mosquito sleeping nets. Despite a huge infusion of research funding in recent years from the Gates Foundation, the best medical minds in the world have yet to come up with an effective malaria vaccine.

Malaria is a protozoal parasite that spends part of its life cycle in our blood cells. It is transmitted by the female *Anopheles* mosquito, which, upon biting, first spits under your skin, as a way of preparing for an easier blood feast. It is through that saliva that malaria-laden mosquitoes spread disease.

There are four types of malaria, but traveling surfers will mainly be dealing with two major kinds: (1) vivax malaria, which is the most common one, is not often fatal, but can be chronic and harder to eliminate by treatment; and (2) falciparum malaria, which is less common, more easily eliminated by treatment, but can go to the brain and cause seizures and death (called cerebral malaria). The symptoms of malaria are similar to a really bad flu, with extreme fatigue, recurrent fever (often quite high, but not always), a really bad headache, and severe abdominal pain, as well as aching muscles and joints (but realize that not every malaria sufferer has all these symptoms). For vivax and falciparum malaria, the symptoms begin about five to eight days after being bitten by the mosquito, but can be delayed as long as three months. The malaria parasite has the ability to rapidly evolve and has continued to develop resistance to every medication so far developed to treat or prevent it (prophylaxis). No single drug works to treat or prevent all types

## Countries with a Risk of Malaria

Malaria always present

Malaria sometimes present

of malaria, nor for any one type of malaria from country to country, nor for many years before resistance sets in, so do not depend on your physician to be up to date on which medications to take to prevent malaria when you travel—it is best to go online for that information (wwwnc.cdc .gov/travel), or to go to a travel medicine clinic.

At present, the most commonly prescribed medication worldwide for preventing malaria is a combination product of antimalarial drugs called Malarone (a combo of atovaquone 250 mg and proguanil 100 mg). Malarone is taken daily, beginning one to two days before entering a malarial area and continued for seven days after leaving the malarial area. You start it early in case you have a bad reaction (not common) and need to try an alternative medication. You continue it for an extra week due to how long the malarial life cycle lasts. Forgetting to take it on the back end is a surprisingly common way to get malaria despite having otherwise dutifully taken your pills. Malarone is often confused with earlier antimalarials such as Fansidar and Lariam (mefloquine), which often have side effects, including rashes, upset stomach, and strange and unpleasant dreams, leading many to not ever want to take antimalarials again. Malarone has fewer side effects—most people have none. An easy alternative to any of the malarial prevention medications is daily use of the widely available antibiotic, doxycycline 100 mg per day, which doesn't have many side effects—just watch out for added sun sensitivity, vaginal yeast infections, and remember to take it after you return, for a full month (longer than for Malarone).

## Case Study

Bill is a devoted Indo surf explorer, but due to prior bad reactions to malaria-prevention pills, one year he decided to wing it, pledging to stay on the boat the whole time, reasoning that mosquitoes had rarely found their way offshore to boats he had been on in the past. One night, anchored in a bay near a remote town, his buddies all having gone ashore to find somewhere to eat, and dutifully having stayed on board to avoid mosquitoes, he was awakened by a mosquito buzzing around his ears. He spent considerable time trying to find it in his cabin and kill it but couldn't, and eventually went back to sleep. When he woke up in the morning, he found the mosquito dead on his pillow, plump with his blood. About one week later, the high fevers began, but with a twist—it felt like his brain was going to explode. Fearing that he would die, his buddies got him back to Bali and on to Singapore, where he was hospitalized with cerebral malaria. Even with good treatment, it took weeks to recover. Months later he could barely surf.

The most common question asked by traveling surfers is whether they need antimalarial medications for a trip to Indonesia. In a nutshell, here's the answer: it depends on *where* in Indonesia you are going and also *how* you are going (land or sea). Bali supposedly doesn't have malaria (but we surf docs have seen surfers who caught malaria in Bali); if you are on a boat, say, in the Mentawais, your risk of getting malaria if not on preventive medications is quite low (but not zero). If you are staying on land, for instance in Sumbawa, Java, the Mentawais, or Nias, you definitely should be taking antimalarials.

Being a die-hard surfer takes on a different connotation when you have an active case of malaria but are nevertheless intent on going surfing. Know this: if you truly have malaria, you won't feel well enough to go surfing, no matter how good it looks. If it seems pretty certain you have malaria and not a flu or dengue fever (see below), it's time to bail and go to a modern medical clinic that can diagnose and treat you. The traditional way to diagnose malaria is, in a properly equipped medical center, for a thick smear of blood to be examined under a microscope. But in the field, quick tests have more recently been developed, requiring only that a drop of blood be placed on a specially treated card (called the LDH card test, which is pretty good for diagnosing all types of malaria) or a dipstick (the PfHRPC test, but is only good for diagnosing falciparum malaria). Surfers particularly concerned about malaria could purchase these in-field tests, but should have a health professional teach them how to use such test kits.

Although the CDC does not recommend self-treatment for malaria, if you are test-kit positive or have classic malaria symptoms and it is not possible to get to a medical facility within twenty-four hours, self-treatment is actually not hard to do: just take four tablets of Malarone for three consecutive days—but only if you didn't catch malaria while using Malarone for malaria prophylaxis (obviously that malaria type is resistant to Malarone).

What this option also means is that even if you chose to forego taking Malarone preventively, you absolutely should bring enough Malarone tablets to treat yourself in case you get malaria: bring twelve tablets, at least!

## Dengue Fever

Though dengue is caused by a virus—a very different organism than the malaria protozoa—it, too, is spread by mosquitoes and causes many of the same symptoms as malaria. One key difference between the two diseases is that the dengue-transmitting mosquitoes are of a different type (*Aedes aegypti*), and they more often feed during the day (hiding indoors and in shadowed areas). Malarial regions overlap with dengue, extending over much of the tropical surf locations in the Pacific and Indian

## Countries with a Risk of Dengue Fever—2014

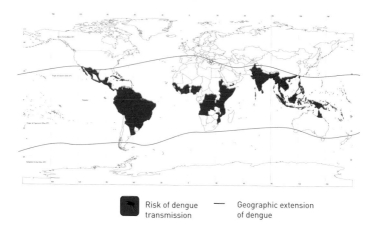

Risk of dengue transmission

Geographic extension of dengue

oceans, but dengue is a far more common cause of high fever and flu-like illnesses among travelers returning from closer to the United States, such as the Caribbean (including Puerto Rico), Mexico, and Central America. There are even occasional cases in southern US states and Hawaii. There are four subtypes of the dengue virus. As with malaria, there is no vaccine for dengue, but another key difference between the two diseases is that with dengue there aren't any medications to prevent it, nor to stop the infection once it begins. At best, treatment is limited to symptom care, to help lower the fever and to relieve the pain of aching bones and muscles. Note, though, with dengue there is a tendency toward bleeding (under the skin, in the gut), so medications that in any way thin the blood, such as aspirin, Pepto-Bismol, or ibuprofen-type drugs, should not be used. Acetaminophen/Tylenol would be safer.

Dengue is often called break-bone fever, so extreme is the pain in the bones and muscles and also in the head (especially behind the eyes). It comes on about two to seven days after being bitten by a mosquito carrying the virus, and the symptoms last three to seven days. A rash—consisting of tiny red bumps that begin on the chest and back and then spread to the face, arms, and legs—often appears as the infection is ending. There are recently developed quick DNA-based tests to diagnose dengue, and conceivably these could be taken along for surf trips to high-risk dengue areas, but as with the rapid-malaria kits, a health professional should teach you how to use these kinds of test kits.

Despite millions of dengue infections worldwide annually, it is seldom a fatal disease. Very few surfers are known to have died from it. Generally, less than 5 percent of dengue sufferers go on to develop the sometimes fatal secondary dengue condition, which is called dengue hemorrhagic fever or, more broadly, dengue shock syndrome. Untreated, with a dengue shock syndrome, there is an up to 20 percent fatality rate (highest in children), but with treatment, even in out of the way hospitals, the fatality rate is as low as 1 percent. Treatment is supportive—primarily intravenous fluids, sometimes transfusions. Dengue hemorrhagic fever is a bizarre internal bleeding, shocklike syndrome that usually only lasts one to two days. It is largely an autoimmune process, seen most often in dengue sufferers who had dengue earlier in life. One of the specific subtypes of dengue more often develops into a shock syndrome. Also, different parts of the world, such as in Puerto Rico, report a higher percentage of dengue sufferers going on to develop a shock syndrome (up to 20 percent).

Many surfers have faced the dilemma of whether to bail out on a surf trip to seek medical help in case they have malaria, even though it might be dengue and probably not needing medical attention. There is no foolproof way to tell, but here are the chief considerations: dengue symptoms are consistent every day until winding down after a weeks' time, but malaria symptoms will continue to worsen though often appearing only every three to four days and usually at night. Note, too, how long from when you were bitten by the mosquito that symptoms develop: if under five days, it's more likely to be dengue. Finally, dengue sufferers often have more extreme pain behind their eyes and can't tolerate bright light as well as malaria sufferers. If you have ever had dengue before and think you may again have dengue, you are at higher risk for developing a dengue shock syndrome and should relocate yourself to be close to a proper hospital. If there are any signs of major bleeding or shock setting in (light-headedness, low blood pressure, a weak and rapid pulse, or depressed consciousness), head for the hospital.

## Yellow Fever

Also mosquito-transmitted, it is caused by a virus that can cause massive liver damage (yellow jaundice), but fortunately it isn't nearly as common worldwide as it once was, with most cases occurring in the jungle regions of South America and Africa—not places surfers tend to frequent. Fortunately, there is a generally safe vaccine against it, but it is only effective about half the time. Nevertheless, many countries around the world require that you be vaccinated for yellow fever (and will turn

## Countries with a Risk of Yellow Fever

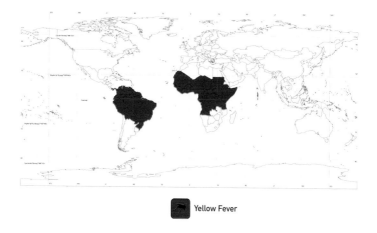

Yellow Fever

you away without a yellow fever vaccination certificate), particularly if your passport reveals you are from or have previously traveled in countries that have reports of yellow fever and if you haven't been vaccinated for it within the past ten years.

# Rift Valley Fever

A mosquito-transmitted virus causing flulike symptoms that can lead to organ failure, which is present throughout Africa, but is also being reported with greater frequency in surf zones among campers along the coastal areas of South Africa and Madagascar. Interestingly, it is worse during El Niño (rainy) years. No vaccine yet for it and no actual treatment, other than symptom care.

# Chikungunya Virus Infection

Another mosquito-transmitted viral infection causing severe flulike symptoms, dominated by painful joints as well as bizarre rashes. It is present in Africa and southern Asia (India through Thailand and in some parts of Indonesia), with increasing case reports in the surf-filled islands of Reunion, Mauritius, and the Seychelles. There's an experimental vaccine but no actual treatment, other than symptom care. The painful joints can continue for weeks and months, leading doctors to misdiagnose it as an autoimmune disease, such as rheumatoid arthritis.

## Japanese Encephalitis and Zika Virus

Again, a mosquito-transmitted virus, with a predilection for the central nervous system, which can lead to permanent neurological problems, even death. It is present throughout Asia, China, Japan, Southeast Asia, and in many of the western Pacific Islands. Fortunately, there is a pretty good vaccine against it, and for some countries with frequent outbreaks of it, the vaccine may be strongly recommended, if not required. Know that vaccination requires three shots over thirty days, so plan accordingly.

Zika virus deserves mention, because it too is carried by mosquitoes in a large number of tropical surf locations, including Tahiti and many other parts of the Tropical Pacific, Brazil, and upward through Central America and the Caribbean. While the viral infection from Zika virus is not typically severe, it can cause fetal abnormalities, so female surfers traveling in Zika virus regions should ensure they are not pregnant.

There are a host of other mosquito-transmitted illnesses, but the ones above are what traveling surfers need to keep in mind.

### Case Study

Upon returning home to New Jersey from an epic surf trip in Nicaragua, Jimmy Moscone noticed an itchy mosquito bite on his back that just wouldn't go away. The bite grew bigger, began to hurt and drain pus, so he went to a walk-in clinic where they diagnosed him with a boil and prescribed an antibiotic. The antibiotics didn't help at all and the red bump grew yet bigger. At night he had occasional stabbing pains and swore he felt something moving under his skin. Pus started staining his clothes and he couldn't take the pain anymore, so he finally went to an ER. They thought it was an abscess (and that Jimmy was nuts) and did a bedside ultrasound. Much to everyone's disgust, a fat maggot was seen wriggling on the screen!

*The Diagnosis:* Botfly infestation. *Range:* Southern Mexico to South America.

*The Treatment:* Cover the botfly larva's breathing hole to suffocate it and ease its removal. A dab of Vaseline covered by duct tape for 24 hours usually does the job. Next, gently extract the dead larva with tweezers.

*Fun Facts:* Botflys use mosquitoes to carry their eggs. The drainage wasn't pus, but worm excrement!

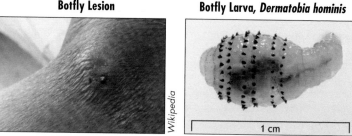

**Botfly Lesion**

*Wikipedia*

Note central breathing hole.

**Botfly Larva, *Dermatobia hominis***

1 cm

*Wikipedia*

Black spines anchor it in place.

# Funky Food and Water

Though the need for clean water and food sanitation in developing countries continues to be a priority of local governments and international health organizations, those efforts can't yet match the twin burdens of poverty and lack of education in poor countries.

When we surfers travel in the developing world, we don't as often (as in years past) grunge it, but also, we aren't usually going first class. But by whichever means of travel in the developing world we choose, the problems of gastrointestinal diseases cannot be escaped.

Contaminated water is the major culprit, more so than food. Any number of gut-wrenching bacteria, viruses, and parasites are passed on through water, usually originating from shit-contaminated lakes and rivers. To dramatically reduce your chance of getting a gut infection, drink only bottled water, even if you are in a first-class hotel or restaurant and have been reassured that the water is safe. Similarly, avoid ice cubes, despite reassurances to the contrary.

One sure way to disinfect water is to boil it, which will kill viruses and bacteria, as well as parasites such as giardia. But boiling requires fuel and time and it doesn't remove particulates from silty water. Water filters with a pore size smaller than one micron will remove everything from water, except viruses. To kill those, add a tablet of iodine or chlorine disinfectant (available in camping stores). Then to counteract the lousy taste these disinfectants impart, consider adding an iced tea mix or vitamin C, or use a charcoal filter.

There are also battery-powered ultraviolet light devices to sterilize water, but they don't work well for cloudy water.

**Wise surf travelers know to:** *boil it, cook it, peel it, or forget it.*

Raw vegetables and unpeeled fruits are high-risk. Poor handwashing practices should be assumed to be present among farmers, food preparers, and handlers; if you are reassured that the vegetables or fruit have been thoroughly washed, remember that wash water may be contaminated. Watch out for fruit juices that have been reconstituted. Boiled or steamed vegetables should be okay. Baked items and breadstuffs are usually fine. Poultry, pork, and beef can be contaminated—meat stuffs may contain various parasites, so should be eaten with caution (well done recommended over rare). Fish is generally okay, but shellfish represent a hazard, particularly in regions with cholera.

# Traveler's Diarrhea

Traveler's diarrhea is by far the most common illness among surfers traveling in underdeveloped countries, with attack rates of 30–70 percent, depending upon the destination. The major cause is poor hygiene practices in food growers, restaurants, and street vendors. About 90 percent of the time the culprit is a bacteria (*E. coli, Shigella, Salmonella, Campylobacter*); the other 10 percent are viruses and parasites such as the protozoa giardia, less often amoebas (*Entamoeba histolytica* is not so common). Once they get into your system, bacteria and viruses usually take six to forty-eight hours to cause symptoms, while with parasites, it is longer, up to one to two weeks. Traveler's diarrhea usually has an abrupt onset, with urgent repeated diarrhea (can be watery or bloody), mild to severe cramps and abdominal pain, vomiting or not, and some fever. Untreated bacteria-caused traveler's diarrhea usually lasts for three to five days, but viral-caused diarrhea is shorter, at two to three days. Parasite-related symptoms from giardia and other bugs can persist for weeks, to months, to years.

Since about 90 percent of traveler's diarrhea is caused by bacteria, antibiotics can help quite a lot, both in reducing symptoms and shortening the course of the illness. For traveler's diarrhea, the CDC recommends oral antibiotics in the fluoroquinolone class, which includes ciprofloxacin (Cipro) and levofloxacin (Levaquin)—Cipro is given twice daily, and Levaquin once daily, and though a single dose will often suffice, a three day course is generally recommended. An alterative antibiotic is

SURF TRAVEL-RELATED INFECTIONS

**283**

azithromycin (Zithromax), which is taken once daily. Treatment of parasites will depend upon the results of a stool culture.

Symptoms can be substantially helped with bismuth subsalicylate (Pepto-Bismol), two ounces or two chewable tablets four times per day. Don't be alarmed if your stools turn black from it, but recognize that upper gut bleeding can also turn your stools black—so if you are on Pepto-Bismol but continue to have a lot of abdominal cramping and pain, you probably need to see a doctor. Young children shouldn't be given Pepto-Bismol, since it is an aspirin product.

The diarrheal symptoms can also be markedly helped with drugs that slow the gut down, such as over-the-counter loperamide (Imodium), two 2 mg capsules followed by one additional 2 mg capsule per unformed stool, up to eight capsules per day. Imodium can be used at the same time as Pepto-Bismol. Also effective at slowing down diarrhea is the prescription medication, diphenoxylate/atropine (Lomotil), 5 mg four times per day.

There have been a number of studies that showed that traveler's diarrhea can be prevented about 80 percent of the time with daily use of Pepto-Bismol or prescribed daily oral antibiotics, particularly with rifaximin (Xifaxan), but the CDC is not yet recommending use of preventive antibiotics for traveler's diarrhea. There are also studies supporting daily use of an oral probiotic (over-the-counter capsules or powders containing healthy gut bacteria, including Lactobacillus GG) to prevent traveler's diarrhea.

## Food Poisoning

Traveler's diarrhea is different from food poisoning, which is due to bacterial toxins, often from *Staphylococcus, Salmonella, Shigella,* or *Campylobacter* growing in unrefrigerated foods such as potato salad, mayonnaise, custard, and meats. The onset of symptoms can be as little as one hour after ingestion, but may be delayed for up to one day. In addition to vomiting and diarrhea, with food poisoning there is often a more toxic all-body illness. The treatment principles are similar as for traveler's diarrhea.

## Typhoid

This continues to be a significant problem in the world, with 200,000 people a year dying from it worldwide. It is caused by a bacteria in the *Salmonella* family and is transmitted by the fecal-oral route—which means contaminated water and food. It is not uncommon along coastal Mexico in various out-of-the-way rivermouth surf spots. The incubation period is six to thirty days, and it comes on slowly, over a number of days, with fatigue, fevers building through the day, loss of appetite, bad headache, often a reddish rash around the trunk. The infection can last up to a month, with the worst symptoms in the second or third week. Antibiotic treatment with a fluoroquinolone (i.e., Cipro of Levaquin) can be lifesaving, but may not dramatically turn things around for three to five days.

## Cholera

Fortunately this isn't as common as it once was, but the world is far from rid of it; cholera keeps creeping around the planet, triggering local epidemics. There are ongoing epidemics in Asia, Indonesia, Africa, Eastern Europe, and parts of Latin America (in the early '90s, coastal Peru had an epidemic) and the Caribbean (Haiti, since the 2010 earthquake). Cholera is caused by toxins produced by *Vibrio* bacteria, which lives freely in fresh and brackish water and infects people via contaminated drinking water, fish, shellfish, and vegetables. Cholera may only cause mild stomach upset—you'd not believe you had cholera, but it can also lead to profuse watery diarrhea that quickly leads to severe dehydration (see below) and for which rehydration is essential therapy, along with recommendations as for traveler's diarrhea. There are various cholera vaccines of varying effectiveness, but in recent years they have been made more effective and are oral. The two major oral vaccines are CVD-103 (a live vaccine, brand name Vaxchora), which is what is available in the US, and WC-rBS (an inactivated virus, brand name Dukoral), available without a prescription in Canada and in use throughout Europe and Scandinavia.

## Severe Diarrhea and Vomiting

In general, if one has vomited and is having diarrhea, it means the stomach and gut have rejected what was in it and needs a rest, particularly the stomach, from food—if not fluids—for up to six hours, to lessen the chance of triggering more vomiting. If one is not becoming dehydrated from repeated vomiting (less than six times per day) and diarrhea (less than six times per day), then withholding water or any fluids for at least two, if not six, hours after an episode of vomiting will often give the stomach and gut a rest. However, if the rate of vomiting and diarrhea are excessive, and there are signs of dehydration, such as dry lips and mouth, dry eyes (no tears), sagging skin, rapid pulse, not urinating, light-headedness when standing, one should begin powering the fluids, even if it triggers more vomiting. Despite the vomiting, enough will get absorbed to shift the balance. The best fluid to use is called oral rehydration solution (ORS). Basically it is water with some salt and sugar added and can be easily made up in an emergency (see chart). Preprepared oral rehydration packets are available in most pharmacies in the developing world, so you just need to add boiled or treated water. If you don't have the ingredients for an oral rehydration solution, or, for that matter, don't have water you know to be particularly clean, it is still better to get *any* type of fluid in when facing life-threatening, severe dehydration.

## SURF-SURVIVAL DRINK

## Oral Rehydration Solution for Severe Diarrhea

- **Water (boiled or bottled), 8 oz.**
- **Sugar, 2 teaspoons**
- **Salt (sodium chloride), a pinch**
- **Baking soda, ¼ teaspoon (if available)**

## Hepatitis

Surfers have historically been more vulnerable to acquiring hepatitis A in their travels, sometimes from surfing rivermouths in undeveloped countries (due to people with hepatitis shitting in the water upstream) but more often from hepatitis-contaminated food and water. It can also be sexually transmitted. Fortunately, there is a good vaccine for hepatitis A, and off-the-beaten-path traveling surfers should strongly consider getting it. Hepatitis B and C are not generally transmitted by fecal-oral routes but are rampant in the developing world from intravenous drug use, needles, and scalpels or other instruments that pierce the skin, and transfusions. There is an excellent vaccine for hepatitis B, which all surfers should receive.

# STIs and HIV

For traveling surfers, sexually transmitted infections aren't nearly as big a problem as might be imagined, or as used to be the case, when surfers might vagabond around the world for months or even years, finding love on the road wherever they could. The STI prevention drill that surfers use at home applies to travel: condom use is a must.

These days the risk of HIV infection to international travelers is quite low, with geography (i.e., countries with high infection rates) far less of an issue compared to the behaviors of the travelers. However, if you engage in high-risk, unprotected sexual activities and/or high-risk drug use, your risk of acquiring HIV is considerable. Countries with high HIV and hepatitis rates, as in much of Africa, are *not* places to elect to have surgical procedures or blood transfusions, except in an absolute emergency.

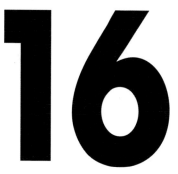

# 16

## The Surfer's Medical Kit

**W**hen it comes to dealing with medical problems, surfers pride themselves on being self-sufficient, both in and out of the water. Even when they should probably belly up to an emergency room, most surfers will rummage around with what they have at hand—famously, duct tape—and try to make do. This chapter will

help them do an even better job at avoiding a visit to the doctor.

**The following tips for creating a complete surfer's medical kit will undoubtedly come in handy if kept in the car for local surf trips as well as at home.**

When the Surfer's Medical Association (SMA) was formed, in 1986, there ensued a series of intense debates and whole conferences devoted to coming up with the ultimate traveling medical kit for surfers. The arguing was over the extent to which a typical surfer could be expected to function as a barefoot doctor, from dealing with something simple like when to start on an antibiotic, to trickier medical tasks such as flushing out a plugged-up ear, to technical skills like suturing and dealing with fractures. It was decided to trust in surfers' innate ability to know their limits and to not hold back on providing sophisticated information and actual medical tools for them to use in even the heaviest of medical situations. The medical advice in this chapter has been worked and reworked many times through the last twenty-five years by SMA members (both surf docs and barefoot docs), with a particular eye to practical matters such as the cost, size, and weight of the kit. It's easy and relatively affordable if you're willing to put in the time to assemble it. For those going to remote places and into the developing world, bear in mind you may be the *only* doctor around for hundreds of miles. Be prepared!

## General Travel Items for Personal Health

The following items are for personal health and hygiene when traveling. Carry them separately from your medical kit, but expect that their uses may overlap.

- Condoms
- Dental floss
- Duct tape
- Earplugs (for surfing and for loud boat engines)
- Emergency phone/Internet numbers
- Health insurance (evacuation insurance if traveling)
- Health record (vaccination history, allergies, etc.)
- Insect repellent (DEET, picaridin, oil of lemon eucalyptus, or IR 3535)
- Leatherman knife or Swiss Army knife type of multitool

THE SURFER'S MEDICAL KIT

- Malaria-preventive drugs (if going into malarial regions)
- Mosquito netting, permethrin-treated (if going to the tropics)
- Nail clippers
- Needle and thread
- Personal prescription drugs, with written prescriptions (on bottle okay)
- Skin lotion (Skin So Soft by Avon helps repel no-see-ums)
- Sunscreen
- Sunglasses (100 percent UV)
- Thermometer
- Toothbrush and toothpaste
- Vision correction (if needed: extra glasses/contacts/lens solution, copy of prescription)
- Visor/hat
- Water (if needed)
- Women's health (tampons/pads, birth control, pregnancy test kit)

# The Surfer's Traveling Medical Kit (a.k.a. the Barefoot Doctor Kit)

Basic but comprehensive, this compact kit will enable you to take care of the vast majority of medical problems a surfer may encounter. Use of this kit presupposes a modicum of common sense and some basic health knowledge. Almost everything can be bought over the counter. A physician, especially a surf doc (contact the SMA at surfersmedicalas -sociation.org or SMAcentral@aol.com to find a surf doc near you), should be happy to prescribe the few prescription items once they realize the degree of responsibility you are demonstrating. If they are reluctant, let them know where you are traveling to and show them a copy of this book, with this list of recommendations—which should reassure them that you're not just a drug fiend.

# Container

This kit will easily fit into a nylon toiletry soft pack or small camera bag measuring at least 12 × 8 × 4 inches or into a one-tray fishing tackle box or a similar case. Ideally, try to find a waterproof container or keep it in a dry bag. To save room, ask the pharmacist for the smallest possible pill containers (and keep the pills in those containers with the prescription on them, unless you want to run afoul of a Customs Officer); over-the-counter medications can be mixed together in pill containers, but use Marks-A-Lot on outside the container to indicate which pill is which, e.g., white = aspirin, red = ibuprofen, etc.

# Knowledge

- Knows how to use a digital thermometer
- Can clean and dress a simple wound
- Can use butterfly Band-Aids or Steri-Strips (ideally with benzoin)
- Can take a person's pulse
- Can use a digital blood pressure cuff
- Can use a wound-closure staple gun
- Can devise and apply a basic splint
- Can stop bleeding (i.e., with direct pressure)
- Can recognize an eye infection
- Can recognize an ear infection (and use an earscope)

# Tools (All Nonprescription)

- Duct tape, 10 yards, wrapped on itself
- Leatherman/Swiss Army knife (with scissors)
- Thermometer (oral, unbreakable, battery powered, with extra battery)
- Eyedropper (plastic, if not part of ear antibiotic bottle cap)
- Earscope (lay variety otoscope, with extra battery [inspect ear canals])
- Blood pressure/pulse cuff (digital), with extra battery (assess for shock/dehydration, screen locals in third world, use as tourniquet)
- Bulb syringe (the type used for baby care) 35 cc (to flush ear canals)
- Safety pins, four (small and large) (make slings, use to dig out splinters)
- Tweezers, standard drugstore type (Swiss Army knife tweezers usually too small)
- Razor blades (one-sided) or X-Acto blades, three
- Strike-anywhere matches (twenty) or disposable lighter (if allowed on plane)
- Headlamp (with extra batteries)
- Pen and sheet of paper (record meds used, so know what to replace; keep notes)

- Applicators (cotton Q-tips), 10 (not for ears!)
- Tongue blades, 2
- Unbreakable small mirror (compact)
- Water-filtration straw or pump, 1 (to purify water in a hurry)
- Soap (small bar)
- Gloves, latex or vinyl—6 (for working with pus/wounds, surfboards)
- Alcohol, isopropyl (rubbing), 25 ml
- Vinegar (any kind), 25 ml (mix with alcohol, for ear flushing)
- Eye patch, 1
- Dental: oil of cloves (Eugenol), 5 cc (for tooth pain or sores in mouth)
- Elastic wrap (Ace bandage), four inches wide, 1 (for sprains)
- Bandages/wound cover
  - adhesive tape (1" × 5 yd, waterproof), 1 roll
  - Band-Aids (1" × 3", waterproof), 30
  - extralarge sheer plastic Band-Aids (2" × 2"), 10
  - 4" × 4" sterile gauze pads, 8
  - Opsite (5.5 "), clear/waterproof wound cover, box of 10 ($25) or
  - Opsite Spray, only comes in 100 ml size ($25)
- Wound closure
  - Benzoin tincture, 10 ml (helps Steri-Strips stay on, even in the water)
  - ¼" Steri-Strips, 3 packs
  - DermaBond (2-octyl cyanoacrylate), in 0.5 ml sealed vial, 1 ($13)
  - 3M 5 staple gun (contains 5 staples—be sure comes with staple remover), ($8)
- Stethoscope, lightweight/nursing variety—if experienced in use (assess lungs/heart)

## Medications Not Requiring a Doctor's Prescription (in the United States)

- Aspirin 325 mg/5 gram tablets, 50 (pain, fever, inflammation, possible heart attack)
- Acetaminophen/Tylenol 325 mg tablets, 50 (pain, fever)
- Ibuprofen/Advil 200 mg tablets, 50 (pain, fever, inflammation)
- Melatonin 3 mg tablets, 10 (for sleep and to prevent jet lag)
- Antacid tablets (Mylenta, DiGel), 10 (indigestion)
- Bismuth subsalicylate (Pepto-Bismol), 20 tabs (diarrhea, nausea)
- Loperamide (Imodium) 2 mg capsules, 30 (acute diarrhea)

- Laxative pills (cascara or senna—Nature's Remedy, Senokot), 20 (constipation)
- Diphenydramine (Benadryl) 30 mg, 30 tabs (itch, insect bites, allergic reactions, hives, sleep) (also may want 2 percent diphenydramine/Benadryl cream, 15 grams)
- Antibiotic ointment (Bacitracin, Polysporin), one 15-gram tube
- Antifungal cream (Micatin, Tinactin), 15 grams
- Pseudoephedrine (Sudafed) 30 mg, 30 tabs (nasal, sinus, ear conditions)
- Eye drops (artificial tears, Refresh), 15 ml (dry eyes)

## Medications Requiring a Prescription (in United States)

- Cephalexin (Keflex) 500 mg, 20 tablets (general infections: skin, sinus, throat, ear, urinary tract, one tablet four times a day)
- Doxycycline 100 mg, 40 tabs (dose/use as with cephalexin twice daily, especially good for sinus infections, and if allergic to Keflex or penicillin; also for resistant-*Staph* and malaria prevention)
- Ciprofloxacin (Cipro) 500 mg, 20 tabs (especially good for traveler's diarrhea: two tab/day for three days; also for urinary tract infections.)
- Vicodin (hydrocodone 5 mg / acetaminophen 500 mg), 20 tabs (for severe pain)
- Sulfacetamide sodium 10 percent eyedrops, 10 cc (for eye infections)
- Antibiotic ear drops (Otobiotic), 15 cc (for painful ear infections)
- 1 percent silver sulfadiazine cream (Silvadene), 50 grams (burns, skin infections)
- Lindane lotion 1 percent (Kwell), 60 cc (if going where there may be crabs/lice)
- Fluconazole (Diflucan) 150 mg tablet, 3 (single dose for women with vaginal yeast infection)
- Injectable epinephrine (Ana-Kit, EpiPen), 1 kit (if you have or you are traveling with someone with a history of allergic/anaphylactic reactions)

## Holistic Remedies (Optional)

- Vitamin C 500 mg, 50 tablets (for colds, low immunity)

- Echinacea/goldenseal tincture or capsules, 1 cc or 20 caps (viral/colds, sore throats, gut infections)
- Garlic capsules, 30 or gloves (prevent/treat general infections)
- Cayenne capsules, 15 (prevent colds/flu)
- Aloe vera gel, 100 ml (sunburn)
- Royal jelly (bee pollen), 15 gram (burns, wounds)
- Arnica, 30C homeopathic tablets (for traumatic injuries, splinters)
- Probiotic capsules or powder (if need to be on antibiotics and as diarrhea preventive)
- Tea tree oil, 15 cc (antiseptic)

## Additional Items/Medications for Health Professional Surfers a.k.a. the Big Kahuna Kit

Physicians, nurses, medics/EMT-trained—to add to the above kit, particularly if you may be the only doctor at a surf camp or with a large group in a remote place or may be called upon to see patients in developing world villages.

- Ear speculums, metal, 2 (small and large)
- Wax-remover curette, 1
- Bayonet tweezers, 5" Lucae or Wilde (disimpacts earcanal, removes hard-to-grasp debris)
- Ophthalmoscope, with batteries
- Flurorescein strips, 3 (put in sterile red-top blood-draw tube)
- Urine dip sticks—5 (put in red-top tube)
- Xeroform dressing, five 5" × 9" (burns)
- Nu Gauze, 1 bottle (to pack drained abscess)
- Silver nitrate sticks, 5 (in red-top tube) (to cauterize)
- SAM Splint 4.25" × 36", rolled ($12)
- Sterile field (eye drape), three 16" × 16"
- Suturing Kit
  - 3.0 and 6.0 nonabsorbable nylon sutures, 3 packs each
  - 4.0 absorbable sutures, 2 packs
  - Needle holder, pickups, scissors (that can be resterilized by boiling)
  - 1 percent lidocaine with epinephrine, 5 ml vials, 5 (one without Epi)
  - 3 cc syringes, 5
  - 27 gauge 1½" needles, 5

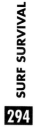

- Needles, gauges 18 and 23 (many uses)
- Viscous lidocaine 2 percent, 30 cc (before cleaning wounds, suture; mouth sores)
- Syringes, 10 cc, 2; and 60 cc. 1 (for flushing)
- Scalpels, 5 (blades of choice, one should be resterilizable by boiling)
- EpiPen auto injector, Ana-Kit 0.3 mg epinephrine (severe allergic reactions/anaphylaxis)
- Alcohol pads, 20
- Prednisone 5 mg tabs, 30
- Asthma inhaler (albuterol), 1
- Nitroglycerin 0.4 mg tabs, 100 (in unopened bottle)
- Furosemide (Lasix) 20 mg, 20
- Prochlorperazine (Compazine) 5 mg, 10 tabs and 5 suppositories (for severe vomiting)
- Diazepam 5 mg, 30 tabs (muscle relaxant, severe anxiety, seizures)
- Fluociniolone solution .01 percent, 5 cc (for severe ear infection)
- Fluocinolone cream (Lidex) .05 percent, 15 gram tube (severe skin conditions/rashes)
- Hydrocortisone cream 1 percent, 15 gram tube (less severe rashes/ skin conditions)
- Chloramphenical ophthalmic ointment 0.1 percent, 3.5 gram tube (severe eye infections)
- Metronidazole (Flagyl) 500 mg, 30 tabs (specific infections)
- Dicloxicillin 500 mg, 40 capsules (specific infections)
- Ciprofloxacin 500 mg, 40 tabs (specific infections)
- More cephalexin + doxycycline + Cipro tablets than for above barefoot doctor kit
- C-A-T tourniquet

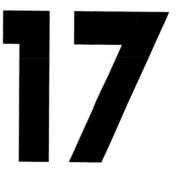

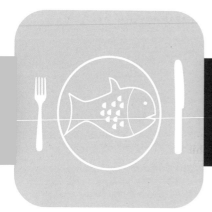

# Seafood Poisonings

Fish is good for you. It is an excellent source of lean protein and contains a number of essential nutrients. Fish is one of the few dietary sources of Vitamin D and can be rich in omega-3 fatty acids which are major components of your cell membranes and brain. Additionally, numerous studies have found that eating fish on a regular basis is linked to reduced mortality from stroke and coronary artery disease. Fortunately, as surfers we have ample opportunity to eat seafood because it is usually plentiful in coastal areas and often a dietary staple on small islands. Furthermore, fishing is a perfect companion to surfing when the waves go flat or you're on a boat trip. Few things are more rewarding than reeling in a nice fat yellowfin, filleting it onboard, and enjoying fresh sashimi with your mates.

 However, some fish species have the potential to harbor toxins and eating those fish can lead to a wide variety of symptoms ranging from mild diarrhea to strange neurologic symptoms and even sudden death. The various illnesses caused by seafood poisonings are highly regional, sporadic, and species-specific. Chances are good that as a waterman you have heard of some of these diseases, and may even know someone who has been stricken, but are somewhat hazy on the details. With hard-to-pronounce names like ciguatera and scombroid and a dizzying array of often overlapping and peculiar symptoms (e.g. loose-feeling teeth), it is no wonder that most are left scratching their heads thinking "what the fugu?" Even most doctors have trouble keeping these illnesses straight.

The goals of this chapter are to clear up some of the confusion surrounding fish poisonings, help you decide if someone's seafood-related illness is minor and self-limited or warrants significant concern, and to help you avoid toxic fish altogether.

## Scombroid

The most common fish poisoning in the United States and Europe is scombroid, which occurs when eating improperly refrigerated fish in the *scombridae* family. The flesh of these tasty pelagic fish such as blue-fin tuna and wahoo is rich in the amino-acid histidine which gets converted by bacteria to histamine as the fish begins to spoil. Within twenty to thirty minutes of ingesting tainted fish, the victim develops a sunburn-like rash of the face and chest, diarrhea, and a throbbing headache (see photo). This is often accompanied by heart palpitations, sweating, and less commonly by light headedness and a weak pulse (signs of low blood pressure), blurred vision, and wheezing. A flushing rash to the face and chest combined with a headache, diarrhea, and stomach cramps shortly after eating fish in the *scombridae* family essentially clinches the diagnosis. Interestingly, while some individuals may have severe symptoms, others eating the same meal might get lucky and experience few if any symptoms because the histamine is unevenly distributed throughout the fish. Often, but usually after it is too late, people will note that the fish they ate had a "burning, peppery, or bubbly" after-taste.

**Scombroid Rash**

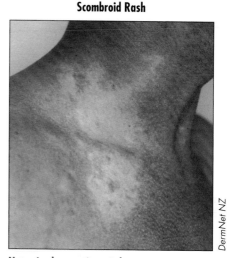

**Not raised, sometimes itchy.**

The treatment, you guessed it, is an *anti*histamine such as Benadryl, Claritin, or Tagamet which will rapidly resolve the symptoms. If nausea and vomiting are prominent features, antiemetics such as Zofran or Phenergan should be administered. Scombroid poisoning can also trigger wheezing and shortness of breath among asthmatics, which responds well to asthma inhalers such as albuterol. Fortunately, even without treatment, symptoms generally resolve within twelve hours. Rarely does an individual develop such severe symptoms that they require IV fluids or hospitalization. You will undoubtedly impress your mates with your surf-doc knowledge by noting that this is not a true seafood allergy (because histamine is not released by the immune system, but ingested), and therefore affected individuals are free to eat seafood in the future without fear of recurrence.

The most commonly implicated species of fish in the *scombridae* family are tuna and mackerel, though non-scombroid open-ocean fish such as mahi-mahi (dorado) and swordfish can also cause the illness (see box).

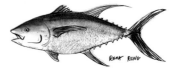

**Yellowfin tuna (*Thunnus albacares*).**

## Fish Linked to Scombroid

- Amberjack
- Anchovy
- Atlantic Bluefish
- Australian salmon
- Blue Fin tuna
- Bonito (Kahawai)
- Herring
- Mackerel

- Mahi-mahi (Dorado)
- Marlin
- Needlefish
- Sardine
- Saury
- Skipjack
- Wahoo
- Yellowfin tuna

It is important to note that these large fish, once caught, may have traveled thousands of miles and may have passed through many hands before reaching your dinner plate. For example, a tuna steak sandwich you order in San Blas, Mexico might have been caught off the coast of Costa Rica, processed in Miami, and sold to a wholesale restaurant distributor in Puerto Vallarta. If anywhere along that journey the fish is allowed to reach a temperature above 40°F (4.5°C), it may begin to decay, resulting in high levels of histamine in its flesh. The toxin, once formed, is resistant to cooking, freezing, smoking, or pickling.

# Ciguatera

Ciguatera is caused by consuming reef-fish tainted by a naturally occurring toxin and can be encountered in tropical surfing destinations worldwide, although it is particularly common in the Caribbean and French Polynesia. This fascinating disease is characterized by gastrointestinal symptoms, followed by bizarre neurologic symptoms which can last from days to weeks, or even longer.

Ciguatoxin, the causative agent of the disease, is produced by *Gambierdiscus toxicus*, a unicellular plankton which often makes its home on the surface of algae growing on damaged coral reef. The toxin is introduced into the food chain by small herbivorous fish which peck on the surface of coral reefs, ingesting the toxic plankton. Those smaller fish are then gobbled up by carnivorous reef-fish which in turn are gobbled up by larger carnivorous fish such as grouper or barracuda which accumulate the toxin. Humans then eat these reef fish and fall ill.

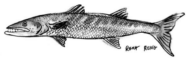

Great barracuda (*Sphyraena barracuda*).

## Fish Linked to Ciguatera

- Amberjack
- Barracuda
- Grouper
- Hogfish
- Jacks
- Moray eel
- Parrot fish

- Snapper
- Spanish mackerel
- Surgeon fish
- Trevally
- Triggerfish
- Wrasses

The initial symptoms of ciguatera fish poisoning are nausea and abdominal pain followed by diarrhea, but in contrast to scombroid first appear six to twelve hours after a fish meal. The GI symptoms generally last from one to three days, and as these are subsiding the real fun begins. Ciguatoxin is a potent neurotoxin which has the opposite effect of the numbing medicine your dentist uses. Instead of deadening sensory nerves by blocking sodium channels in nerves, it opens up the spigots, causing uncontrolled firing of sensory nerves triggering tingling sensations of the lips, arms, and legs as well as temperature reversal; ice-cold beer feels scalding hot, while a hot mug of coffee feels freezing cold. As if that were not enough, intense muscle aches, weakness, apathy, and dizziness are common. But wait, there's more . . . itching of the skin is reported by most victims, many develop a bad headache and about a third complain that their teeth feel loose. These neurologic symptoms begin within the first two days of ingestion and usually fade away within a week or so but can last for months to years. On occasion the toxin has cardiac effects and patients can develop a slow heart rate and low blood pressure. With modern medical care the mortality rate is 1 to 2 percent. Anyone who does not appear to be recovering quickly or who looks really ill from presumed ciguatera poisoning should seek medical care.

The treatment is what we doctors call "supportive," which really means that there is no specific treatment. If the patient is dehydrated, we give fluids, if they are vomiting, we give anti-nausea medications, for low blood pressure, we administer adrenaline-like medications. An IV medicine called mannitol has been used with some reported success for the neurologic symptoms, but not all experts agree that it works. The best solution is to avoid toxic reef fish to begin with.

Because ciguatoxin has no effect whatsoever on the health, appearance, or taste of the fish, without sophisticated testing contaminated fish can't be identified before eating. Since this disease is so highly regional, talking to local fishermen is one good way to avoid it. For example, coral reefs on the south side of an island which have been damaged by a hurricane or runoff might harbor high levels of harmful algae, causing fish feeding there to be poisonous, whereas reefs on the north side of the island may be healthy, and fish caught there perfectly safe to eat. Unlike the migratory fish causing scombroid, reef fish such as parrot fish and snapper tend to stay put in a fairly confined area. Because these fish are relatively small and not caught in huge numbers, they are rarely sold on the international market, which is why ciguatera is seldom encountered in temperate climates.

It is said that savvy mariners of yesteryear used an old-fashioned technique called a CAT-scan to see if a fish was in fact safe to eat. That is, they would remove the fish's liver (where toxins are most highly concentrated) and feed it to a cat. If the cat refused to eat it or died, the fish was deemed unsafe for human consumption. In some parts of the world, the fish is left out and if ants don't avoid it, the fish is considered safe; in other parts of the world they look to see if flies land on it. But we can't

## Ciguatera Survival Story

In a letter titled "An account of some poisonous fish in the South Seas, 1774," ship's surgeon William Anderson documented the symptoms of shipmates who had eaten a large fish aboard Captain Cook's HMS *Resolution* off Vanuatu:

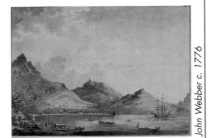

*John Webber c. 1776*

Capt. Cook's *Resolution*.

"Immediately after eating, nothing was felt. About 2 in the afternoon some felt an uneasiness in the stomach, with an inclination to vomit; but it was near the evening before those who suffered most were affected. The symptoms at first were a universal lassitude and weakness, followed by a retching; and in some, by grippings and looseness. To these succeeded a flushing heat and violent pains in the face and head, with a giddiness and increase of weakness; also, a burning heat in the mouth and throat. Some imagined that their teeth were loose...The pulse all this time was rather slow and low." *4 days later:* "Another, in particular, had the pains in his knees so increased that they made him cry out. The uneasiness at the stomach and the heat of the throat in all had nearly ceased. A hog, which had eaten the offals died the third day, as did a parrot."

recommend these techniques. (Who wants to eat a fillet with flies and ants all over it?) Ciguatera testing kits exist, but the ones available to the general public are inaccurate, and chances are good you won't have one the next time you catch a reef-fish. Unfortunately cooking with an extra high flame doesn't help either, because like scombroid, this toxin is heat-stable, and unaffected by cooking, smoking, or freezing.

In endemic areas, the larger and older the fish, the higher the concentration of toxin. As a general precaution, many experts recommend avoiding the consumption of reef-fish bigger than a dinner plate caught in unfamiliar waters, and steering clear of certain high-risk species like barracuda, grouper, and moray eel altogether. Individuals that have suffered from ciguatera poisoning are cautioned to avoid alcohol, nuts, and all fish (even freshwater fish) for at least a year as these foods can cause a return of neurologic symptoms long after the disease has resolved. Strange indeed.

## Fugu

Puffer fish or fugu ("river pig" in Japanese) are small, boxy, slow-moving fish, which ward off predation by inflating themselves like a balloon with water, exposing porcupine-like spines. If the porcupine impersonation isn't enough to keep predators at bay, they also are laden with tetrodotoxin, a lethal nerve agent a thousand times more potent than cyanide which has no known antidote. Of the approximately 190 species of puffer fish, the majority are poisonous.

Unfortunately, it also happens to be a fairly tasty fish, and when properly prepared with the most toxic parts removed, the diner gets just enough tetrodotoxin to experience numbness and tingling of the lips and mouth, as well as a mild euphoria. Fugu has been considered a delicacy for many centuries in Japan and Korea where part of its allure, no doubt, is the culinary thrill of knowing that you are eating what could be your last meal. Indeed, the consumption of fugu was banned in Japan from 1620–1856 after a large group of samurai warriors preparing for battle died after a fugu meal. Currently, however, there are over two thousand fugu restaurants in Tokyo alone where the fish is served as part of an elaborate and expensive meal prepared by specially trained chefs, but don't try this at home, folks. A single large torafugu, the most prized (and poisonous) species in Japan, has enough toxin to kill as many as thirty people. Chefs licensed to serve fugu are required to take a three-year course where they learn how to carefully remove the most toxic parts without contaminating the meat. The final exam includes eating a fish that you have prepared—the passage rate is only 35 percent.

Tetrodotoxin is produced by bacteria in the fish and is most concentrated in the liver, ovaries, eyes, and skin with lesser amounts in the muscle. It acts by blocking electrical signals in motor nerves by disrupting the flow of sodium ions, resulting in muscular weakness which can progress to paralysis and death from asphyxia. Onset of symptoms is rapid, beginning with tingling of the mouth and lips within fifteen to thirty minutes after ingestion. As the facial muscles begin to weaken, victims develop difficulty swallowing, speaking, and double vision. With severe intoxications the muscles of the arms, legs, and most importantly diaphragm become weak and the person is no longer able to breathe and dies of hypoxia. The toxin does not cross the blood-brain barrier, so victims remain alert and awake as they become paralyzed. Victims of severe poisonings die six to twenty-four hours after ingestion.

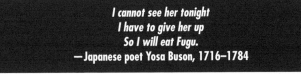

> I cannot see her tonight
> I have to give her up
> So I will eat Fugu.
> —Japanese poet Yosa Buson, 1716–1784

Every year a dozen or so people a year die from fugu poisoning and almost all of them are recreational fishermen who consume the liver, ovaries, or other parts of the fish where the heat-stable toxin is most highly concentrated. Though there is no antidote to tetrodotoxin, if ventilatory support is provided via mouth-to-mouth resuscitation, a bag-valve-mask, or a ventilator, the prognosis is excellent. Usually after about twelve hours the effects of the toxin begin to wear off and the patient is able to breathe spontaneously with no residual after-effects. The bottom line is to never eat any small, boxy, bug-eyed, spiny fish unless you are at a reputable fugu restaurant in Asia.

## Shellfish Poisonings and "Red Tides"

Just as fish can be poisonous, so too can shellfish. The cause of these diseases is similar to that of ciguatera, in that mollusks and crabs filter out toxic algae and concentrate those toxins causing human disease when eaten. Most shellfish poisonings occur when favorable environmental conditions allow toxic dinoflagellates to bloom in great quantities forming so called "red tides." Like ciguatera the toxins do not affect the health or taste of the shellfish and are heat-stable, but unlike ciguatera they can also occur in colder waters—think Ocean Beach, Raglan, and Hossegor. It is important to note here that "red tide" is somewhat of a misnomer, because "harmful algal blooms," as they are properly known, have nothing to do with the tide, and may turn water yellow or brown, and yes, even red, or may not discolor water at all. The species of harmful algae and their concentration determine the type of disease and its severity. In the United States, Europe, and Australia, health departments routinely monitor seawater and shellfish to determine levels of these naturally occurring algal blooms. If levels of toxins in shellfish are determined to be too high, then commercial fisheries are closed and warning signs posted on the beach. Shellfish beds once closed, are often reopened a few months later, after the clams have "detoxed" themselves, but beware that Alaskan butter clams are known to retain toxins for at least two years. Most poisonings occur when recreational harvesters are unaware of or ignore these warnings. Shellfish beds in developing countries may not be closely monitored, so once again, local knowledge is important.

## Paralytic Shellfish Poisoning

Paralytic Shellfish Poisoning (PSP), caused by the ingestion of mollusks contaminated by the potent neurotoxin, saxitoxin, is a potentially serious disease, with fatality rates as high as 10 percent. Clams, mussels, and oysters harvested in areas exposed to harmful algae blooms of the genus *Alexandrium* (and others) accumulate saxitoxin, which acts by blocking our newfound friend the sodium channel, inhibiting nerve conduction and muscular contraction. As the name implies, in severe cases, it results in muscular paralysis, respiratory failure, and death.

Symptoms occur rapidly, usually within thirty minutes of ingestion. Nausea, vomiting, diarrhea, and tingling of the lips are early symptoms of disease. The GI symptoms are short-lived and tend to be relatively minor in nature. Tingling of the lips may later spread to the neck and chest. In moderately severe cases, numbness and tingling involves arms and legs and the victim develops muscular weakness, double vision, difficulty swallowing, and slurred speech. Any of these signs of weakness or muscular incoordination after a meal including bivalves should ring alarm bells because any further weakness could lead to complete paralysis of the breathing muscles and, unless respiratory support is provided, death. If victims are provided ventilatory support via mouth-to-mouth respirations, bag-valve-mask, or a mechanical respirator, the prognosis is excellent. Symptoms peak at twelve hours and begin to subside over the next twenty-four hours, with complete neurologic recovery the rule in survivors. The critical actions here are early recognition that numbness and tingling of the lips, double vision, or weakness after a tasty mussel stew might in fact be PSP and then formulating a plan to provide ventilatory support to the victim for at least the next twelve hours. Other, less severe shellfish poisonings associated with harmful algal blooms are described in the table below.

## Table of Shellfish poisonings

| Disease | Toxin | Distribution | Symptoms |
| --- | --- | --- | --- |
| Neurotoxic Shellfish Poisoning | Brevitoxin | US Gulf States, New Zealand | Tingling of lips and tongue. Temperature reversal, muscle aches. Similar to ciguatera, but less severe. With on-shore winds causes wheezing and eye irritation. Non-Fatal |
| Amnestic Shellfish Poisoning | Domoic Acid | Northern latitudes, US Pacific NW, Eastern Canada | Nausea, vomiting, and diarrhea at first. 1–2 days later: Headache, dizziness, blurred vision, confusion, permanent short-term memory loss. Rarely seizures. Mortality 4% |
| Diarrhetic Shellfish Poisoning | Okadaic Acid | Europe, Japan | Onset rapid, <30 minutes. Severe diarrhea, abdominal pains. Self-limited 1–2 days. Non-Fatal |

# *Vibrio* Infections from Shellfish

Unlike the diseases described above which are caused by toxins, these seafood poisonings are caused by infections from bacteria of the genus *vibrio*. Many *vibrio* species are natural inhabitants of near-shore salt and brackish waters and populate the same waters where filter feeding

## Fishhook Removal Tip

There are two techniques for removing fishhooks. One is to advance the hook through the skin, cut off the barb, and then back the hook out. This is painful but almost always successful. A lidocaine injection or a cube of ice on the skin will provide some pain relief.

The other is the string yank technique, best for hooks not too deeply embedded. Wrap a strong line (>30 lbs. test) around the midpoint of the bend in the fishhook. Depress the shank of the hook as shown to re-open the hook's entry wound and partially disengage the barb. Quickly and firmly yank the line in a direction parallel to the shank while applying downward pressure on the shank. Count to three, but yank on two before the victim flinches. For both techniques protective glasses should be worn so no one gets a hook in the eye. If a treble hook is the culprit, apply tape to the two exposed barbs. Once the hook is removed, wash the area with soap and water and monitor for signs of infection.

**Advance and Cut**     **String Yank**

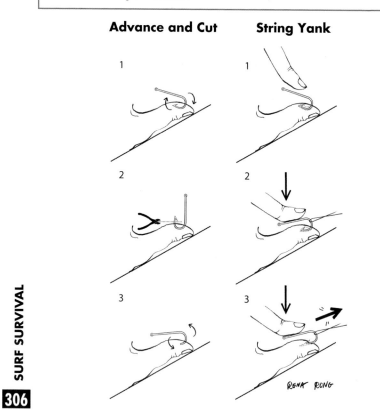

RENA RONG

bivalves such as oysters also thrive. These bacteria are taken up by mollusks and concentrated to up to 100-fold, yet have no ill effect on shellfish beds. However, people eating these contaminated shellfish *can* get sick, almost invariably from raw or undercooked oysters, and usually during the summer months when bacterial levels are highest. Note that in contrast to ciguatera, scombroid, or PSP, cooking completely eliminates risk of these bacterial food-poisonings, because high temperatures kill bacteria, and heat-stable toxins play no role in the disease process.

Mostly, the vibrioses, as these illnesses are collectively known, cause nothing more than a bad case of diarrhea, and fortunately for oyster-loving surfers around the world are quite rare. To surfers accustomed to taking small, calculated risks, we say order a dozen on the half-shell and enjoy. The reason we bother to discuss *vibrio* infections at all, is that in very rare cases, and even then, only among individuals with pre-existing medical conditions, *vibrio* can cause severe, rapidly progressing infections with high fatality rates. Early recognition of those life-threatening infections is important.

Oysters tainted with high levels of bacteria look, taste, and smell normal, so you can't tell a "bad" one from a good one. Raw oysters contaminated with *V. parahaemolyticus* and other strains cause abdominal cramps and diarrhea, sometimes accompanied by vomiting, typically beginning within twelve to twenty-four hours after ingestion. The diarrhea can be explosive, and may be bloody and accompanied by fevers, but is usually self-limited with the vast majority of people recovering in one to three days without antibiotics. This is by far the most common type of food-poisoning from raw oysters.

*Vibrio cholerae*, which can be harbored by shellfish in heavily polluted waters causes cholera, resulting in a profuse "rice water," chronic diarrhea which can cause severe, and occasionally fatal dehydration if left untreated (discussed in detail on page 285).

The most feared *vibrio* by far, however is *V. vulnificus*. This particularly virulent bug is coated with a special cell membrane to help it evade the immune system and secretes enzymes that dissolve tissue, so it can rapidly spread through the body. Heard of flesh-eating bacteria? Well this is it. Fortunately, healthy people exposed to *V. vulnificus* are typically able to fight off these infections and only get standard-issue abdominal cramps and gastroenteritis as with *V. parahaemolyticus*. However, in individuals with liver disease or weakened immune systems, the infection can spread from the digestive system into the blood stream, causing overwhelming and often fatal sepsis within forty-eight hours. Victims start out with vomiting and diarrhea and then develop high fevers, blood-filled blisters on the limbs, and low blood pressure.

*V. vulnificus* can also enter the body through open wounds exposed to contaminated waters, or puncture wounds from fishhooks or marine animals. In these cases, a red rash will begin near the wound, spread rapidly, and then develop those tell-tale blood-blisters. Again, among healthy people skin infections will usually resolve, though often require treatment with antibiotics such as ciprofloxacin or doxycycline. However, among those with conditions that weaken the immune system, such as alcoholic liver disease, diabetes, immunosuppressant medications, and AIDS, these wound infections can cause rapid tissue destruction, not infrequently requiring amputations. Those folks *should* avoid eating raw seafood, or exposing open cuts to warm, silty water.

Infections from *V. vulnificus* require treatment in an intensive care unit setting with broad spectrum antibiotics, IV fluids, blood pressure support, and aggressive surgical debridement. Key to diagnosis and treatment is the early recognition that someone who has eaten raw oysters in the last forty-eight hours and has fever, a blistering rash, and is immunocompromised, needs medical care right away.

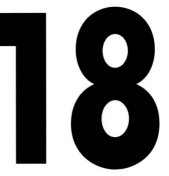

# 18

*Everything about him was old except his eyes,
and they were the same color as the sea
and were cheerful and undefeated.*
        —**Hemingway, The Old Man and the Sea**

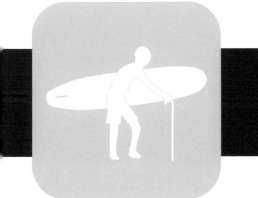

# Surfiatrics

**S**urfiatrics is a newly coined term that combines the words
"surfing" and "geriatrics." While these may seem like contradictory
concepts to many in the outside world, we aging surfers know
better. Surfiatrics focuses on optimizing a surfer's ability to surf in
every decade of life and on using a variety of tactics to "maintain

the stoke." Although the natural, inevitable changes that occur with the aging process can be delayed, they cannot be prevented. All of them affect surfing ability. The degree to which they affect our surfing life is highly variable, and can be managed, slowed, or minimized. In this chapter we discuss how to maximize your time and enjoyment on the water by adapting your goals, equipment, and attitude to meet the inevitable challenges that come along with aging. The key objectives are to preserve and prolong both the *how* and the *why* of surfing.

## The "Stoke"

Surfing is a highly addictive activity. After dialing into what is literally a moving band of energy, we experience the feeling of mastery over nature; the adrenaline rush we get from the speed and power of the wave leaves us craving more. The sense of being a part of the beauty and majesty of the ocean, while not part of the adrenaline experience, is to feel at one with the essence of nature. Surfing is something we love.

For those of us fully addicted, it is something that we don't ever want to give up. Though surfing is undeniably healthy for mind and body, it can be as addictive as drugs or alcohol, sometimes with as much collateral damage. Relationships and careers can be damaged by surfing. The "last wave" syndrome is real. How many important activities are missed or delayed because we just can't quite get out of the water until we catch one last wave?

Compare that with sports like football and baseball. How many football players do you see wanting to play one last down before they leave the field? How many baseball players want to play just one more inning? The difference with surfing lies in the concept of Stoke. Here we discuss the preservation of Stoke, even when one can no longer physically surf, and share examples of how Lifelong Stoke is attainable and can endure until our very last breath.

"Wait until you hit fuggin seventy! Happened to me last month and off I toddled to South Shore Oahu to celebrate . . . commiserate? Nice head-high waves as clean as a whistle. Caught a few, missed plenty. Mostly long or at least longer boards on the outer reefs like Pops and a good vibe with a lot of older guys and really talented women in the water. The first thing that you really start to lose is a fast pop-up to get you on your feet and into a wave super quick, especially when they're on the dribbly side. But once you're up and going the moves still come pretty naturally—top and bottom turns, decent cutbacks, down the line trimming, and even a bit of nose time. You come to appreciate what you are—not what you were, or thought you were— and it's still the best fun you can have standing up even if you climb out of bed every morning and ask yourself *what bit's gonna hurt today?"* —Mike Safe, Bondi Beach on swellnet.com

# Elisabeth Kübler-Ross meets the Surfing World

Many years ago, well-known physician Elisabeth Kübler-Ross published a now-famous book, *On Death and Dying,* in which she identified five stages of transition experienced by those with terminal diseases. Those stages are: Anger, Denial, Depression, Bargaining, and Acceptance. What she did not discuss, but is now widely recognized, is that any significant change in our lives—whether physical or emotional; sudden or gradual; terminal or merely degenerative—will propel us through some variant of these stages. For the aging surfer, the analogous version of these stages is: Recognition, Understanding, Acceptance, Adaptation, and Celebration.

# Recognition

## You Start Aging before You Know It

The effects of aging on the surfer are inevitable, continuous, and relative. The issues we may face in our forties and fifties differ from the problems that plague us in our sixties, seventies, and beyond. How we react and adapt to these changes is determined by our age, our health, our fitness, and our attitude.

It comes as little surprise that objective measures of physical performance peak between the ages of twenty-five and thirty-five, after which they begin to decline. No matter which parameter is examined, be it strength, endurance, balance, or reaction time, all begin a gradual decline starting in the mid-thirties. At first these changes are subtle, and hardly noticeable. But at a certain point, every surfer becomes aware that something is a little different. Pop-ups once made fluidly, are now more often bobbled; waves that should have been caught slip by despite maximum paddling efforts. Reflexes and timing are slowed, leading to botched takeoffs on what should have been easy waves. Fatigue sets in during a session sooner than before. Recovery from injury isn't as fast as it used to be. Keeping off extra weight is harder, no matter how much we exercise or watch our diet. The list goes on and on.

# Understanding

# Aging and Physical Performance

But the story of aging and human performance is more complicated (and less depressing) than a continuous and inevitable downward spiral. As an example, let's take a look at VO2 max, widely regarded as the gold standard of aerobic fitness. VO2 max measures one's capacity to burn oxygen and turn it into energy, thus incorporating the lungs' ability to oxygenate blood, the heart's ability to pump that blood, and the muscles' ability to burn that oxygen and turn it into power. Among the general population, there is a linear decline in VO2 max of about 10 percent per decade after age thirty, with a steeper decline after eighty. The average sixty-year-old, therefore, has about 30 percent less aerobic capacity than the average thirty-year-old. Some of this decline, no doubt, is due to the increasingly sedentary lifestyle of a sixty-year-old "couch potato" as compared to his younger, more active peers. However, these data reflect the *average* population, not we surfers who by our own estimates are well above average! When well-conditioned master-age athletes are studied, the news is not as bad. Competitive swimmers, cyclists, and runners (data is lacking on surfers) only lose about 5 percent of their VO2 max per decade. Better yet, no matter what your age, unless you are already supremely fit, you can increase your VO2 max by 15 to 20 percent with a vigorous exercise regimen, effectively turning back the clock on time. By way of example, the fittest seventy-year-old cyclists and runners have a VO2 max of equal to the average, more sedentary thirty-five-year-old. Though a portion of your VO2 max is genetically pre-determined, the takeaway here is that if you put in the effort, it really is possible for you to move the needle significantly.

A review of muscle strength and power, which are measures of anaerobic capacity, tells a similar story. As we age, we tend to lose strength, power (quick delivery of force), and muscle mass. The make-up of the muscles changes as well, with muscle fibers being replaced by fat and connective tissue, and fewer small blood vessels (capillaries) feeding those muscles. At the microscopic level, there is a drop in the size and number of "fast-twitch" muscle fibers (type II) which generate power, though the number of "slow-twitch" (type I) endurance fibers remains relatively constant. The upshot of these changes is that for sports requiring large amounts of power such as weight-lifting, performance drops more precipitously after age forty than it does for endurance athletes such as runners and cyclists. However, strength training can slow or even partially reverse some of the age-related changes that occur in muscle. A vigorous resistance training program (weights, resistance bands) can increase capillary density of muscle by 20 percent, increase muscle mass by about 10 to 15 percent, and increase force production by 30 to 100 percent. With anaerobic training programs, significant increases in strength and power have been demonstrated into the ninth decade and beyond.

Fortunately for senior surfers, all is not lost with age. Good surfing is not solely a function of one's strength and endurance, but also involves a high degree of knowledge, judgment, and skill—traits that, like a good bottle of wine—can improve over time. A modest physical decline does not adversely affect our positioning, nor the skill to pick the best waves and the patience to wait for them. Top competitive surfers such as Kelly Slater, Mark Occhilupo, Shane Dorian, and others have shown that world-class surfing is possible well past one's physical prime. For those who picked up the sport as adults, many report that their surfing improved with additional water-time such that they experienced their best surfing in their early sixties.

## Acceptance

## Play the Hand of Cards That You Have Been Dealt

At any given juncture, whether relating to surfing or other aspects of life, we have no choice other than to play the hand of cards we've been

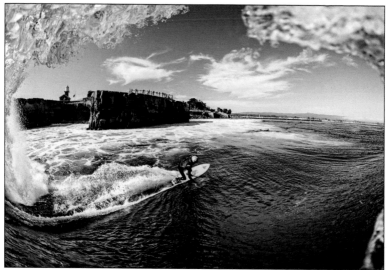

**Rym Partridge, age seventy, in perfect form at Steamer Lane.**

dealt. But how we play this hand of cards is highly variable. Aging surfers often waste significant amounts of precious time in anger and frustration over declining function. Sometimes this anger and frustration causes older surfers to quit the sport altogether. What a waste! The most successful surfers recognize and accept the inevitable changes of aging, and utilize training, judgment, and experience to offset overall net declines in ability and wave count. They make the effort to maximize current abilities, and keep enjoying the sport. At the extremes of adaptation, consider legendary surfer Gerry Lopez. While he is clearly aging, and no longer charging Pipeline, Gerry still carves gorgeous, stylish lines in sizeable surf. At seventy (as of this writing) he's deeply involved with SUP, yoga, and snowboarding, and he's still stoked. He has accepted the changes of aging, and has chosen to play his hand of cards very well indeed.

Consider, also, other benefits that come with age. Aside from wisdom, additional perks that may come in the latter stages of life are a more open schedule, and some disposable income. Now you can surf your home break late on a Tuesday morning—just as the dawn-patrol crowd is leaving—and nod knowingly at your fellow grey-hairs in a less crowded lineup. If you planned well you should also have some extra money at your disposal with which you can travel to uncrowded breaks that match your abilities. Maldives, Tavarua, Baja, Central America? Your time is much better spent on maximizing these opportunities than by being angry about what you can no longer do. To move ahead and make the most of surfing capabilities at any age, Acceptance is a critical stage of evolution. Bring on the Stoke!

## Adaptation

### Resilience: The Net Goal

"Surf today to surf tomorrow," a saying borrowed from Gerry Lopez, has long been the mantra of the Surfer's Medical Association, the organization that brought us authors together. This maxim can be interpreted in a number of ways. To younger surfers it serves as a gentle warning: an injury today might keep you out of the water tomorrow. Viewed through the longer lens of surfiatrics, it takes on a related but slightly different meaning: "we're in this for the long haul."

For older surfers, staying in the game requires a can-do attitude and a good deal of resilience to overcome any obstacles aging throws our way. Resilience, in turn, requires adapting to new realities. Not only must we stay fit, but it becomes increasingly important that we adapt our equipment, mindset, and tactics so that we can continue to "surf tomorrow."

### Fitness: Spigot for the Fountain of Youth

Once retired or semi-retired, you should have more free time on your hands that can be devoted to surfing and to getting in better shape. Hopefully you have maintained a reasonable degree of fitness through middle age, but it's likely that you have gained some extra ballast, lost some strength and agility, and perhaps developed some joint aches and pains or other health issues.

Regardless of your current level of fitness, it is unlikely that you have reached your full genetic potential. With fewer excuses and a more open schedule, now is the time to pump up the volume of your workouts. Not only will improved fitness increase your wave count and decrease frustration and risk of injury out on the water; it is absolutely fundamental to maintaining your health and independence into old age.

While the health benefits of exercise are often touted, they cannot be overstated. It is well established that regular, moderate to high-intensity exercise decreases your risk of heart disease, stroke, type-2 diabetes, peripheral vascular disease, osteoporosis, falls, dementia, and depression, while increasing your sense of well-being and self-esteem. Viewed as a treatment for staving off disease, it is far more powerful than any medication.

As an older surfer, job number one is to ward off frailty and preventable disease through regular exercise and a healthy diet. While the average lifespan in industrialized countries has almost doubled in the last 200 years, the average healthy years of life, termed "health span" has not kept pace, such that the years of ill-health and disability are increasing. A well-rounded fitness program will slow and can even reverse age-related declines in flexibility, balance, and strength, which will serve you well as you advance into old age.

Before embarking on a more rigorous exercise regimen in your golden years, however, it is prudent to consult your physician for "medical clearance." This may involve an EKG and an exercise stress test, or simply a review of your medical records. While surfing is the best and most specific workout for surfing, lack of swell, or an inland location, make it unlikely that surfing can be your primary means of exercise. Even if fortunate enough to live near a surfable coast with consistent, year-round swell, you can prolong your surf sessions and improve surfing performance with land-based training.

To get the most out of your workouts and to avoid injury from poor technique, consider hiring a trainer to design a fitness program that meets your needs. Try to focus on strengthening your weakest links, for example, your left shoulder, stiff neck, or poor balance. Work on functional movements such as pop-ups, and visualize surfing maneuvers as you work out. Ideally, you can find a trainer with the expertise to design a program with surfing in mind. Traditional gym workouts rarely emphasize flexibility, balance, and stability, all of which are key ingredients to good surfing. These assets can be maintained and even improved with a focused training program. If going to the gym does not appeal to you, swimming (aerobic, sport-specific) and yoga (balance, flexibility, core strength) are two other time-tested activities that can go a long way toward improving your surfing fitness. For more comprehensive and detailed surf-specific training techniques, please refer to Chapter 2.

Be mindful that with advanced age, recovery between workouts and from minor overuse injuries requires more time than when you were younger. Be sure to take days off for rest and regeneration. Mild to moderate discomfort is normal when stretching, lifting, or endurance training. However, if it *really* hurts, listen to your body and stop. If pain from a particular activity endures for more than a few days and/or you have arthritis, modify your training activities, for example, yoga poses or ballistic exercises (jumping), accordingly. If you have had orthopedic injuries or surgery (and by this age who hasn't?), incorporate your physical therapy routine into your fitness regimen, even after that injury has healed up. We call this life-long preventive rehab strategy "pre-hab." See Chapter 4 for more details.

That being said, there is no evidence that once medically cleared, older athletes need to "take it easy" when performing exercise. Indeed, with improved training techniques, world-records for many events have been falling more rapidly among older age groups than their younger peers. The results for timed events demonstrate that sport performance can be preserved at a remarkably high level even among older age-groups.

For the few younger surfers actually reading this don't wait until you are old to fight getting older. The effects of a sedentary lifestyle are cumulative. Although there is a reversible component to muscle atrophy, decrease in VO2 max, etc., it requires little effort to get or stay in great shape if you put the work into it during middle age. While not insurmountable, the physical and mental efforts required to get back in shape are far greater once you are significantly deconditioned. Stay ahead of the curve.

## Equipment: Evolving the Board to Suit the Surfer

For those who have been surfing since their teens, there is a certain pride in being able to ride a modern, high-performance shortboard. These boards are favored for their maneuverability, acceleration, and ability to generate speed, but they also require significant paddling power to catch waves, mandate a late take-off, and must be pumped aggressively to generate speed. The challenge of catching waves on these low-volume "potato chips," particularly in less than ideal conditions, has led many a middle-aged surfer to quit surfing.

Shortboard ego aside, wave count matters. If the water is crowded, regaining a competitive advantage against younger surfers by riding a more forgiving board with additional volume is a must. More volume = greater paddling speed = more waves caught.

An increase in volume and paddling power can be achieved in a number of ways; shorter, wider, and thicker as in a fish, slightly longer, wider, and thicker as in an egg/mini-mal, or significantly longer, wider, and thicker as in a traditional longboard. Many aging shortboarders gravitate toward "step-ups," traditional thruster shapes that are considerably longer and floatier than the average thruster. Fortunately, the surf industry has recognized this growth market of aging surfers, and is producing stock boards that address the needs of older/heavier surfers. If you prefer to work with a custom shaper, find one that clearly

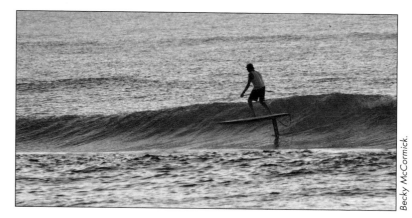

Gene Bagley, cutting edge and fully stoked at sixty-seven.

understands your needs and abilities as an older surfer. Someone who shapes for WSL contest surfers may have a hard time creating a board that works for you. Let the shaper know your goals, and try various shapes and sizes until you find a board or boards you really like.

What if surfing on a traditional board of any shape is no longer practical? A loss of flexibility in your neck or back or a bum shoulder may make prone paddling painful, difficult, or impossible. If this is the case, it may be time to move to a stand-up paddle board. With its more ergonomic paddling stance and greater volume, the SUP has been an epiphany for many an aging surfer. The advantages of increased paddling-power, an improved vantage point for spotting approaching sets, and elimination of the pop-up are all but guaranteed to boost your wave count. We know many excellent older surfers that were ready to quit surfing altogether and completely regained their stoke after taking up SUP, extending their surf careers by decades.

If pop-ups are your issue, and you don't want to lug around a SUP, how about a bodyboard or kneeboard? The pop-up is eliminated, swim fins provide added paddling power, and late-takeoffs are less hairy. Both bodyboards and kneeboards make catching hollow waves much more realistic for the average surfer, yielding the kind of tube-time you may have only dreamed about in your earlier years.

**"I'm not afraid of death; I just don't want to be there when it happens."**
**—Woody Allen**

# Dealing with Specific Medical Issues

Most of the adaptive strategies outlined in this chapter assume an essentially healthy aging surfer. However, it is not uncommon for many of us to deal with one or more diseases which are not directly caused by or related to surfing. Common medical conditions that impact the individual aging surfer include heart disease, diabetes, stroke, arthritis, degenerative neurologic diseases such as Parkinson's, and even mental illness. While it is beyond the scope of this book to address every chronic medical condition, the aging surfer must be aware of the additional adaptations needed to minimize the impact of these illnesses on surfing ability and safety. In-depth discussions with a specialist, personal physician, and other similarly afflicted surfers should be integrated into the overall adaptive plan. Below are a few examples of how you can adapt to specific medical issues.

Like other older adults, some surfers may require joint replacements of the knee or hip. Many older surfers have had one or both of these joints replaced and, with the right adaptive techniques, continue to shred! Pacemakers are not uncommon in older adults. Consult your physician, but keep on surfing. On anticoagulants (blood thinners) for abnormal heart rhythm? Wear a helmet and stay away from sharp or shallow reefs so as to avoid head trauma, cuts, and bruises. However, taking these medications does not mandate an end to your surfing days. Again, consult your physician about the risks (you know the benefits!). We know a committed lifelong surfer who developed significant, volatile insulin-dependent diabetes. He wears a waterproof insulin pump. He also limits the length of his sessions and is careful about maintaining consistent calorie intake before and after surfing. Just in case, he tucks a candy bar in his wetsuit. A lot more is possible than you may think if you have the right attitude.

## Mental Adaptation

Mental adaptation to age-related changes and abilities is a crucial pathway to Celebration and Lifelong Stoke. One of the key elements is to reconcile physical realities with expectations. If your expectations are unrealistic, you are certain to be disappointed with your surfing. Some recommendations:

*Acknowledge that your reflexes will slow over time.* A wave that builds steadily and breaks at a predictable pace is much easier to catch than one that hits a ledge and throws over quickly. In the latter case, there is a narrow window to catch the wave, pop up, and manage the drop. The steeper wave may go hollow, offer a huge adrenaline rush, and be a "thing of beauty," but it is a younger man's wave, so get over it.

*Gain pleasure from other surfers' waves.* If you do call another surfer into a wave, take pleasure in their wave as well as the ones that you ride. If they score a good wave, enjoy watching them and let them know about it. Good karma has a way of paying dividends.

*Appreciate quality over quantity.* Older surfers sometime kid each other about going "bobbing" rather than surfing, since much of the time we seem to be bobbing around watching others catch waves. Consider another, more positive perspective: Maybe we are *"Steelheading."* When steelhead fishermen go out, they are not seeking to catch large numbers of fish. They are patient, and happy if they catch a few really great fish. How many good waves are enough? Even if you used to catch fifteen to twenty waves in a session, maybe three good waves are enough, especially if it is a beautiful day and you are out with good friends. It is no longer about the biggest waves or the highest wave count. Instead of being angry or frustrated, think how cool it is that you are paddling out and catching any waves at all.

*Don't be a hero.* If the surf is too big and breaking in shallow water, maybe you need to surf another day, or find a smaller, gentler break to minimize the risk of injury.

*Stay connected with the ocean.* Even if you can't surf, go to the beach for a walk. If there is a swell, watch others ride waves and "talk story" on shore. Just looking out at the ocean is therapeutic if you are a waterman. Consider surf photography, flat-water SUP, or fishing. If you can't get to the water, track the surf forecast online and follow the WSL.

## Tactics: Savvy Surfing for Seniors

Equipment adaptation and fitness are not the only secret weapons available to older surfers. Now well off your physical prime, making the most out of your time on the water increasingly depends upon surfing smarter rather than harder. Here are some surfiatric tips from a few old Kahunas:

| | |
|---|---|
| Schedule your sessions | Figure out which times of day and breaks are least crowded, even when there is a good swell. The fewer people in the water, the more waves for you. |
| Get limber | Even when the surf is firing, take the time to do a pre-surf warm-up. Allow your muscles to lengthen, and joints to loosen up. We discuss this in Chapter 4 but mention it again here, because being older and wiser, you might actually listen. |
| Find your own zone | Avoid breaks with narrow takeoff zones which focus crowds and maximize competition for set waves. Instead, look for a gap in the lineup where there are fewer surfers nearby. Find a break with shifting peaks and wait for the waves to come to you. |
| Anticipate | If you want to be in the ideal spot, learn to time sets, be patient, and paddle to the spot where the set is likely to peak before other surfers get there. |
| Minimize late takeoffs | Regardless of the break and the conditions, if a wave appears to be a late takeoff, maybe you want to call someone else into the wave. |
| Know your breaks | Closely monitor the forecasts including period, swell direction, wind, and tide. |
| Use your quiver | Use the right board for the conditions. Don't hesitate to ride a longboard when the surf is small, mushy, or sloppy. Switch boards routinely to adapt to various breaks, conditions, and crowds. |
| Conserve energy | When possible keep a steady pace and take time to recover after waves. Always leave a little in reserve. Surfers who are too tired increase risk of injury to themselves and others. |
| Avoid marathon sessions | Super-long sessions are unnecessary and increase risk of overuse injuries. Length of session should match your fitness-level and the conditions. |

# Celebration

## Looking at the Glass Half-Full

We have discussed that there is no point in being angry about what you can no longer do. It gets you nowhere. While humans have a natural tendency to find the "dark spots" in every situation, as we age, we need to work hard on finding the "bright spots." And there are plenty of them. Staying active is something to celebrate. Newfound "assets" like more wisdom and a more open schedule are key bright spots. Knowing that we have adapted successfully is also worth celebrating. Respect in the lineup is another bright spot that may come as a pleasant surprise.

## Respect

As we evolve into older surfers, one of our greatest fears is to be disrespected in the water. Beyond being embarrassed by obvious declining performance, no one wants to be viewed as being "in the way." However, respect among your younger peers can be a surprising bright spot. As an aging surfer, you likely will never get much respect at unfamiliar breaks. But at your home break—where you are known—a high degree of respect is likely. Forget about the groms. Bless their hearts, they are somewhat brain dead, even with their peers. But with the older "younger guys" (30–55), you will be seen as a survivor, someone who refuses to give up. While all the locals will want their share of waves, they will call you into waves, and issue compliments if you get a good one. They will remember when you were a better surfer than you are now. If they know that you are being respectful, they likely won't get pissed if you "kook" a takeoff or accidentally takeoff in front of them. Most of them also want to keep surfing for many years to come, and will view you as an inspiration, a reminder that there is hope of staying in the water as they, too, get older. Once in a while you will totally nail a drop, a bottom turn, or power through a long fast section. One of the greatest pleasures of being an older surfer is when our younger peers hoot and yell shouts of encouragement. For those shouts of encouragement, we are grateful. And for just a moment, we feel nineteen again, still as stoked as ever!

## Experiences and Memories

Over time, experiences take on a changing nature and meaning. And all experiences (good and bad) produce memories. A lifetime of surfing means a lifetime of memories. Nothing (barring dementia) can take away great memories. No illness or infirmity can keep us from enjoying the ocean and the wonders of nature on a beautiful day, both in the present and in memory. How about the lifelong friends we have made in the water and on surf trips? How about the adventures, the great waves, the shared experiences? Forget the dark spots. It's time to celebrate the things we have earned, and that no one can take away from us. These are the keys to Lifelong Stoke. We need to stay positive, no matter our chronologic age or condition.

# Summary: The Secret Is Lifelong Stoke

During the period of transition into older age, it is essential that we spend considerable time and effort to continue doing whatever it is that we love. And for surfers, that means continuing to surf for as long as we can. A long list of veteran surfers has paved the road for us. That list includes John "Doc" Ball, LeRoy Grannis, Woody Brown, Dorian "Doc" Paskowitz, Fred Van Dyke, Gwyneth Haslock, Albert "Rabbit" Kekai, John Kelly, Peter Cole, Eve Fletcher, and many others who've surfed into their eighties and beyond.

However, the real question is how do we maintain a positive outlook when we can no longer surf? Brian Lowdon, the Australian physiologist who published the earliest landmark articles on the physiology of surfing, developed a neuro-degenerative disease that affected his ability to surf. He adapted and maintained his Stoke by switching to bodyboarding. When he could no longer body board, he continued to write and to follow competitive surfing.

The Malibu legend, Terry "Tubesteak" Tracy, was famous in the surfing community for giving Gidget (a real person, and the inspiration for the movie of the same name) her nickname. He lost the ability to surf due to peripheral neuropathy and balance problems. When asked how he maintained his Stoke despite being unable to surf, he said, "I felt bad about having no shoes until I met a man who had no feet." He adapted. He maintained a positive attitude. He started judging contests, and kept in close contact and "talked story" with fellow legends of surf such as Bing Copeland, Tom Morey, Greg Noll, and *Surfer's Journal* publisher, Steve Pezman. He also followed the exploits of his grandson, Hawaiian big-wave surfer, Josh Tracy.

The pathway to Lifelong Stoke rests with each individual surfer. The answer is found not only in fitness and savvy, but in attitude and expectations. Blake Wylie, DO, who did a profile of Tubesteak Tracy for the Surfer's Medical Association, produced an elegant summary of Lifelong Stoke:

> **Stoke is not a place, or a wave ridden, or a trip to a world-class resort.**
>
> **Stoke is a state of mind.**
>
> **Stoke is a commitment to continue the lifestyle, the relationships, and the involvement in something that you love.**

No matter what your age, keep on surfing.

# Additional Reading
# and Online Resources

## General Surfing Information

*The Encyclopedia of Surfing* by Matt Warshaw, Harcourt Press, 2005

Surfline.com

*Surfing Illustrated a Visual Guide to Wave Riding,* by John Robinson, McGraw-Hill, 2010

*The Stormrider Guide North America* by Drew Kampion, Low Pressure LTD, 2002

## Travel Medicine

CDC.gov/travel

The International Society of Travel Medicine. istm.org

The American Society of Tropical Medicine and Hygiene. astmh.org

usembassy.org

The International Association for Medical Assistance to Travellers. iamat.org

## First-Aid

*A Comprehensive Guide to Marine Medicine 2nd Edition,* by Eric Weiss and Michael Jacobs, Adventure Medical Kits, July 2012

Wilderness Medical Society. *Practice Guidelines for Wilderness Care, Fifth Edition.* Edited by William Forgey, MD, The Globe Pequot Press, 2006

*Wilderness Medicine 7th Edition*, Edited by Paul Auerbach, Mosby Elsevier, 2016
*A Medical Guide to Hazardous Marine Life, 2nd Edition* by Paul Auerbach, Mosby Year Book, Inc., 1991

# Surf Medicine

The Surfer's Medical Association. Surfersmedicalassociation.org
P.O. Box 1295
Capitola, CA 95010
Surfing Medicine International. Surfingmed.com
*Surfing Medicine*—the online journal of the SMA. journal.surfersmedicalassociation.org
*Sick Surfers Ask the Surf Docs & Dr. Geoff* by Mark Renneker, Kevin Starr, and Geoff Booth, Bull Publishing Co, 1993.
*Surfing and Health* by Joel Steinman, Meyer & Meyer Sport (UK) Ltd, 2009

# Fitness and Sports Medicine

*Fit to Surf* by Rocky Snyder, Ragged Mountain Press, 2003
*Faster, Better, Stronger* by Eric Heiden, Massimo Testa, and DeAnne Musolf, HarperCollins Publishers, 2009
*Surf Flex* by Paul Frediani, Hatherleigh Press, 2001
Surf Stronger DVDs by Scott Adams (surfstronger.com)

# Aid and Environmental Organizations

Surfrider Foundation USA. Surfrider.org
P.O. Box 6010
San Clemente, CA 92674-6010 tel. (949) 492-8170
Surfrider Foundation Australia. Surfrider.org/au
681 Barrenjoey Road
Avalon NSW 2107
Surf Aid International. Surfaidinternational.org

# Index

90-90 stretches, 40–41

**A**

acne, 135–136
actinic keratoses, 118, 131
acupuncture, 27
aerobic conditioning, 26, 57–60, 65, 312
A-frame peak, 21
agility, 51–53
aging
    acceptance of, 313–315
    adaptation to, 315–321
    celebration of, 321–322
    equipment and, 317–318
    fitness and, 315–317
    medical issues in, 319–321
    mental adaptation in, 319–321
    physical performance and, 312–313
    recognition of, 311–312
    reflexes and, 319–320
    resilience and, 315
    respect in, 322
    understanding, 312–313
AIDS, 287
algal blooms, harmful, 303–304
Allen, Woody, 318
allergic reactions, 205–206
aloe, 122–123
amberjack, 299, 300
anaerobic conditioning, 57–60
anatomy, shoulder, 101
anchovy, 299
Andersen, Doug, 68–69
ankle injury, 83, 111–112
antibiotics, 146–147, 195–196, 283–284
antihistamine, 298
antioxidants, 131–132
aquagenic pruritus, 137
arm circles, 27–29
arthritis, 54, 60, 108, 109, 280, 316, 319
assessment, of conditions, 12–13
Atlantic bluefish, 299
aural toilet, 149–150

**B**

back flush, 107
back pain, 105–108
Bagley, Gene, 318
bailing, 91–92
balance, 51–53, 260
barracuda, 300
basal cell skin cancer, 133, 134
baseball, 73
basketball, 73
bathymetry, 5, 7
beach breaks, 13–15
beginners, 17–23
biceps curls, 105

biceps stretch, 105, 259
big surf
    allure of, 236–237
    defining, 233–235
    equipment, 245–247
    fear of, 236–237
    risk of, 237–239
    surviving, 240–244
    working up to, 239
bird dogs, 108
bleeding, 76–77,184–185
board control, 21–22
bodyboarding, 17–18
bodyboard injuries, 77
bodysurfing, 17–18
body-weight training, 54–57
Bonine, 270
bonito, 299
booties, 89–90
botfly infestation, 281, 282
box jellyfish, 219–224
Bradshaw, Ken, 240
breath holding, 4, 80, 244
brevitoxin, 305
Brown, Tim, 68–69, 103
Brown, Woody, 238
buddy system, 22–23
burpees, 54–55

**C**

calf stretch, 42
car accidents, 265–266
carbohydrates, 65–66, 67–68
cardiopulmonary resuscitation (CPR), 173–175
cellulitis, 139
Centers for Disease Control and Prevention (CDC), 264
cerebral malaria, 275
chest compressions, 175
chest stretch, 41–42
Chicama, 25
chikungunya virus, 280
children, 23
chin tucks, 100
chiropractic manipulation, 27
chocolate milk, 68
cholera, 285, 307
cholesterol, 67
ciguatera, 299–302
cinnarizine, 270
clam exercise, 255
cliffs, 15–16
cold urticaria, 137–138
cold water hives, 137–138
concussion, 76, 253
condition assessment, 12–13
conjunctivitis, 157

conscious victim rescue, 164–166
contact lenses, 159–160
control of board, 21–22
coral reef, 78, 218–219
core region circuit training, 47–50
corneal sunburn, 158
costochondral separation, 114
Couto, Danilo, 246
CPR, 173–175
crime, 266
crocodiles, 230–231
Cross, Dickie, 238
crowds, 94
currents, 5, 8–11,164, 240. *See also* rip
      currents
cuts, 81–82, 187–189

## D

DEET, 272, 273
dehydration, 70, 241, 269, 285, 286, 307
dengue fever, 277–279
dermatitis, 136
diarrhea
      severe, 285–286, 307
      traveler's, 283–284
diet 64–67
dimenhydrinate, 270
disc herniation, 106–107
dislocations, 84, 102, 202–205
domoic acid, 305
Dorian, Shane, 313
Doudt, Kenny, 209
Downward Dog (yoga pose), 44
Dramamine, 270
drop in, 20, 21
drowning, 172–175
Duhaime, Phillipe, 173
Dungeons, 235

## E

ear
      plugged-up, 153–155
      surfer's, 143–145
      swimmer's, 145–149
eardrum injuries, 152–153
earplugs, 148–149
eel, 300
elbow injury, 97, 112–113
electrolytes, 70
Emerich, Markus, 155
energy reserves, 4. *See also* fitness
entering water, 13–16
etiquette, 2, 19–23
evacuation, in travel, 266–267
exercise. *See* fitness
exiting water, 13–16
eye cancer, 159
eye trauma, 161
eyewear, 159–160

## F

falciparum malaria, 275
falls, 80

Fansidar, 276
fats, 67
fin cuts, 75–76, 85–86, 187–189
finger dislocation, 84, 204–205
first aid kit, 290–295
fishhook removal, 306
fish stings, 226–228
fitness
      aerobic conditioning in, 57–60
      after surf, 40–46
      agility in, 51–53
      aging and, 315–317
      anaerobic conditioning in, 57–60
      balance in, 51–53
      body-weight training in, 54–57
      core region circuit training in, 47–50
      Hawaiian Lifeguard standards for,
            61–62
      overtraining in, 62–63
      program, 26, 60–62
      regenerative training in, 51–53
      stability in, 51–53
      strength training in, 47
      stretching and, 40–46
      warm-ups in, 26–39, 99
Fitzpatrick skin classification,127
Flat Back (yoga pose), 44
flexibility, 40–46
Florida, 16
flotation vests, 241–242
fluids, 70
fluorouracil, 131
foiling, 261
folliculitis, 141
food contamination, 282–283
food poisoning, 284, 297–308
football, 73
forecasting, 11–12
fractures, 84, 197–201
freestyle stroke, 3
fruits, 66
fugu, 302–303

## G

ginger, 269–270
glasses, 159–160
gluteal stretch, 108, 256
gluteal syndromes, 256–257
glycemic index 66, 68
golfer's elbow, 112
grains, 66
groin stretch, 42
grouper, 300
Gulf of Mexico, 16

## H

hamstring stretch, 42
hamstring tree stretch, 110, 255
Hands Up (yoga pose), 43, 46
handwashing, 283
harmful algal blooms, 303–304
Hawaiian Lifeguard fitness standards, 61–62
head injury, 77, 180–181

Head to Knees (yoga pose), 44, 46
healing, 98–99
heartburn, 69
heart rate, 4, 27, 58–59, 62, 92,
    176–177, 243, 300
heat rash, 136
helmets, 23, 90, 91, 160, 245, 261, 319
hepatitis, 184, 264, 286, 287
herniated disc, 106–107
herpes, 138
herring, 299
Hetzler, Douglas, 151
hip bridges, 33–39, 49
hip circles, 29
hip injury, 108–109
histamine, 297–298
histidine, 297–298
HIV, 287
hives, 137–138, 206
hogfish, 300
holistic remedies, 293–294
homicide, 266
horizontal abduction, 104
hydration, 70, 178
hyperventilation, 244
hypothermia, 70, 176–180

**I**

iliotibial band stretch, 255
iliotibial band syndrome, 254–256
Indicators, 80
indigestion, 69
Indonesia, 16, 276–277
infections, 139, 185–186, 196–197, 208–209,
    271–287
injuries
    ankle, 111–112
    chronic, 95–115
    dislocation, 84
    eardrum, 152–153
    elbow, 112–113
    eye, 161
    from falls, 80
    fracture, 84, 197–201
    head, 77, 180–181
    hip, 108–109
    knee, 109–111
    laceration, 81–82
    minimization of risk of, 84–94
    neck, 79, 94, 99, 173, 183
    in other sports, 73
    protective gear in prevention of, 89–91
    rib, 113–115
    seafloor, 77–79
    spine, 181–183
    sprain, 82–83, 97–98
    in stand-up paddling, 249–261
    strain, 82–83, 96–97, 99–100
    surfboard-related, 75–77, 85–88
    wave-force, 79–80
insurance, travel medical evacuation, 267
IR3535, 272, 274
Iron Cross, 40–41
Irukandji jellyfish, 222

Irwin, Steve, 215
isokinetic shoulder rotation, 104
isometric shoulder protraction, 30–31
isometric shoulder rotations, 104

**J**

jacks, 300
Japanese encephalitis, 281
Jaws, 7, 235
jellyfish, 219–224
Jet Ski, 152, 171, 172, 233, 235, 241, 245–247
Johnson, Jack, 90
Joyeux, Malik, 90

**K**

Kahanamoku, Duke, 164
Keaulana, Brian, 246
keratoses, 131–132
kicks, 109
kneecap dislocation, 205
knee injury, 109–111
knobbies, 141
Kübler-Ross, Elisabeth, 311

**L**

lacerations, 81–82, 187–189
Lariam, 276
lateral epicondylitis, 259–260
latissimus stretch, 42
leash. See also surfboard leash
leg lift, 110
leg raise, 109, 110–111
lice, sea, 225
ligaments, 83
lightning, 16–17
localism, 19
logs, 94
Long, Greg, 246
Lopez, Gerry, x–xi, 314, 315
low-back pain, 105–108
Lowden, Brian, 72, 323
Low Plank (yoga pose), 44

**M**

mackerel, 297–298, 299, 300
mahi-mahi, 299
malaria, 274–277
Malarone, 276
marlin, 299
massage, 27
Mavericks, 7, 73, 235, 242
McAleer, Chris, 78, 79
meal
    post-surf, 68–69
    pre-surf, 67–68
meclizine, 270
medical clearance, 316
medical kit, 290–295
medications, for medical kit, 292–293
melanoma, 132–134
mid-trap exercise, 105, 115, 258
miliaria rubra, 136

milk, chocolate, 68
mitochondria, 58–59
mosquito, 272–282
motion, of ocean, 4–11
motion sickness, 268–270
motor vehicle accidents, 265–266
Mountain (yoga pose), 43, 46
mountain climbers (exercise), 57
multidirectional instability, 102
murder, 266
muscle fibers, 313
muscle soreness, 61
myelopathy, 108
myofascial release, 27

**N**

Nathanson, Andrew, 72, 91
nausea, 122, 196, 222, 269, 292, 298, 300,
    304, 305
Nazare, 235
neck circles, 29–30
neck flexion, 100
neck injury, 79, 94, 99, 173, 183
neck rashes, 134–135
neck strains, 99–100
neck stretches, 29–30
needlefish, 299
Noll, Greg, 237
nutrients, 65–67
nutrition 65–68

**O**

Occhilupo, Mark, 313
ocean, motion of, 4–11
oil of lemon eucalyptus, 272, 274
okadaic acid, 305
omega-3 fatty acids, 67
O'Neill, Jack, 87
oral rehydration solution (ORS), 286
otitis externa. *See* swimmer's ear
Outer Reefs, 235
overtraining, 62–63
oxygen levels, in exercise, 58–59
oysters, 307

**P**

PABA, 123
paddling 4, 9–12, 20–22, 25–27, 52, 59, 60,
    99, 102–103, 112–113, 249–259
pain, low-back, 105–108
Paralytic Shellfish Poisoning (PSP), 304–305
Parmenter, Dave, 250
parrot fish, 300
Partridge, Rym, 314
patella dislocation, 205
patellar tendon syndrome, 254–256
pectoralis stretch, 115
Perry, Tamayo, 90
personal protective gear, 89–91
Phenergan, 270
physical therapy (PT), 98–99
pica pica, 225
picaridin, 272, 273–274

pinguecula, 158–159
Pipeline, 8, 73, 90, 314
piriformis stretch, 108
piriformis syndrome, 256–257
Plank (yoga pose), 45
planning, pretrip, 263–264
plantar fasciitis, 110
points of reference, 3
popped rib, 114
Portuguese man-of-war jellyfish, 219–224
pressure immobilization technique, 229
pre-surf meal, 67–68
pretrip planning, 263–264
prickly rash, 136
promethazine, 270
prone hip extension, 257
prone plank to duck dive, 50
protective gear, 89–91
proteins, 66
PSP. *See* Paralytic Shellfish Poisoning (PSP)
pterygium, 158–159
Puerto Escondido, 8
puncture wound, 184, 190, 195, 196, 208,
    214, 216, 228, 231, 308
push-up plus, 105
push-ups, 57
push-up superman alternating arms, 48

**Q**

quadruped arm/leg raise, 257
quad sets, 110

**R**

rashes, 134–135, 136–137
rash guard, 18, 89
Raynaud's phenomenon, 138
red eye, 157
red tide, 136, 303–304
reef cuts, 78, 218–219
reflux, 69
refraction, 7
regenerative training, 51–53
rehabilitation, 97, 98–99, 111–112, 258–259
rehydration 285, 286
Reliefband, 269
rescue, 164–172
resilience, 315
resuscitation. *See* CPR
Retin A, 131
retinal detachment, 160
rib injury, 113–115
Rift Valley fever, 280
right of way, 21
rip currents, 8–10, 14, 164
rocks, 94
rocky shorelines, 15–16
rotational mobility, 30–33
rotator cuff injury, 102, 257–258
rugby, 73

**S**

Safe, Mike, 311
salmon, 299

saltwater crocodiles, 230–231
San Onofre, 8
sardine, 299
saury, 299
saxitoxin, 304
scalene stretch, 114
scaption, 259
scapular retraction squeezes, 32
scapular squeezes, 100, 104, 115, 258
sciatica, 107
*scombridae* fish, 297–298
scombroid, 297–299
scopolamine, 270
scorpion stretches, 109
sea anemones, 219–222
Sea-Band, 269
seabather's eruption, 225
seafloor injuries, 77–79
seafood, 297–308
sea lice. *See also* sea bather's eruption
seasickness, 268–270
sea snakes, 228–229
seasonal affective disorder (SAD), 117
sea ulcers, 139–140
sea urchins, 215–218
seborrheic dermatitis, 134
seborrheic keratosis, 131
secondary drowning, 172
sexually transmitted infections (STIs), 287
shake outs, 30
shallow-water wipeout, 92–93
shape, wave, 8
sharks, 209–213
shellfish poisoning, 303–305
Shonan Beach, 16
shore break, 13, 14, 94, 250
shoulder anatomy, 101
shoulder dislocation, 84, 202–204
shoulder protraction, 30–33
shoulder strain, 100–101
side-lying external rotation, 104
side-lying leg lift, 110, 256
side-shore current, 10–11
single-leg split squat, 49
sinus problems, 153–155
skiing, 73
skin
    cancers, 132–134
    infections, 139, 307–308
    keratoses in, 131–132
    trauma, 139–141
    wet suit-related problems in, 134–136
skin stapler 194
skin adhesives, 190–195
skin type, 127–129
skipjack, 299
Slater, Kelly, 313
slings, 200–201
SMA. *See* Surfer's Medical Association
    (SMA)
snakes, 228–229
snaking, 22
snapper, 300
sneaker waves, 15

snowboarding, 73
soccer, 73
softball, 73
solar urticaria, 137
Spanish mackerel, 300
SPF, 125–126
spine flutter, 47
spine injury, 181–183
splints, 189, 199–201, 229
spondylolisthesis, 107
spondylolysis, 107
sprains, 82–83, 97–98
squamous cell skin cancer, 133, 134
squat jumps, 54
squat thrusts, 56
stability, 51–53, 260
stand-up paddling (SUP)
    elbow, 259–260
    getting into water in, 249–250
    injuries in, 249–261
    offshore, 251–252
    overuse injuries, 254
*Staph*, 139
Steamer Lane, 314
stingrays, 214–215
stings, 208–209, 215–218, 219–224
STIs. *See* sexually transmitted infections
    (STIs)
stitches, 194–195
stoke, 310–311, 323
stonefish, 226–228
straight leg raise, 109, 110–111
strains, 82–83, 96–97
    neck, 99–100
    shoulder, 100–101
strength training, 47
stretching, 40–46
Stugeron, 270
sun
    benefits of, 117
    damage, 118–123
sunblock, 123–126
sunburn, 121–123, 158
sunglasses, 159–160
sun rash, 137
sun salutation, 43–46
sunscreen, 123–126
supermans, 48
surfboard-related injuries, 75–77, 85–88
surfboard leash, 3, 13–15, 18, 84, 88–89,
    166, 185, 204, 241–246, 250–253
surfer's ear, 143–145
surfer's knots, 141
surfer's lip, 138
Surfer's Medical Association (SMA), 289,
    315, 323
surfer's myelopathy, 108
surfer's red eye, 157
surfer's rib, 114
surf forecasting, 11–12
surfing etiquette, 2, 19–23
surf rescue, 164–172
surgeon fish, 300
swimmer's ear, 145–149

swimming
as aerobic exercise, 60
importance of, 2–4

**T**

talon noire, 140–141
Teahupoo, 91
tendinitis, 60, 102, 257
tennis elbow, 259–260
tetanus vaccine, 186
tetrodotoxin, 302–303
thoracic extension, 100, 105, 115, 258
thoracic outlet syndrome (TOS), 103–105
Tibetan Rite 1, 29
Tibetan Rite 2, 33–35
Tibetan Rite 3, 36–37
Tibetan Rite 4, 37–38
Tibetan Rite 5, 38–39
tide, 12
time interval, between wave crests, 6
Todos Santos, 235
TOS. See thoracic outlet syndrome (TOS)
tourniquets, 184–185
Transderm-Scop, 270
travel
crime in, 266
evacuation in, 266–267
infections in, 271–287
items for personal health, 289–290
medical care in, 266–267
medications in, 264
motor vehicle accidents in, 265–266
pretrip planning for, 263–264
traveler's diarrhea, 283–284
Trent, Buzzy, 236
tretinoin, 131
trevally, 300
triangulation, 11, 246
triceps stretch, 42
triggerfish, 300
trunk twists, 29–30
tuberculosis, 264
tube-riding wipeout, 93
tuna, 297–298, 299
typhoid, 284–285

**U**

ulcers, sea, 139–140
unconscious victim rescue, 167–171
underarm rashes, 134–135
undertow, 8
UPF, 126
upper-crossed syndrome, 103–105
upper trapezius stretch, 100
Upward Dog (yoga pose), 45
urine, 209
UVA, 119
UVB, 119

**V**

V02 max, 312–313

vaccinations, 264
van Dyke, Fred, 237
vegetables, 66
VHF Radio, 252
*Vibrio,* 305–308
*Vibrio cholerae,* 307
*Vibrio parahaemolyticus,* 307
*Vibrio vulnificus,* 307–308
vision correction, 159–160
vision loss, 160
vitamin A, 67
vitamin B$_{12}$, 66
vitamin D, 67, 117
vitamin E, 67
vitamin K, 67
vivax malaria, 275
vomiting, 285–286

**W**

wahoo, 299
Waikiki, 8
Waimea Bay, 235
warm-ups, 26–39, 99
Warrior (yoga pose), 45
Watanabe, Moto, 90
water, entering and exiting, 13–16
water contamination, 282–283
water itch, 137
wave-force injuries, 79–80
wave formation, 5–7
wavelength, 6
wave period, 6, 7
wave shape, 8
wax folliculitis, 141
wet suit, 18, 89, 126, 177–180
wet suit acne, 135–136
wet suit dermatitis, 136
wet suit-related skin problems, 134–136
white fingers and toes, 138
wipeout, 77, 84, 86, 91–94, 99, 114, 152, 154, 160, 181, 182, 202, 204, 208, 218, 239–241, 245, 249, 251–253
Wise, Bob, 233
wound care, 184–197
wound cleansing, 185–186
wound closure, 190
wound closure strips, 190–195
wound dressings, 195–196
wound evaluation, 187–189
wounds, puncture, 184, 190, 195, 196, 208, 214, 216, 228, 231, 308
wrasses, 300

**Y**

yellow fever, 279–280
yellowfin tuna, 299
yoga, 43–46

**Z**

Zika virus, 281

# About the Authors

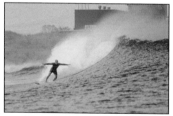

*Freight Trains, Nicaragua*

Andrew Nathanson, MD, FACEP, FAWM, is a longtime surfer and clinical professor of emergency medicine at Alpert Medical School of Brown University. He trained at Los Angeles County–USC medical center and has continued his clinical career at Rhode Island Hospital, a busy level 1 Trauma center in Providence, Rhode Island. His academic interest has always involved marine medicine, and he has published numerous peer-reviewed studies of surfing, wind-surfing, and sailing injuries. As an active member of the Wilderness Medical Society, he organizes their biennial Travel, Dive, and Marine Medicine conference. He has surfed all over the world but most enjoys surfing with his wife and son at a secret spot in Little Compton, Rhode Island.

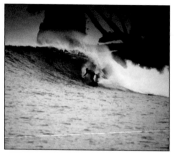

*Burger World, Indonesia*

Clayton Everline, MD, CSCS, FAWM, practices as a sports physician for both athletes and watermen at the Straub clinic on Oahu. He is founder of Waves of Health, LLC: Ocean Sports, Environmental, and Outreach Medicine. He is board-certified in both sports medicine and internal medicine and is a fellow of the Academy of Wilderness Medicine (FAWM). Additionally, he is clinical assistant professor of orthopedic surgery at Seton Hall University, a strength and conditioning Specialist (CSCS), has been featured as Top Doctor in *Men's Health* magazine, and a columnist in *Surfline Health and Fitness*. Dr. Everline has been a medical director at many professional surfing events, including Hawaii's renowned Triple Crown of Surfing, and is program chair for the annual Waves of Health Pipeline Masters Medical Conference. He lives on the North Shore of Oahu with his gorgeous wife, Kristina. www.everlinemd.com www.boardsportsdoc.com www.thewavesofhealth.org

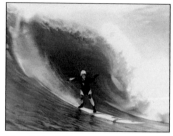

*Maverick's, California*

Mark Renneker, MD, is the founder of the Surfer's Medical Association, co-wrote the "Ask the Surf Docs" column for *Surfer* magazine for a number of years, and is the co-author of *Sick Surfers Ask the Surf Docs*. He is a board-certified family physician and specialist in medical advocacy and is an associate clinical professor in the Department of Family and Community Medicine, at the University of California, San Francisco, where he teaches medical students about advocacy medicine. He has been surfing for fifty-five years, on all seven continents (including Antarctica), lives, works, and surfs at Ocean Beach, San Francisco, and is a longtime Maverick's regular.

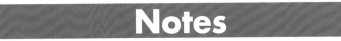

# Notes

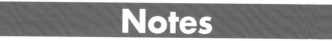

# Notes

...........................................................................

...........................................................................

...........................................................................

...........................................................................

...........................................................................

...........................................................................

...........................................................................

...........................................................................

...........................................................................

...........................................................................

...........................................................................

...........................................................................

...........................................................................

...........................................................................

...........................................................................

...........................................................................

...........................................................................

...........................................................................

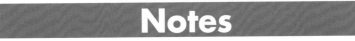

# Notes

# Notes

.............................................................................

.............................................................................

.............................................................................

.............................................................................

.............................................................................

.............................................................................

.............................................................................

.............................................................................

.............................................................................

.............................................................................

.............................................................................

.............................................................................

.............................................................................

.............................................................................

.............................................................................

.............................................................................

.............................................................................

.............................................................................

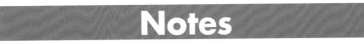

# Notes